Nephrology and Hypertension

FOURTH EDITION

D1371965

The House Officer Series is based on Weiner and Levitt's *Neurology for the House Officer*, first published in 1973.

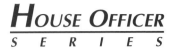

Nephrology and Hypertension

FOURTH EDITION

Editors

C. Craig Tisher, M.D.

*Professor of Medicine and Pathology
and Anatomy and Cell Biology
Senior Associate Dean, College of Medicine
Folke H. Peterson/Dean's Distinguished Professorship
Division of Nephrology, Hypertension and Transplantation
University of Florida College of Medicine
Gainesville, Florida*

Christopher S. Wilcox, M.D., Ph.D.

*George E. Schreiner Professor of Nephrology
Chief, Division of Nephrology and Hypertension
Vice-chair for Academic Affairs,
Department of Medicine
Georgetown University Medical Center
Washington, D.C.*

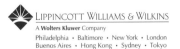

LIPPINCOTT WILLIAMS & WILKINS
A **Wolters Kluwer** Company
Philadelphia · Baltimore · New York · London
Buenos Aires · Hong Kong · Sydney · Tokyo

Acquisitions Editor: Paula Callaghan
Developmental Editor: Mary Beth Murphy
Production Editor: Thomas Boyce
Manufacturing Manager: Kevin Watt
Cover Designer: Diana Andrews
Compositor: Circle Graphics
Printer: R R Donnelley

© 1999 by LIPPINCOTT WILLIAMS & WILKINS
227 East Washington Square
Philadelphia, PA 19106-3780 USA
LWW.com

All rights reserved. This book is protected by copyright. No part of this book may be reproduced
in any form or by any means, including photocopying, or utilized by any information storage and
retrieval system without written permission from the copyright owner, except for brief quotations
embodied in critical articles and reviews. Materials appearing in this book prepared by individuals as part of their official duties as U.S. government employees are not covered by the above-
mentioned copyright.

Printed in the USA

Library of Congress Cataloging-in-Publication Data

Nephrology and hypertension / editors, C. Craig Tisher, Christopher S.
   Wilcox. — 4th ed.
      p.   cm. — (House officer series)
      Rev. ed. of: Nephrology. 3rd ed. c1995.
      Includes bibliographical references and index.
      ISBN 0-7817-2077-X
      1. Nephrology Handbooks, manuals, etc.   2. Kidneys—Diseases
   Handbooks, manuals, etc.   3. Hypertension Handbooks, manuals, etc.
   I. Tisher, C. Craig, 1936–   .   II. Wilcox, Christopher S.
   III. Nephrology.   IV. Series.
      [DNLM: 1. Kidney Diseases Handbooks. 2. Hypertension Handbooks.
   WJ 39 N4385 1999]
   RC903.N45   1999
   616.6′1—dc21
   DNLM/DLC   99-38983
   for Library of Congress   CIP

Care has been taken to confirm the accuracy of the information presented and to describe
generally accepted practices. However, the authors, editors, and publisher are not responsible for errors or omissions or for any consequences from application of the information in
this book and make no warranty, expressed or implied, with respect to the currency, completeness, or accuracy of the contents of the publication. Application of this information in a
particular situation remains the professional responsibility of the practitioner.
    The authors, editors, and publisher have exerted every effort to ensure that drug selec-
tion and dosage set forth in this text are in accordance with current recommendations and
practice at the time of publication. However, in view of ongoing research, changes in government regulations, and the constant flow of information relating to drug therapy and drug
reactions, the reader is urged to check the package insert for each drug for any change in
indications and dosage and for added warnings and precautions. This is particularly important when the recommended agent is a new or infrequently employed drug.
    Some drugs and medical devices presented in this publication have Food and Drug
Administration (FDA) clearance for limited use in restricted research settings. It is the responsibility of the health care provider to ascertain the FDA status of each drug or device planned
for use in their clinical practice.

10   9   8   7   6   5   4   3   2   1

To Audrae Tisher and Linda Wilcox

Preface

The fourth edition of this clinical text that is part of the House Officer Series has been expanded to include additional information on hypertension; hence, it has been retitled *Nephrology and Hypertension*. The presentation of the content is intended to assist both the house officer and the medical student as they evaluate and treat patients with kidney disease and hypertension and the many associated complications. The editors believe this text can also be of value to individuals beginning their subspecialty training in nephrology or as a reference guide for physicians trained in other specialties and subspecialties. Recent information suggests that previous editions of the text have been used successfully as textbooks by individuals receiving training as physician assistants and nurse practitioners.

Both nephrology and hypertension encompass a wide variety of disciplines that include physiology, anatomy, pathology, biochemistry, immunology, molecular biology, pharmacology, and cell biology. Despite the fact this handbook is intended primarily to represent a practical clinical manual, it is occasionally necessary to include information derived from research conducted in the clinical and basic sciences that aids directly in our ability to correctly diagnose and treat kidney dysfunction, kidney disease, and hypertension.

This fourth edition, now titled *Nephrology and Hypertension,* contains 32 chapters, each written in a concise yet lucid manner, to facilitate the management of ill patients. In a departure from previous editions, the text is organized into six sections that include: Approach to the Patient with Renal Disease; Glomerular, Tubulointerstitial Diseases, and Vasculitis; Disorders of Water, Electrolytes, and Acid-Base Regulation; Diseases of the Urinary Collecting System and Bladder; Hypertension: Diagnosis and Management; and Renal Failure: Diagnosis and Management.

Chapter 1 provides a brief overview of the structural and functional features of the kidney. Chapters 2 through 4 outline a practical approach to the functional and radiologic evaluation of the kidney, including the clinical indications for a kidney biopsy. Chapter 5 discusses the clinical significance of hematuria and identifies those clinical settings in which thorough evaluation is a necessity. In Chapter 6 the etiology, pathophysiology, and method of evaluation of proteinuria and the nephrotic syndrome are presented.

Chapter 7, the initial chapter in the second section of the book, "Glomerular, Tubulointerstitial Diseases, and Vasculitis," reviews the very important entity of diabetic nephropathy. Chapter 8 discusses several forms of renal disease that are glomerular in type including minimal change disease, focal segmental glomerulosclerosis, membranous glomerulonephritis, post-infectious proliferative glomerulonephritis, rapidly progressive glomerulonephritis, anti-GBM glomerulonephritis, membranoproliferative glomerulonephritis, IgA nephropathy, and fibrillary glomerulonephritis. Chapter 9 describes the various types of glomerulonephritis observed in patients with systemic lupus erythematosus. In Chapter 10 the problem of vasculitis is addressed in its many forms including Wegener's granulomatosis, polyarteritis nodosa, microscopic polyarteritis, and Schönlein-Henoch purpura. Chapter 11 provides descriptions of the renal manifestations of the thrombotic microangiopathies, progressive systemic sclerosis, multiple myeloma, and amyloidosis. Chapter 12 discusses tubulointerstitial nephritis, a disease process of varied etiology that can present with either acute or chronic renal failure. In Chapter 13 there is a review of the more frequently encountered familial and cystic forms of renal disease. This section ends with a discussion of HIV infection and the kidney including HIV-associated nephropathy. The appropriate management of HIV-infected patients with acute as well as chronic renal failure also is presented in Chapter 14.

Four chapters are contained within the section of the handbook entitled "Disorders of Water, Electrolytes, and Acid-Base Regulation." These include "Disorders of Water Balance," Chapter 15; "Potassium Disorders," Chapter 16; "Acid-Base Disorders," Chapter 17; and "Calcium, Phosphorus, and Magnesium Disorders," Chapter 18.

Just two chapters comprise the section on "Diseases of the Urinary Collecting System and Bladder." In Chapter 19 renal stone disease is reviewed and a scheme presented to aid in the identification of the many causes of this entity, also termed renal lithiasis. Chapter 20 reviews the extremely common problem of urinary tract infection.

The fifth section, "Hypertension: Diagnosis and Management," contains four chapters devoted exclusively to common hypertensive problems while the last chapter, Chapter 25, focuses on the use of diuretics in clinical practice.

The last section of the handbook, "Renal Failure: Diagnosis and Management," begins with Chapters 26 and 27 which provide detailed discussions of acute and chronic renal failure, respectively. Each chapter contains a wealth of practical clinical information on the identification and management of these two common entities. Chapters 28 and 29 chronicle the many forms of dialysis as renal replacement therapy for the management of both acute and chronic renal failure. Chapter 30 discusses the proper management of the renal transplant patient. This chapter is followed by a discussion in Chapter 31 of the important role of adequate nutrition in both acute and chronic renal failure. The final chapter of this handbook, Chapter 32, outlines the use of various drugs in renal failure and provides an extensive set of tables to aid the clinician in the proper dosing of drugs.

This text was written and reviewed by faculty and fellows in the Division of Nephrology, Hypertension and Transplantation at the University of Florida and the Division of Nephrology and Hypertension at Georgetown University. Every effort has been made to provide a concise yet sufficiently detailed text so that the user can easily derive highly useful, accurate, and up-to-date information to aid in the care of patients with nephrological problems and hypertension. The editors have reviewed and revised each chapter extensively in an effort to achieve these goals.

Contributors

From the Division of Nephrology, Hypertension and Transplantation at the University of Florida College of Medicine, Gainesville, Florida:

Koshy O. Abraham, M.D.
Instructor in Medicine

Anupam Agarwal, M.D.
Assistant Professor of Medicine

Janet M. Crabtree, M.D.
Assistant Clinical Professor of Medicine

David T. Lowenthal, M.D., Ph.D.
Professor of Medicine, Pharmacology and Exercise Science

Kirsten M. Madsen, M.D., Ph.D.
Associate Professor of Medicine

Marnie J. Marker, M.D.
Senior Clinical Fellow in Nephrology

R. Tyler Miller, M.D.
Associate Professor of Medicine

G. Edward Newman, M.D.
Senior Clinical Fellow in Nephrology

Edward A. Ross, M.D.
Associate Professor of Medicine

John R. Silkensen, M.D.
Assistant Professor of Medicine

C. Peter Spies, M.D., Ph.D.
Senior Clinical Fellow in Nephrology

C. Craig Tisher, M.D.
Professor of Medicine and Pathology and Anatomy and Cell Biology
Senior Associate Dean, College of Medicine
Folke H. Peterson/Dean's Distinguished Professorship

Jill W. Verlander, D.V.M.
Associate Scientist in Medicine

I. David Weiner, M.D.
Associate Professor of Medicine

Charles S. Wingo, M.D.
Professor of Medicine and Physiology

Leonid V. Yankulin, M.D.
Senior Clinical Fellow in Nephrology

From the Division of Nephrology and Hypertension at Georgetown University Medical Center, Washington, D.C.:

Abdul R. Amir, M.D.
Senior Renal Fellow

David S. Amrose, M.D.
Senior Renal Fellow

Nicolas J. Guzman, M.D.
Associate Professor of Medicine

Wen-Ting Ouyang, M.D.
Senior Renal Fellow

Thomas A. Rakowski, M.D.
Associate Professor of Medicine

Christopher S. Wilcox, M.D., Ph.D., F.R.C.P., F.A.C.P.
George E. Schreiner Professor of Nephrology
Chief, Division of Nephrology and Hypertension

James F. Winchester, M.B., Ch.B.
Professor of Medicine

Contents

Section C: Disorders of Water, Electrolytes, and Acid-Base Regulation

Section D: Diseases of the Urinary Collecting System and Bladder

Section E: Hypertension: Diagnosis and Management

Section F: Renal Failure: Diagnosis and Management

Chapter 1

Renal Structure in Relation to Function

Kirsten M. Madsen
Jill W. Verlander

GROSS ANATOMY

The kidneys are located retroperitoneally from the T-12 to the L-3 vertebra. The right kidney is positioned slightly lower than the left. Each kidney is approximately 11 to 12 cm long, 5 to 7.5 cm wide, and 2.5 to 3 cm thick. Kidney weight in adult men is 125 to 170 g and in adult women is 115 to 155 g. On the medial margin is a cleft, the hilus, through which the renal pelvis, the renal artery and vein, lymphatics, and a nerve plexus pass into the sinus of the kidney (Fig. 1.1). The renal pelvis, an expansion of the upper end of the ureter, continues into funnel-shaped tubes called the calyces that connect with the renal papillae. The kidney is covered by a tough fibrous capsule that is normally smooth and easily removable.

The kidney can be divided into cortex and medulla. In humans, the medulla forms 8 to 18 renal pyramids, the bases of which are located at the corticomedullary junction (Fig. 1.1). The apices of the pyramids extend toward the renal pelvis, each forming a papilla. From the base of the pyramids, medullary rays consisting of collecting ducts and the straight portions of proximal and distal tubules extend into the cortex. Based on segmentation of the nephron (Fig. 1.2), the medulla can be divided into an outer medulla, which in turn can be subdivided into an outer and inner stripe, and an inner medulla, which includes the renal papilla. The functional unit of the kidney is the nephron, which consists of a renal corpuscle or glomerulus and its associated tubule (Fig. 1.2). The tubular portion of the nephron is composed of three major subdivisions: the proximal convoluted tubule (PCT), the loop of Henle, and the

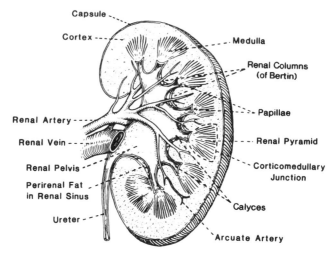

FIGURE 1.1   Cut surface of a bisected kidney.

distal convoluted tubule (DCT). The latter continues into the collecting duct system, which is derived from the ureteric bud and, strictly speaking, is not part of the nephron. The loop of Henle includes the proximal straight tubule (pars recta of the proximal tubule), the thin limb segments, and the thick ascending limb (TAL) (pars recta of the distal tubule).

Each human kidney contains approximately 1.2 million nephrons. Those originating from outer and midcortical glomeruli have short loops of Henle that bend in the inner stripe of the outer medulla. Juxtamedullary nephrons originating from glomeruli located near the corticomedullary junction have long loops of Henle that reach into the inner medulla. In the human kidney, 10% to 15% of the glomeruli belong to long-looped nephrons.

MICROSCOPIC ANATOMY

Glomerulus

The glomeruli are located in the cortex. The human glomerulus measures approximately 200 μm in diameter, and it includes a capillary tuft and the surrounding parietal epithelium of Bow-

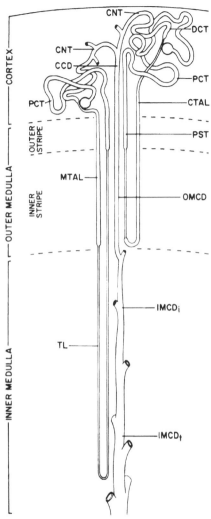

FIGURE 1.2 Relationships among various segments of the nephron and zones of the kidney. CCD, cortical collecting duct; CNT, connecting segment; CTAL, cortical thick ascending limb; DCT, distal convoluted tubule; IMCD$_i$, initial inner medullary collecting duct; IMCD$_t$, terminal inner medullary collecting duct; MTAL, medullary thick ascending limb; OMCD, outer medullary collecting duct; PCT, proximal convoluted tubule; PST, proximal straight tubule; TL, thin limb of Henle's loop.

man's capsule. The glomerulus is responsible for the formation of an ultrafiltrate of plasma. It consists of a capillary network lined by a thin fenestrated endothelium, a central mesangial region, and the visceral epithelium with its associated basement membrane (Fig.1.3A). The filtration barrier between the blood and the urinary space is composed of the fenestrated endothelium, the peripheral glomerular basement membrane, and the slit pores between the foot processes of the visceral epithelial cells (Fig. 1.3B). The thin *endothelium* is perforated by pores or fenestrae measuring approximately 70 to 100 nm in diameter. It constitutes the initial barrier to the passage of blood constituents but is not believed to represent a significant barrier to the passage of macromolecules.

The glomerular basement membrane is located between the endothelium and the visceral epithelium and is approximately 300 nm thick. It is composed of three layers: a central dense layer, the lamina densa, and two electronlucent layers, the lamina rara externa and lamina rara interna. The glomerular basement membrane is believed to constitute a size-selective as well as a charge-selective barrier to the passage of macromolecules. It is composed of various glycoproteins, including type IV and type V collagen, laminin, fibronectin, and negatively charged glycosaminoglycans rich in heparan sulfate. These anionic sites appear to be important in establishing the charge-selective characteristics of the filtration barrier.

The *visceral epithelial cells* (or podocytes) have long cytoplasmic processes that divide into foot processes or pedicles that are in close contact with the glomerular basement membrane. The space between adjacent foot processes is called the filtration slit or slit pore, and it is closed by a thin membrane, the slit diaphragm. The foot processes possess a negatively charged surface coat that is rich in sialic acid and is important for maintaining the normal structure and function of the filtration barrier. Removal of the anionic surface coat causes the foot processes to disappear and to be replaced by a continuous band of cytoplasm along the glomerular basement membrane. Similar changes called "foot process fusion" or "efface-ment" are observed in various proteinuric conditions.

The *mesangium* is separated from the capillary lumen by the endothelium and consists of mesangial cells and surrounding mesangial matrix. The mesangial cells provide structural support for the capillary loops. They contain numerous filaments and have contractile as well as phagocytic properties. Cell contraction is believed to limit filtration, perhaps by reducing the area of the

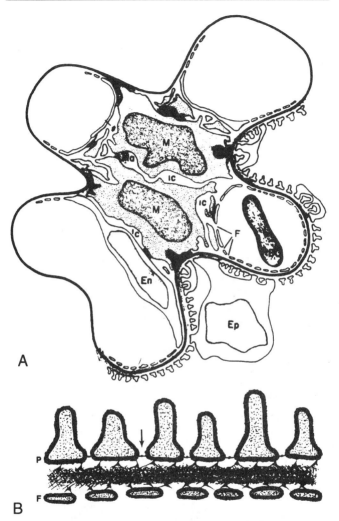

FIGURE 1.3 **A.** Relationship among endothelial cells (En), epithelial cells (Ep), and mesangial cells (M) of the glomerulus. F, endothelial fenestrae; Ma, mesangial matrix; IC, intercellular channels. (From Latta H. Ultrastructure of the glomerulus and juxtaglomerular apparatus. In: Geiger SR, ed. *Handbook of physiology*. Bethesda: American Physiological Society, 1973:1–30.) **B.** Glomerular basement membrane with adjoining endothelial fenestrae (F) and epithelial foot processes (P) with slit pores (*arrow*). (From Kanwar YS, Farquhar MG. Anionic sites in the glomerular basement membrane: in vivo and in vitro localization in the lamina rarae cationic probes. *J Cell Biol* 1979;81:137.)

glomerular filter. It is stimulated to contract by angiotensin II, arginine vasopressin, and thromboxane, a response that is inhibited by prostaglandin E$_2$. Mesangial cells are phagocytic, and in certain forms of glomerulonephritis they appear to be involved in the sequestration of immune complexes from the glomerular tuft.

The *parietal epithelium* of Bowman's capsule is continuous with the visceral epithelium at the vascular pole. At the urinary pole there is an abrupt transition from the parietal epithelium to the epithelium of the proximal tubule.

Juxtaglomerular Apparatus

The juxtaglomerular apparatus located at the vascular pole of the glomerulus has tubular and vascular components. The vascular components include the terminal portion of the afferent arteriole, the initial portion of the efferent arteriole, and the extraglomerular mesangium between the arterioles. The tubular component is a specialized part of the TAL called the macula densa. Some cells in the vascular portion of the juxtaglomerular apparatus contain numerous granules. These granular cells secrete renin, which, by forming angiotensin, is involved in regulation of tubuloglomerular feedback and in control of aldosterone-stimulated sodium and potassium transport. Therefore, the juxtaglomerular apparatus is important in the control of renal hemodynamics and salt excretion.

Proximal Tubule

The proximal tubule includes an initial pars convoluta, or PCT, and a pars recta, or proximal straight tubule, that is located in the medullary ray (Fig. 1.2). The PCT has numerous lateral cell processes that extend from the apical to the basal surface of the cell and interdigitate with similar cell processes from adjacent cells (Fig. 1.4). Mitochondria are located in these processes in close proximity to the cell membrane. The presence of these lateral cell processes and interdigitations gives rise to a complex extracellular compartment between the cells. This intercellular space is separated from the tubule lumen by the tight junction or zonula occludens. A prominent endocytic–lysosomal system is present in the cells and is important in the reabsorption and catabolism of proteins from the tubule fluid. Based on morphologic differences, the proximal tubule can be subdivided into

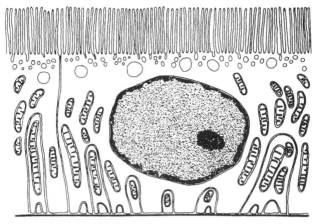

FIGURE 1.4 Proximal tubule cell.

three distinct segments. The S_1 segment corresponds to the initial PCT; the S_2 segment corresponds to the terminal PCT and the initial proximal straight tubule; and the S_3 segment constitutes the remainder of the proximal straight tubule.

The main function of the proximal tubule is the reabsorption of sodium, chloride, bicarbonate, potassium, phosphate, water, and organic solutes, such as glucose and amino acids, and the secretion of organic acids and bases, including common drugs such as salicylates, barbiturates, penicillin, and many diuretics. Much of the sodium reabsorption is an active process mediated by the Na^+/K^+-ATPase or sodium pump located in the basolateral plasma membrane. The transport of the various anions and organic solutes across the luminal membrane is coupled to the reabsorption of sodium down its concentration gradient. Fluid reabsorption is accomplished primarily by isosmotic water flow through the cell and the intercellular spaces.

Thin Limb of Henle's Loop

The thin limb of Henle's loop extends from the proximal tubule to the TAL (Fig. 1.2). Short-looped nephrons have only a short descending thin limb segment that is located in the inner stripe of the outer medulla. Long-looped nephrons have both a long descending and a long ascending thin limb. Four morphologically distinct segments can be identified in the thin limb. All are lined by a flat epithelium containing few cell organelles.

The thin limb of Henle's loop is important in the counter-current multiplication mechanism. The descending limb is permeable to water but impermeable to sodium, whereas the ascending limb is almost impermeable to water but highly permeable to sodium and modestly permeable to urea. Accordingly, water diffuses out of the descending limb, and subsequently sodium exits the ascending limb down its concentration gradient. Thus, the countercurrent mechanism is involved in the maintenance of a hypertonic medullary interstitium and in the formation of a dilute tubule fluid.

Distal Tubule

The distal tubule includes the TAL, which can be subdivided into a medullary and a cortical segment, the macula densa, and the DCT (Fig. 1.2). The transition from the TAL to the DCT occurs shortly after the macula densa. Cells of the TAL and the DCT possess extensive invaginations of the basolateral plasma membrane and interdigitations of cell processes between adjacent cells. Numerous elongated mitochondria are located in the lateral cell processes in close proximity to the plasma membrane. In contrast to the proximal tubule, the luminal membrane of the distal tubule does not possess a brush border (Fig. 1.5). The ultrastructural composition of the distal tubule is characteristic of an epithelium involved in active transport. Both the TAL and the DCT are responsible for active reabsorption of sodium chloride, which is important in the countercurrent multiplication process and the urinary concentrating and diluting mechanisms. Because the TAL is relatively impermeable to water, the active reabsorption of sodium chloride creates a hypertonic interstitium and ensures the delivery of a hypotonic tubule fluid to the DCT. The TAL is the site of action of the loop diuretics (e.g., furosemide), whereas thiazide diuretics exert their effect mainly on the DCT.

The *connecting segment* is located between the distal tubule and the collecting duct (Fig. 1.2). It is a transition region where a mixture of cells from adjacent regions can be encountered including DCT cells, connecting tubule cells, and collecting duct cells (intercalated and principal cells).

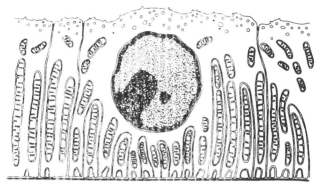

FIGURE 1.5   Distal tubule cell.

Collecting Duct

The collecting duct system can be divided into the cortical, outer medullary, and inner medullary collecting duct (IMCD) (Fig. 1.2). The cortical collecting duct includes the initial collecting tubule and the segment located in the medullary ray. The epithelium of both the cortical collecting duct and the outer medullary collecting duct is composed of two distinct cell types, principal cells and intercalated cells, the latter constituting approximately one-third of the cells. Principal cells have a light cytoplasm with few cell organelles and a relatively smooth luminal surface (Fig. 1.6), whereas intercalated cells have a dark-staining cytoplasm with many mitochondria and numerous small tubulovesicles (Fig. 1.7). The luminal surface of intercalated cells is covered with microprojections that are either microvilli or microplicae. Two different configurations of intercalated cells have been observed: type A cells, which are involved in hydrogen ion secretion; and type B cells, which secrete bicarbonate. A main function of principal cells in the cortical collecting duct is potassium secretion.

    Intercalated cells gradually disappear in the early portion of the IMCD and are absent in the papillary portion. Cells in the terminal two-thirds of the IMCD are believed to constitute a distinct cell type that is called the IMCD cell. The IMCD cells have a very light cytoplasm and few organelles. They increase in height as the collecting duct descends toward the papillary tip. The principal cells and the IMCD cells are responsive to antidiuretic hormone.

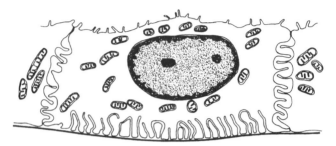

FIGURE 1.6 Principal cell.

In the presence of antidiuretic hormone, water is reabsorbed from the collecting duct, which leads to the formation of a hypertonic urine. In the absence of antidiuretic hormone, the collecting duct is relatively impermeable to water, and a hypotonic urine is formed.

Interstitium

The interstitium is composed of interstitial cells and a loose flocculent extracellular material rich in glycosaminoglycans. Interstitial tissue is sparse in the cortex where two types of interstitial cells have been described: one that resembles a fibroblast and another less common mononuclear cell. In the medulla there is a gradual increase in the amount of interstitial tissue from the outer

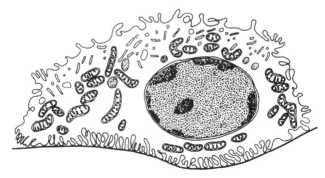

FIGURE 1.7 Intercalated cell.

medulla to the papillary tip. Three different types of interstitial cells have been described in the medulla: type I, the typical reno-medullary interstitial cell; type II, a mononuclear cell; and type III, a pericyte. The renomedullary (type I) cells are very prominent in the inner medulla, where they are arranged in rows between adjacent tubules and vessels resembling rungs on a ladder. These cells have numerous lipid inclusions or droplets, whose function is not known with certainty. The renomedullary cells are important sites of prostaglandin E_2 production.

Vasculature

The blood flow to the kidneys is large, amounting to approximately 1,200 ml/min (20–25% of cardiac output). The renal artery divides into anterior and posterior segmental branches at the hilus of the kidney (Fig. 1.1). From the segmental arteries, lobar arteries run toward the papillae, where they divide into interlobar arteries that ascend along the sides of the renal pyramids. At the cortico-medullary junction, they continue into the arcuate arteries, which run parallel to the surface of the kidney. From the arcuate arteries, interlobular arteries ascend into the cortex, where they give off afferent arterioles to the glomeruli. Blood leaves the glomeruli through the efferent arterioles that form the peritubular capillary networks in the cortex. The efferent arterioles from juxtamedullary glomeruli descend into the outer medulla, where they form vascular bundles containing the vasa recta through which the outer and inner medulla is supplied. Blood from the capillaries drains into the interlobular, arcuate, and interlobar veins, which accompany arteries of the same name, and finally leaves the kidney through the renal vein. Networks of lymphatics are present in the renal cortex and the renal capsule, but lymphatics have not been described in the medulla. In the cortex they follow the arteries and are embedded in the periarterial interstitial tissue.

Innervation

The kidneys are innervated mainly via the celiac plexus and the greater splanchnic nerves. Adrenergic nerve fibers follow the blood vessels throughout the cortex and outer stripe of the outer medulla. Nerve endings have also been described in contact with both proximal and distal tubules in the cortex and with various components of the juxtaglomerular apparatus.

Suggested Readings

Clapp WL, Abrahamson DL. Development and gross anatomy of the kidney. In: Tisher CC, Brenner BM, eds. *Renal pathology with clinical and functional correlations, 2nd ed.* Philadelphia: JB Lippincott, 1994:3–59.

Kriz W, Kaissling B. Structural organization of the mammalian kidney. In: Seldin DW, Giebisch G, eds. *The kidney: physiology and pathophysiology.* New York: Raven Press, 1992:707–777.

Madsen KM, Brenner BM. Structure and function of the renal tubule and interstitium. In: Tisher CC, Brenner BM, eds. *Renal pathology with clinical and functional correlations, 2nd ed.* Philadelphia: JB Lippincott, 1994:661–698.

Tisher CC, Brenner BM. Structure and function of the glomerulus. In: Tisher CC, Brenner BM, eds. *Renal pathology with clinical and functional correlations, 2nd ed.* Philadelphia: JB Lippincott, 1994:143–161.

Tisher CC, Madsen KM. Anatomy of the kidney. In: Brenner BM, ed. *The kidney, 5th ed.* Philadelphia: WB Saunders, 1996:3–71.

Chapter 2

Clinical and Laboratory Evaluation of Renal Disease and Fluid Status

Wen-Ting Ouyang
Thomas A. Rakowski

HISTORY AND PHYSICAL EXAMINATION

Kidney diseases may be part of a systemic, inherited, or drug-induced disease. Therefore, a comprehensive history and physical examination are essential. Physical examination is unreliable in complex ICU situations where invasive procedures may be required to assess a patient's volume status.

Clinical Assessment of Volume Status

Orthopnea is a sensitive symptom of volume overload. Jugular venous distention (JVD) is useful in assessing volume status and left ventricular failure. Distension of the internal or external jugular vein more than 3 cm above the sternal angle indicates an abnormal JVD. This is supported if there is abdominal–jugular reflux (hepatojugular reflux) or Kussmaul's sign. The JVD must be differentiated from pure right-sided heart failure such as occurs in cors pulmonale. These patients often give a history of smoking or recurrent pulmonary emboli and have an accentuated pulmonary second heart sound. An echocardiogram may be helpful for diagnosis. A third heart sound can be a normal finding in persons below age 45 years or may indicate congestive heart failure (CHF) and fluid overload, idiopathic hypertrophic subaortic stenosis (IHSS), or regurgitation of the mitral or tricuspid valves. In chronic renal failure or end-stage renal disease (ESRD), hypertension is a valuable clue to the presence of fluid overload. The finding of fine rales at the end of inspiration on chest examination suggests pulmonary edema, fibrosis, or atelectasis. Peripheral edema indicates renal fluid retention. It suggests CHF, nephrotic syndrome, cirrhosis, cors pulmonale, or malnutrition. Postural hypotension (fall in systolic BP >10%) with reflex tachycardia indicates intravascular volume depletion. More severe dehydration reduces skin turgor and axillary sweating.

Clinical Diagnosis of Uremia

Uremic encephalopathy alters mental status and may cause grand mal seizures. Uremic pericarditis causes a pericardial friction rub. Initial symptoms of renal insufficiency are often nonspecific. Nocturia suggests a failure to concentrate the urine. Shortness of breath may indicate CHF, anemia, or metabolic acidosis. Anorexia, nausea, vomiting, diarrhea, and confusion are uremic symptoms that, in the presence of established renal insufficiency, point toward advanced uremia.

EXAMINATION OF THE URINE

A urine specimen obtained within the last 2 hours should be tested with dipstick for pH, protein, glucose, hemoglobin, leukocyte esterase, nitrites, and specific gravity. The sample should be centrifuged at 3,000 rpm for 3 to 5 minutes, and the sediment placed on a slide under a coverslip and examined under the microscope.

Color

Urine should be clear and yellow. A dark brown color suggests bilirubinuria; a red color suggests hemoglobinuria, myoglobinuria, porphyria, or drugs such as rifampin and pyridium. A turbid white color suggests pyuria or crystalluria.

Specific Gravity

The normal range is 1.005 to 1.030. A specific gravity of 1.010 normally corresponds to a urine osmolality of 285 mmol/kg. Radiocontrast, protein, or glucose and urine concentration as a result of dehydration raise the specific gravity.

pH

The normal urine pH is 4.5–7.5. A persistent acid pH is a normal finding. A persistent alkaline pH is found in vegetarians or in patients with classical, type II distal renal tubular acidosis (RTA), urinary tract infection with urease-producing proteus organisms, or administration of alkali or acetazolamide.

Glucose

Urine glucose suggests either diabetes mellitus or decreased glucose reabsorption from the proximal tubule (renal glycosuria or proximal renal tubular acidosis).

Leukocyte Esterase and Nitrite

A positive reaction of leukocyte esterase indicates pyuria. Nitrite suggests gram-negative bacteriuria. These tests lack sensitivity.

Protein

A positive test should be followed by a 24-hour urine collection for measurement of protein or microalbumin. Excretion of >150 mg/24 hr of protein or >30 mg/24 hr of microalbumin is abnormal. Pure tubular dysfunction should not result in proteinuria above 1.5 g/24 hr. Greater quantities of proteinuria indicate a glomerulopathy. Proteinuria above 3.5 g/24 hr is termed nephrotic range. The dipstick test does not detect Bence Jones protein, which requires testing with sulfosalicylic acid. A false-positive test for protein occurs with pyridium, gross hematuria or a high pH.

Examination of the Urinary Sediment

More than three red blood cells (RBCs) per high-power field (hpf) is abnormal. Dysmorphic RBCs indicates a glomerular source for bleeding. The presence of white blood cells (WBCs) suggests urinary tract infection or inflammation. Pyuria with a negative bacteria culture suggests prostatitis, chronic urethritis, renal tuberculosis, renal stone disease, or papillary necrosis. Wright's or Hansel's stain can identify eosinophils in the urine. This suggests drug-induced allergic interstitial nephritis. Renal tubular epithelial (RTE) cells are often seen in acute tubular necrosis, glomerulonephritis, or pyelonephritis. Table 2-1 details the types of casts.

BIOCHEMICAL ANALYSIS OF URINE

Biochemical tests of glomerular filtration rate, including assessment of blood urea nitrogen, serum creatinine, creatinine clearance, and nuclear medicine tests, are described in Chapter 3.

Urinary Sodium Concentration

A level <10 mEq/L in patients with oliguric azotemia indicates a prerenal cause for the acute renal failure. A U_{Na} >40 mEq/L in an azotemic patient indicates acute tubular necrosis (ATN), diuretic use, or adrenal insufficiency. Intermediate levels require the calculation of the fractional excretion of sodium (FE_{Na}).

$$FE_{Na}(\%) = (U_{Na}/S_{Na}) \times (S_{creat}/U_{creat}) \times 100$$

The use of FE_{Na} to diagnose acute renal failure is detailed in Table 2-2.

Urinary Chloride Concentration

This is valuable to diagnose the cause of metabolic alkalosis. A U_{Cl} <15 mEq/L suggests chloride-responsive metabolic alkalosis. This is characteristic of extrarenal Cl^- loss, prior diuretic use, or severe volume depletion leading to contraction alkalosis. A U_{Cl} >15 mEq/L indicates chloride-resistant metabolic alkalosis.

TABLE 2.1   Urine Casts

Type	Description and clinical relevance
Hyaline	Mucoprotein matrix without cellular elements; does not indicate renal disease
Red cell	Indicates glomerular bleeding
Leukocyte	Common in pyelonephritis but also observed in interstitial nephritis and glomerulonephritis
Renal tubular epithelial	Observed with acute tubular necrosis, glomerulonephritis, and tubulointerstitial disease
Granular, waxy	Represents degenerative cellular elements
Broad	Characteristic of chronic renal failure

TABLE 2.2   Fractional Excretion of Sodium in Acute Renal Failure

$FE_{Na} > 1\%$	$FE_{Na} < 1\%$
Diuretic use	Prerenal azotemia
	Dehydration
Mineralocorticoid deficiency	Congestive cardiac failure
Chronic renal failure	Renal vasoconstriction or ischemia:
Acute tubular necrosis	Ischemic nephropathy
Acute interstitial nephritis	Bilateral renal artery stenosis
Severe ischemic nephropathy	Hepatorenal syndrome
Nonreabsorbable solutes	Sepsis
Mannitol	Early phase of rhabdomyolysis
Glucose	Nonsteroidal antiinflammatory agents
	Thrombotic thrombocytopenic purpura
	Contrast associated nephropathy
Late phase of obstructive uropathy	Acute glomerulonephritis
	Some patients with nonoliguric acute tubular necrosis
	Early phase of obstructive uropathy

This is characteristic of Bartter's or Gittelman's syndrome, primary hyperaldosteronism, or current diuretic use (see Chapter 17).

Urinary Anion Gap

This is calculated as:

$$\text{Urinary anion gap} = (U_{Na} - U_K) - U_{Cl}$$

The anion gap represents unmeasured anions such as phosphate, sulfate or bicarbonate in excess of unmeasured cations such as ammonium (NH_4^+). A normal gap is zero or negative. A positive number in an acidotic patient suggests a failure of NH_4^+ excretion because of renal tubular acidosis or administration of a carbonic anhydrase inhibitor. A negative number indicates extrarenal losses of bicarbonate in diarrhea or pancreatic drainage.

Suggested Readings

Corwin HL. Urinalysis. In: Schrier RW, Gottschalk CW, eds. *Diseases of the kidney, 6th ed.* Boston: Little, Brown, 1997:295–306.

Davidson AM, Grunfeld J-P. History and clinical examination of the patient with renal disease. In: Davidson AM, Camerson JS, Grunfeld J-P, Kerr DNS, Ritz E, Winearls CG, eds. *Oxford textbook of clinical nephrology, 2nd ed.* Oxford: Oxford University Press, 1998:3–19.

Greenberg A. Urinalysis. In: Greenberg A, Cheung A, Coffman T, Falk R, Jennette J, eds. *Primer on kidney diseases, 2nd ed.* San Diego: Academic Press, 1998:27–36.

Levey AS. Clinical evaluation of renal function. In: Greenberg A, Cheung, Coffman, Falk, Jennette, eds. *Primer on kidney diseases, 2nd ed.* San Diego: Academic Press, 1998:20–26.

Chapter 3

Evaluation of Kidney Function: Biochemical and Nuclear Medicine Tests

Christopher S. Wilcox

Laboratory studies are especially important to evaluate kidney disease. This chapter reviews the basic biochemical studies and nuclear medicine tests used to assess renal function.

BIOCHEMICAL TESTS

Assessment of Glomerular Filtration Rate

Blood Urea Nitrogen

The normal range for blood urea nitrogen (BUN) is 7 to 18 mg/dl or 2.5 to 6.4 mmol/L. Urea is freely filtered at the glomerulus, but up to 50% is reabsorbed. Therefore, urea clearance is an imprecise estimate of GFR. Moreover, many conditions may affect BUN independent of the GFR:

- Increased BUN: High-protein diet or increased protein catabolism from gastrointestinal bleeding, corticosteroids, tissue trauma, burns, or tetracyclines.
- Decreased BUN: Low-protein diet or decreased protein catabolism from liver disease or cachexia.

Serum Creatinines (s_{cr})

The upper limit of S_{cr} is 1.2 to 1.5 mg/dl or 106 to 133 μmol/L. Like urea, creatinine is freely filtered at the glomerulus. Creatinine excretion is dependent on filtration, proximal tubular creatinine secretion, and on some tubular reabsorption. However, the S_{cr} normally provides a better estimate of the GFR than does the BUN because the degree of creatinine reabsorption and secretion is relatively small compared to creatinine filtration. Thus, a rise in S_{cr} from 1.0 to 2.0 mg/dl normally indicates a decrease in GFR of roughly 50%. Several factors may affect S_{cr} independently of the GFR:

- Increased S_{cr}: Increased creatine or creatinine intake from a recent meat meal or the use of creatine supplements for body building; a decreased creatinine excretion because of competition for creatinine secretion with ketoacids (in diabetic ketoacidosis), organic anions (in uremia), or drugs (cimetidine, trimethaprim, or acetylsalicylic acid).

- Decreased S_{cr}: Decreased creatinine intake or generation from diminished muscle mass associated with cachexia, aging, or a low protein intake.

Creatinine Clearance and the Estimation of GFR

The GFR is calculated, using the Cockcroft-Gault formula, from the S_{cr} (mg/dl), the age (years), the gender, and the weight (kg):

Man: $GFR = \left[(140 - age) \times \text{lean body weight}\right] / \left(S_{cr} \times 72\right)$

Woman: $GFR = $ value for man $\times 0.85$

However, a better estimate of GFR is obtained by measuring creatinine clearance (C_{cr}):

$$C_{cr}(ml/min) = \text{urine creatinine } (mg/dl) \times$$
$$\text{urine volume } (ml/24 \text{ hr})/$$
$$\left[\text{serum creatinine } (mg/dl) \times 1,440\right]$$

Normal ranges for C_{cr} for adults aged 20 to 50 years follow:

- Men: 97–137 ml/min/1.73 m² or 0.93–1.32 ml/sec/m² IU
- Women: 88–128 ml/min/1.73 m² or 0.85–1.23 ml/sec/m² IU

An improper urine collection results in an inaccurate C_{cr}. The urine creatinine excretion should be 15 to 25 mg/kg/day in men and 12.5 to 20 mg/kg/day in women. These values decline with loss of muscle mass, as occurs in advancing age.

Tubular secretion of creatinine is relatively independent of GFR. At normal values of GFR, tubular secretion accounts for only

15% of creatinine excretion but, as renal function declines, C_{cr} progressively overestimates the true GFR. A C_{cr} of 20 ml/min corresponds to a true GFR of only about 10 ml/min. More accurate assessments of GFR can be achieved with nuclear medicine techniques.

Assessment of Tubular Function

Normally, a decline in GFR is matched by a proportionate decline in tubular function, apparent as a diminished ability to concentrate or dilute the urine or to conserve or eliminate acid, sodium, potassium, and other electrolytes. Therefore, patients with renal insufficiency are at special risk for developing disorders of water, electrolyte, or acid–base status.

Some patients have a more selective defect in tubular function, for example, a renal tubular acidosis. The specialized tests of urine concentration or dilution and of acid excretion are described in Chapters 15 and 17.

NUCLEAR MEDICINE TESTS

Renogram

The renogram is used primarily to assess renal function, although γ-camera pictures provide some information about renal size and shape. Several radiopharmaceutical preparations are available. Technetium diethylenetriaminepentaacetic acid, [Tc^{99m}]DTPA, is freely filtered by the glomerulus and is not reabsorbed. It is used to estimate GFR. Technetium dimercaptosuccinate, [Tc^{99m}]DMSA, is bound to the tubules and delineates the contours of functional renal tissue; it is used to assess cortical scarring from pyelonephritis or vesicoureteral reflux or to diagnose a renal infarct. Radioiodinated orthoiodohippurate (Hippuran) is secreted into the tubules; it is used to assess renal plasma flow. Technetium mercapto-acetyl-triglycine (MAG3) combines the benefits of Tc scanning with many of the characteristics of Hippuran. Currently, it is the agent of choice in most units.

A renogram is obtained by scanning over each kidney for 15 to 25 minutes after an IV injection of radiopharmaceutical. The counts normally rise to a peak (reflecting filtration and/or secretion of the marker) and decline (reflecting elimination of the marker from the nephron). A delay in the time to peak and in elimination occurs in patients with renal parenchymal disease or outflow

TABLE 3.1   Indications for a Renogram

To detect outflow obstruction (furosemide renogram)
To evaluate renovascular hypertension (ACEI renogram)
To evaluate a suspected scar or infarct (DMSA scan)
To quantify individual kidney function

obstruction. In the latter case, IV furosemide, given halfway through the scan, fails to enhance elimination. This "Lasix renogram" is the most sensitive index of outflow obstruction. A similar pattern of delayed time to peak and delayed elimination is seen in kidneys distal to a renal artery stenosis, but these abnormalities are accentuated after blockade of angiotensin II (Ang II) generation with an angiotensin-converting enzyme inhibitor (ACEI). It results from withdrawal of Ang II–dependent tone in the efferent arterioles. This reduces the GFR sharply and thereby reduces the elimination of the tracer from the nephron. The "ACEI renogram" is the most sensitive and specific test available to detect functionally important renovascular hypertension, as discussed in Chapter 22.

Nuclear Medicine Studies of Renal Function

Hippuran or DTPA can quantify the renal plasma flow or GFR, respectively. Both agents are eliminated only via the kidneys. Following IV injection, their plasma levels decline exponentially with a slope that is proportional to their clearances. This "plasma disappearance" method provides a measure of total GFR or renal plasma flow rate. If these methods are combined with scanning over the kidneys, they can estimate the single-kidney GFR or plasma flow rate which is useful to predict the effects on overall renal function of a planned nephrectomy. The indications for renography are summarized in Table 3.1.

Suggested Readings

Dworkin LD, Brenner BM. The renal circulation. In: Brenner BM, ed. *The kidney, 5th ed.* Philadelphia: WB Saunders, 1996:247–285.

Rolin HA, Hall PM. Evaluation of glomerular filtration rate and renal plasma flow. In: Jacobsen HR, Striker GE, Klahr S, eds. *Principles and practice of nephrology, 4th ed.* St Louis: CV Mosby, 1995:8–13.

Wilcox CS. Renovascular hypertension. In: Massry SG, Glassock RJ, eds. *Textbook of nephrology, 2nd ed.* Philadelphia: Lippincott Williams & Wilkins (in press).

Chapter 4

Evaluation of Kidney Structure: Radiology and Biopsy

C. Craig Tisher

The patient with kidney disease will often present with nonspecific signs and symptoms including nausea, anorexia, lethargy, edema, dyspnea, and diminished urine output. Consequently, the physician must rely on laboratory studies to assist the evaluation and diagnosis of kidney disease. This chapter reviews the use of radiologic procedures and the kidney biopsy to aid in the evaluation of the upper urinary tract.

RADIOLOGIC ASSESSMENT

Ultrasonography

Ultrasound resolution is 1 to 2 cm. It can be used to identify the cortex, medulla, renal pyramids, and a distended collecting system or ureter (Table 4.1). A kidney length of <9 cm or a size difference of >1.5 cm between the two kidneys is abnormal in an adult. *Simple cysts* are common and are uniformly benign. They contain no internal echoes, have a sharply defined smooth internal wall, and have increased "through transmission" of sound energy posteriorly. Other hypoechoic renal mass lesions to consider include lymphoma, melanoma, infarct, hematoma, and xanthogranulomatous pyelonephritis. Complex cysts or solid lesions require further investigation with computed tomography (CT), magnetic resonance imaging (MRI), or possibly angiography. Ultrasound has become the procedure of choice in the early diagnosis or screening

TABLE 4.1 Indications for Renal Ultrasound

To quantify renal size
To screen for hydronephrosis
To characterize renal mass lesions
To evaluate perirenal space for abscess or hematoma
To screen for autosomal dominant polycystic kidney disease
To localize kidney for invasive procedures
To assess residual bladder volume in excess of 100 mL
To evaluate for renal vein thrombosis (Doppler)
To assess renal blood flow (Doppler)

of autosomal dominant polycystic kidney disease. *Hydronephrosis* appears as a multiloculated fluid collection within the renal sinus. However, ultrasound does not assess the functional importance of obstruction. An apparent obstruction can occur with anatomic variants such as an extrarenal pelvis, vesicoureteric reflux, and pregnancy. Hydronephrosis may persist after obstruction has been relieved. A furosemide renogram may document functional obstruction.

Intravenous Pyelography

The intravenous pyelogram (IVP) provides an overview of the kidneys, ureters, and bladder. The nephrogram is formed by opacification of the renal parenchyma; its density depends on the GFR, rate of tubular fluid reabsorption, dose of radiographic contrast agent, and rate of intravenous injection. The IVP can demonstrate gross differences in function between the kidneys from the nephrogram phase. Renal insufficiency ($S_{cr} > 2$–3 mg/dl) decreases the diagnostic value of the IVP and greatly increases the danger of causing acute renal failure. Normal renal size as measured by pyelography is approximately 11 cm, which exceeds that measured by ultrasound because of a magnification of approximately 10%. The left kidney is normally larger than the right. The IVP should be examined for renal size and position, calcifications, distorting intrinsic or extrinsic mass lesions, adequacy of parenchymal thickness, abnormalities of cortical contour or papillary appearance, dilation or blunting of calyces, abnormal position or course of the ureters, reflux, congenital variants, and completeness of bladder emptying (Table 4.2).

TABLE 4.2.   Indications for an Intravenous Pyelogram

To assess renal size and contour
To investigate recurrent urinary tract infection
To detect and locate calculi
To evaluate suspected urinary tract obstruction
To evaluate cause of hematuria

Computed Tomography

Computed tomography (CT) is useful for further investigation of abnormalities discovered on ultrasound or IVP. The CT is performed with contrast except when limited to demonstrating hemorrhage or calcification. The contrast media are filtered by the glomeruli and concentrated in the tubules, thus allowing parenchymal enhancement and visualization of neoplasms or cysts. The renal vessels and ureters can be identified. Spiral CT scan with intravenous radiocontrast injection, so-called CT angiography, is an emerging noninvasive procedure to evaluate renal vasculature, especially when renovascular hypertension is suspected. The CT is useful in the evaluation of mass lesions or fluid collections in the kidney or retroperitoneal space, particularly when ultrasound examination is hindered by intraabdominal gas or by obesity (Table 4.3).

Magnetic Resonance Imaging

The loss of the corticomedullary demarcation on magnetic resonance imaging (MRI) is a nonspecific feature of renal disease. Renal cysts are well visualized, but, unlike CT, MRI can not accurately define foci of calcification. In the staging of solid renal lesions, MRI may be superior to CT because it can detect tumor thrombus in major vessels and can distinguish hilar collateral

TABLE 4.3.   Indications for Computed Tomography

To further evaluate a renal mass
To display calcification patterns in a mass
To evaluate a nonfunctioning kidney
To delineate extent of renal trauma
To guide percutaneous needle aspiration or biopsy
To diagnose adrenal causes for hypertension

vessels from lymph nodes. However, some renal neoplasms appear homogeneous with surrounding normal renal parenchyma and therefore may be missed with noncontrast MRI. MRI can help in differentiating adrenal mass lesions because characteristic images may occur in pheochromocytoma; it is also useful to diagnose renal vein thrombosis (Table 4.4).

Arteriography and Venography

Contrast imaging of the arterial and venous vasculature is useful to assess renal artery stenosis, nephrosclerosis, renal vein thrombosis, renal infarction, or a renal mass. It is performed by percutaneous cannulation of femoral vessels, sometimes aided by digital subtraction techniques. *Arteriography* is useful in the evaluation of atherosclerotic or fibrodysplastic stenotic lesions of the renal arteries, aneurysms, arteriovenous fistulas, large vessel vasculitis, and renal mass lesions. It can be combined with selective renal vein renin sampling for evaluation of renovascular hypertension, with percutaneous transluminal balloon angioplasty or stent placement, or with renal ablation. *Venography* is performed to diagnose renal vein thrombosis.

Summary

Radiologic tests can be very valuable diagnostic tools; however, they are expensive and carry a risk of adverse reactions. Proper patient selection and preparation can increase the value of the procedure and diminish toxicity. Even nonionic radiocontrast agents can induce acute renal failure or vascular thrombosis. Prevention and management of radiocontrast-induced renal damage are discussed in Chapter 26. Consultation with the radiologist before selecting the test is often very helpful.

TABLE 4.4   Indications for Magnetic Resonance Imaging

To serve as an adjunct to CT in evaluating renal masses
To serve as an alternative to CT in patients who are intolerant of radiographic contrast agents
To evaluate suspected pheochromocytoma
To assess renal vein thrombosis

RENAL BIOPSY

Percutaneous needle biopsy of the kidney can be useful for establishing a diagnosis, assessing prognosis, monitoring disease progression, or selecting a rational therapy.

Indications

Acute Renal Failure

When the underlying cause of acute renal failure is not evident initially, or recovery of renal function has not occurred after 3 to 4 weeks of supportive therapy, biopsy may be necessary to distinguish acute tubular necrosis from a host of other renal diseases that may require alternative management (see Chapter 26).

Nephrotic Syndrome

Renal biopsy is usually performed in the adult nephrotic patient without evidence of systemic disease to diagnose primary glomerular diseases. The most frequently encountered entities include membranous glomerulonephritis, focal segmental glomerulosclerosis, membranoproliferative glomerulonephritis, IgA nephropathy, amyloidosis, and minimal-change disease (see Chapters 6, 8, and 11).

Proteinuria

In the setting of persistent proteinuria of 2 g/24 hr/1.73 m² or more or when associated with an abnormal urine sediment or with documented functional deterioration, a renal biopsy may detect underlying kidney disease. Patients with orthostatic proteinuria do not require biopsy (see Chapter 6).

Hematuria

Renal biopsy may be helpful in patients with microscopic hematuria persisting longer than 6 months or in those with episodic gross hematuria or a family history of hematuria, particularly when there is an associated abnormal urine sediment or proteinuria. Secondary causes of hematuria must be excluded. Likely pathologic findings include benign essential hematuria, Alport's syndrome, thin basement membrane disease, and IgA nephropathy. Usually biopsy is not helpful in the clinical setting of isolated microscopic hematuria (see Chapter 5).

Systemic Disease

Various systemic disorders may have associated kidney involvement. These include diabetes mellitus, systemic lupus erythematosus, Schönlein-Henoch purpura, polyarteritis nodosa, Goodpasture's syndrome, Wegener's granulomatosis, and certain dysprotein-emias. Biopsy is often performed to confirm the diagnosis, to establish the extent of renal involvement, and to guide management (see Chapters 9–11).

Transplant Allograft

Biopsy of the allograft helps differentiate various forms of rejection from acute tubular necrosis, drug-induced tubulointerstitial nephritis or nephrotoxicity, hemorrhagic infarction, and de novo or recurrent glomerulonephritis (see Chapter 30).

Contraindications

Commonly accepted contraindications to percutaneous needle biopsy include a solitary or ectopic kidney (except transplant allo-grafts), a horseshoe kidney, the presence of an uncorrected bleeding disorder, severe uncontrolled hypertension, small kidneys (usually indicative of chronic irreversible renal disease), renal infection, renal neoplasm, or an uncooperative patient.

Patient Preparation and Complications

Routine laboratory tests before biopsy should include a prothrombin time, partial thromboplastin time, complete blood count, platelet count, blood type, an antibody screen for possible cross-matching should the need for transfusion arise, and urinalysis to exclude a urinary tract infection. If coagulation parameters are abnormal, a bleeding time should be obtained. Patients should avoid ingestion of nonsteroidal antiinflammatory agents or aspirin in the week preceding biopsy. The percutaneous biopsy is usually performed with ultrasound or fluoroscopic guidance. After biopsy, the patient should remain at bed rest for up to 24 hours. Frequent vital signs are recorded to monitor evidence of hypovolemia as a result of hemorrhage. Hematocrits are obtained 4 hours after the biopsy and again the next morning. Aliquots of each voided urine are saved to observe for gross hematuria. Increasingly, percutaneous needle biopsy of the kidney is being performed in the out-patient setting in carefully selected patients.

The most frequent complication is bleeding, but that is usually self-limited. Significant bleeding requiring transfusion, percutaneous arterial embolization of a bleeding vessel, or nephrectomy is uncommon, with an occurrence rate of 2. 1%. The mortality rate of 0.07% is comparable with that of percutaneous liver biopsy or coronary angiography. When percutaneous needle biopsy is technically not feasible, and a histologic diagnosis is imperative, an open biopsy or a laparoscopic biopsy should be considered.

The tissue specimen should be submitted for light microscopy, immunofluorescence microscopy, and electron microscopy and evaluated by a pathologist experienced in interpretation of kidney biopsies.

Suggested Readings

Amis ED. Contemporary uroradiology. *Radiol Clin North Am* 1991;29: 437–650.

Deininger HK, Beil D, Schmidt C, et al. Digital subtraction angiography and other noninvasive methods for evaluation of renal circulation and hypertension. *Uremia Invest* 1985;9:231–241.

Fine EJ, Axelrod M, Blaufox MD. Physiologic aspects of diagnostic renal imaging. *Semin Nephrol* 1985;5:188–207.

Gimenez LF, Micali S, Chen RW, et al. Laparoscopic renal biopsy. *Kidney Int* 1998;54:525–529.

Haas M. A re-evaluation of routine electron microscopy in the examination of native renal biopsies. *J Am Soc Nephrol* 1997;8:70–76.

Olbricht CJ, Paul K, Prokop M, et al. Minimally invasive diagnosis of renal artery stenosis by spiral computed tomography angiography. *Kidney Int* 1995;48:1332–1337.

Tisher CC. Clinical indications for kidney biopsy. In: Tisher CC, Brenner BM, eds. *Renal pathology with clinical and functional correlations, 2nd ed.* Philadelphia: JB Lippincott, 1994:75–84.

Tisher CC, Croker BP. Indications for and interpretation of the renal biopsy: evaluation by light, electron and immunofluorescence microscopy. In: Schrier RW, Gottschalk CW, eds. *Diseases of the kidney, 6th ed.* Boston: Little, Brown, 1997:435–461.

Chapter 5

Hematuria

Nicolas J. Guzman

Hematuria is the presence of abnormal quantities of erythrocytes in the urine. Urine may contain up to three erythrocytes per 10 to 20 high-power fields (or 8, 000 erythrocytes/ml centrifuged urine); the persistent excretion of more than this is an indication for evaluation of the genitourinary tract. Table 5.1 lists some important clinical features associated with hematuria.

DETECTION

Microscopic hematuria is detected by microscopic inspection of the urinary sediment or by *ortho*-toluidine-impregnated paper strips. These give positive results with urine containing as few as three to five erythrocytes per high-power field. This test, however, also detects hemoglobinuria and myoglobinuria. Large numbers of erythrocytes are found in urine samples obtained by urethral catheterization and in voided specimens from menstruating women.

EVALUATION

Initial laboratory studies should include a urinalysis, coagulation tests, and urine cultures. If pyuria is present, a Gram stain of the urine should be performed. Sterile pyuria coupled with hematuria suggests renal tuberculosis.

Once infectious etiologies have been excluded, an intravenous pyelogram should be obtained to exclude renal or pelvic calcifications and masses. Thereafter, a cystoscopy with biopsy of any lesions should be performed, and the material sent for culture

TABLE 5.1 Relationship between Clinical Findings and Origin of Hematuria

Sign or symptom	Renal parenchyma	Urinary tract
Pain	Dull flank pain	Suprapubic pain with dysuria; colicky flank pain
Blood clots	Absent in glomerular diseases; may occur with trauma and vascular anomalies	Common
Cellular casts	Common in glomerular diseases	Absent or mild
Proteinuria	Common >150 mg/dl	Absent
Red blood cells	Usually distorted morphology	Usually normal

and pathologic examination. Selective ureteric urine samples should be inspected for hematuria and sent for culture and cytology. If the intravenous pyelogram reveals a renal mass or calcifications, a renal ultrasound should be performed to determine if the mass is solid or cystic and to identify renal calculi. Further characterization requires retrograde pyelography, a computed tomography scan, an angiogram, or a combination of these studies.

Glomerular causes of hematuria (Chapter 8) should be considered when evaluation fails to provide a definitive diagnosis. Renal biopsy should be considered early in patients presenting with hematuria associated with proteinuria or RBC casts.

The cause of the hematuria will remain unknown in 10% to 15% of all patients.

DIFFERENTIAL DIAGNOSIS

Glomerular Causes

Primary glomerulopathies such IgA nephropathy commonly present with hematuria and/or RBC casts.

Renal involvement in systemic diseases such as SLE, Schönlein-Henoch purpura, and vasculitides commonly causes hematuria. The presence of fever, arthralgias, skin rash, or purpura suggests a systemic disorder. Positive serologic tests for collagen-vascular disease or hypocomplementemia and cryoglobulinemia usually indicate the cause of the hematuria (see Chapter 9).

Wegener's granulomatosis and Goodpasture's syndrome present commonly with pulmonary involvement and hemoptysis. Antineutrophilic cytoplasmic antibodies (ANCA) help in the diagnosis of Wegener's granulomatosis. Antiglomerular basement membrane antibodies are characteristic of Goodpasture's syndrome (see Chapter 8).

Poststreptococcal glomerulonephritis is characterized by a history of recent skin or throat infection and elevated titers of antistreptolysin O, antihyaluronidase, or anti-DNase. Fever associated with the appearance of a heart murmur suggests infective endocarditis, particularly in patients with prosthetic heart valves and a history of recent dental procedures or those who are intravenous drug abusers. Blood cultures will usually demonstrate the causative organism. Echocardiography may disclose the presence of vegetations.

Hereditary nephritis or Alport's syndrome very commonly presents with hematuria. The diagnosis is suggested by a family history of kidney disease, kidney failure, deafness, and ocular abnormalities. Audiometry is abnormal in half of these patients. Benign essential hematuria or thin glomerular basement membrane disease presents as isolated hematuria.

Vascular Causes

Renal vein thrombosis may present with hematuria. These patients will commonly have a history of nephrotic syndrome, and their laboratory evaluation may reveal a hyperchloremic metabolic acidosis, proteinuria, and glycosuria (Fanconi's syndrome). The diagnosis is made by selective renal venography, MRI, or Doppler ultrasound.

Sudden back pain and hematuria, particularly in a patient with an aortic aneurysm, atrial fibrillation, or a recent myocardial infarction, suggest *renal arterial embolism.* Renal angiography is the procedure of choice to identify this condition.

Arteriovenous malformations can present as asymptomatic hematuria. The diagnosis is usually made by angiography.

Cystic Disease

Patients with *polycystic kidney disease* usually have a family history of kidney failure. The diagnosis can be made with renal ultrasound (see Chapter 13).

Tubulointerstitial Disease

Hypersensitivity tubulointerstitial nephritis is suspected when a patient with recent drug exposure presents with hematuria and sterile pyuria, skin rash, peripheral eosinophilia, and eosinophiluria (see Chapter 12).

Papillary necrosis is usually an acute and dramatic condition. It should be considered whenever hematuria occurs in a patient with analgesic nephropathy, sickle cell disease or trait, or diabetes mellitus complicated by acute pyelonephritis with obstruction.

Other Causes

Urinary tract infection is a common cause of hematuria. It usually presents with dysuria and pyuria. Other causes of hematuria are renal cell carcinoma, transitional cell carcinoma, renal calculi, trauma, and prostatic diseases. Systemic coagulation disorders may also present as hematuria.

TREATMENT

Hematuria rarely requires volume replacement. The passing of blood clots can cause severe pain and urinary obstruction, which may require urethral catheterization and saline irrigation. In most patients, the treatment of hematuria is directed toward the primary cause.

Suggested Readings

Fairley KF. Urinalysis. In: Schrier RW, Gottschalk CW, eds. *Diseases of the kidney, 5th ed.* Boston: Little, Brown, 1993:335–359.

Lieberthal W. Hematuria and the acute nephritic syndrome. In: Jacobson HR, Striker GE, Klahr S, eds. *The principles and practice of nephrology, 1st ed.* Philadelphia: Decker, 1991:244–250.

Llach F. Tests, procedures, and treatments: the urine. In: *Papper's clinical nephrology, 3rd ed.* Boston: Little, Brown, 1993:521–568.

Chapter 6

Proteinuria and the Nephrotic Syndrome

Koshy O. Abraham
Anupam Agarwal

A healthy adult excretes less than 150 mg of protein per day in the urine. Excessive amounts of urine protein may denote the presence of a benign disorder or represent evidence of a serious underlying disease. If proteinuria is present, one must be careful not to label a patient with a serious disorder because the prevalence of proteinuria on an initial screening urinalysis in healthy subjects can be as high as 25%, yet only a small percentage of these patients will have underlying renal disease.

PATHOPHYSIOLOGY

The nephron may have several grams of protein delivered to it each day, yet only a minuscule amount appears in the urine. The kidney processes about 150 L of filtrate containing 60 to 80 g/L of protein. This results in the excretion of about 1 to 2 L of urine per day, which contains less than 150 mg of protein. Two factors account for this. First, the glomerular filtration barrier, which comprises an endothelial layer, a basement membrane, and an epithelial cell layer, restricts the filtration of most proteins, and second, the proximal tubule reabsorbs and degrades much of the protein that is filtered.

Glomerular Proteinuria

The glomerulus is a highly efficient filter that restricts the passage of molecules on the basis of size and charge. Neutral dextrans with a radius less than 1.8 nm (18 Å) are freely filtered, whereas those that are 4.2 nm or greater are excluded by the glomerular capillary wall. Molecules within these limits have clearances that decrease progressively as size increases. The glomerular capillary wall also carries a negative charge. This anionic state of the filtration barrier limits the filtration of molecules with a negative charge while molecules carrying a more positive charge have a higher fractional excretion. This explains why albumin (5.5 nm or 55 Å), an anionic molecule, is not filtered across the glomerulus. In certain conditions, such as minimal-change disease, the charge-selective barrier is lost, resulting in a selective proteinuria that leads to loss of albumin as the major filtered protein.

Tubular Proteinuria

Many low-molecular-weight proteins that are filtered by the glomerulus are reabsorbed and degraded by the renal tubules, predominantly the proximal tubule. If the proximal tubule is damaged, proteinuria can occur, but it is rarely greater than 1,500 mg/24 hr unless accompanied by glomerular injury.

Overflow Proteinuria

This is usually seen in patients with no apparent renal disease but results from overproduction of immunoglobulin light chains and heavy chains or other small proteins. The overflow occurs because the amount of filtered protein exceeds the resorptive capacity of the tubules (e.g., multiple myeloma).

INTERPRETATION OF PROTEINURIA

It is essential to determine the presence of albuminuria when protein is present. The presence of a positive dipstick suggests albuminuria and hence glomerular proteinuria. A negative dipstick in the presence of proteinuria suggests tubular or overflow proteinuria. Albuminuria can be further subdivided into several patterns.

Intermittent Proteinuria

This may be a prelude to serious renal disease but is usually seen in patients with a febrile illness, congestive heart failure, stress, or following heavy exercise. There is no long-term risk to developing renal insufficiency.

Orthostatic Proteinuria

This denotes the presence of proteinuria only in the erect position. Protein excretion rarely exceeds 1 g/24 hr, and it is a benign condition. There is no increased risk for developing renal insufficiency or hypertension.

Persistent Proteinuria

This pattern of proteinuria is self-explanatory and denotes a sign of renal disease even with a normal glomerular filtration rate. The renal disease may be a primary glomerular disease or secondary to a systemic disease. Excretion of more than 3.5 g/1.73 m² of body surface area or 50 mg/kg of body weight denotes nephrotic-range proteinuria. On a random spot urine sample, a ratio of urine protein to urine creatinine greater than 3.5 signifies nephrotic-range proteinuria. This determination is helpful in patients unable to collect a 24-hour urine sample.

NEPHROTIC SYNDROME

The presence of nephrotic-range proteinuria with clinical and metabolic derangements denotes the nephrotic syndrome. Diagnostic features include proteinuria (>3.5 g/day/1.73 m² body surface area), hypoalbuminemia (<3.5 g/dl), edema, and hyperlipidemia. The common causes of nephrotic syndrome are listed in Table 6.1. Complications of nephrotic syndrome include increased risk of thrombosis, infections, severe edema, adverse effects of hyperlipidemia, hyponatremia, and acute renal failure. Thrombosis can occur in both the arterial and venous circulations with a predilection for renal veins. Disorders associated with higher risk for this complication include membranous nephropathy, lupus nephritis, and amyloidosis. A sudden increase in the degree of proteinuria, flank pain, hematuria, or worsening renal function in patients with nephrotic syndrome from the above causes should raise a clinical suspicion of renal vein thrombosis.

INVESTIGATIONS

The presence of proteinuria deserves a complete workup, although the investigations are determined by the clinical situation. A

**TABLE 6.1   Common Causes of Persistent Proteinuria
and the Nephrotic Syndrome**

Primary glomerular disorders
  Membranous glomerulonephritis
  Membranoproliferative glomerulonephritis
  Focal segmental glomerulosclerosis
  IgA nephropathy
  Minimal change disease
  Proliferative glomerulonephritis
  Fibrillary glomerulonephritis
Secondary disorders

Hereditary–familial	Diabetes mellitus, Alport's syndrome, sickle cell disease
Autoimmune	Systemic lupus erythematosus, Goodpasture's syndrome, Wegener's granulomatosis, polyarteritis nodosa, pauciimmune glomerulonephritis
Infectious	Postinfectious glomerulonephritis, endocarditis, hepatitis B and C, human immunodeficiency virus
Drug-induced	Nonsteroidal antiinflammatory agents, heroin, gold, mercury, D-penicillamine, captopril
Neoplastic	Hodgkin's disease, lymphomas, leukemia, multiple myeloma
Miscellaneous	Amyloidosis, preeclampsia–eclampsia, interstitial nephritis

24-hour urine collection should be obtained to quantify the protein excretion. To ensure an adequate urine collection, the creatinine excretion should also be measured. Men normally excrete 20 to 25 mg/kg of creatinine per day, and women excrete 14 to 22 mg/kg per day. The calculated and measured creatinine excretion should be compared to ensure a complete collection. The following formulas can be used to estimate creatinine excretion: (a) for men, it is $(140 - \text{age in years}) \times (\text{weight in kilograms})/5,000$; and (b) for women, $[(140 - \text{age in years}) \times (\text{weight in kilograms})/5,000] \times 0.85$. A microscopic analysis of the urine sediment should be undertaken. The presence of hematuria and red cell casts suggests a glomerulonephritis. A renal ultrasound should be performed to evaluate the size of the kidneys, degree of echogenicity, and the presence of both kidneys. Renal vein Doppler studies should be performed for a suspicion of renal vein thrombosis. Basic blood chemistries such as a creatinine, BUN, albumin, and cholesterol should be obtained. In selected patients, one may also obtain complement levels, antinuclear antibody pattern and titer, HIV and hepatitis B and C serology, cryoglobulins, serum and urine electrophoresis, antineutrophil cytoplasmic antibodies (ANCA), and antistreptolysin O and antihyaluronidase titers. In adults, a renal biopsy should be performed in order to confirm the diagnosis or to help in the management of the patient. A schematic approach in the clinical evaluation of proteinuria is shown in Fig. 6.1.

MANAGEMENT

Dietary Protein Restriction and Renin–Angiotensin System Inhibition

Proteinuria *per se* is an independent risk factor for the progression of renal disease, and attempts to lower the level of proteinuria represent an important strategy in delaying progression of the underlying renal disease. The presence of proteinuria is also associated with a higher risk of cardiovascular mortality, as reported in the Framingham study. The management of a patient with proteinuria is twofold. If possible one should treat both the underlying disease process and the proteinuria and/or its complications. The treatment of the underlying disease would depend on the type of renal lesion and may involve the use of corticosteroids and/or cytotoxic agents. Protein loss in the urine leads to hypoalbuminemia, but hypoalbuminemia is not related to proteinuria alone. There is also an increased rate of renal albumin catabolism and an inappropriately low hepatic albumin synthesis rate. Treatment consists of reducing intraglomerular pressure. This can be accomplished by reducing the dietary protein intake, although this may sound contraproductive because of the ongoing protein losses; however, high protein loads will increase intraglomerular pressure and promote the progression of renal insufficiency. In the presence of normal renal function, daily dietary protein intake should be about 0.8 g/kg body weight. With renal insufficiency this should be further reduced to 0.6 to 0.8 g of high-biological-value protein/kg body weight. Allowance should be made for urinary losses, and this amount should be added to the daily protein intake. Angiotensin-converting enzyme inhibitors also reduce intraglomerular pressure and can reduce proteinuria by up to 50%. These agents are

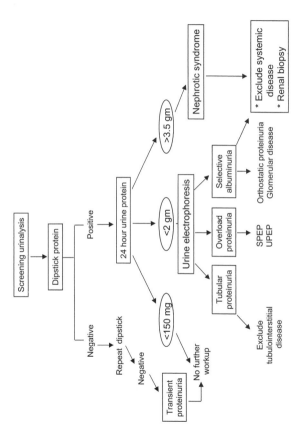

FIGURE 6.1 Approach to the clinical evaluation of proteinuria and nephrotic syndrome. SPEP, serum protein electrophoresis; UPEP, urine protein electrophoresis. Modified from Rosenberg and Hostetter (1992).

now the drugs of choice for the treatment of both diabetic and non-diabetic renal diseases causing proteinuria. Studies in humans, though limited, have shown that angiotensin II receptor antagonists are equally effective in decreasing proteinuria. Drugs considered second-line agents include angiotensin II receptor blockers and the nondihydropyridine calcium channel blockers such as diltiazem.

Edema

Peripheral edema can be a medical as well as a cosmetic problem. Treatment consists of dietary salt and fluid restriction and the judicious use of diuretics. Complete elimination of edema should be avoided because many patients with hypoalbuminemia and edema are intravascularly volume contracted. Diuretics in this setting may cause prerenal azotemia and worsen renal function. The use of diuretics is a delicate balance between providing patients comfort and not worsening their renal function. The combination of a loop diuretic (e.g., furosemide) with metolazone, a quinazoline diuretic with properties similar to a thiazide diuretic has additive effects and can be used in patients not responding to loop diuretics alone.

Hyperlipidemia

Hyperlipidemia increases the risk for cardiovascular disease in the nephrotic patient. There is also evidence that hyperlipidemia may promote progressive renal injury, and hence, it is important to treat this condition. Initially a diet low in saturated fat and cholesterol should be initiated; smoking should be discouraged, and exercise encouraged. If the LDL-cholesterol continues to be elevated despite dietary measures, the patient should begin therapy with a 3-hydroxy-3-methylglutaryl coenzyme A (HMG-CoA) reductase inhibitor.

Hypercoagulability

The presence of thrombotic complications such as acute renal vein thrombosis in patients with nephrotic syndrome requires immediate hospitalization and heparin anticoagulation. Oral anticoagulation with warfarin should be continued for at least 6 months after initial heparin therapy. The treatment of other complications mentioned earlier can be found in the references listed below.

Suggested Readings

Bernard DB, Salant DJ. Clinical approach to the patient with proteinuria and the nephrotic syndrome. In: Jacobson HR, Striker GE, Klahr S, eds. *The principles and practice of nephrology*. Philadelphia: CV Mosby, 1995:110–121.

Lafayette RA, Perone RD, Levey AS. Laboratory evaluation of renal function. In: Schrier RW, Gottschalk CW, eds. *Diseases of the kidney, 6th ed.* New York: Little, Brown, 1997:307–354.

Rosenberg ME, Hostetter TH. Proteinuria. In: Seldin DW, Giebisch G, eds. *The kidney: physiology and pathophysiology, 2nd ed.* New York: Raven Press, 1992:3039–3061.

Chapter 7

Diabetic Nephropathy

John R. Silkensen
Anupam Agarwal

Nephropathy is a serious complication of diabetes mellitus that often leads to end-stage renal failure and is a major cause of morbidity and mortality. In type I or insulin-dependent diabetes mellitus, 30% to 50% of the patients will develop nephropathy and renal failure, whereas in type II or non-insulin-dependent diabetes mellitus, the number is approximately 10% to 20%.

INCIDENCE

Currently about 6% of the United States population or 16 million individuals have diabetes mellitus. The yearly incidence of diabetes, which is the number of new cases diagnosed per year, is approximately 800,000. In 1996, diabetes mellitus ranked seventh in causes of death by disease in the United States. At present, approximately 39% of all patients hospitalized for the treatment of end-stage renal failure have diabetes as the underlying cause. In fact, diabetes is the most common cause of end-stage renal disease in the United States. The prevalence of diabetic nephropathy increases with the duration of the disease. Poor glycemic control, hypertension, and genetic predisposition are all associated with a greater prevalence of renal disease.

CLINICAL PRESENTATION AND PATHOPHYSIOLOGY

Insulin-Dependent Diabetes Mellitus

In 1984, Mogensen and Christensen described the progression of renal disease in insulin-dependent diabetes mellitus (IDDM) and divided this evolution into five stages:

- Stage I. The hyperfiltration–hypertrophy stage is character-ized by an increase in glomerular filtration rate that is 20% to 50% above age-matched control subjects. Hypertrophy of the kidneys, visible on radiologic imaging, is also present. Functionally, glucosuria with polyuria and microalbumin-uria (greater than 20 but less than 200 mg/min) occur in this stage. With insulin treatment of several weeks' duration, the hyperfiltration and hypertrophy correct in most patients, and the microalbuminuria falls below 20 µg/min.

- Stage II. This is a silent stage wherein microalbuminuria is normal or near normal (less than 20 µg/min) and is usually seen from 1 to 5 years following diagnosis in 90% to 95% of pa-tients with IDDM. The GFR is in the normal range in most patients. Features of early structural changes such as glomeru-lar basement membrane (GBM) thickening and mesangial expansion are evident in the kidney on histologic examina-tion. Those patients destined to develop diabetic nephropathy often manifest a persistently elevated GFR (greater than 150 ml/min), early hypertension, and poor metabolic control. From 30% to 50% of diabetic patients will proceed into stage III and beyond and develop structural damage in the kidney.

- Stage III. This is also referred to as the stage of incipient neph-ropathy and occurs after 5 to 15 years of diabetes. There are fur-ther thickening of the GBM and mesangial expansion. The GFR starts to decrease in the later periods of this stage. Micro-albuminuria (20–200 µg/min), which correlates with an excre-tion rate of 30 to 300 mg/24 hr if present, is a poor prognostic indicator. Hypertension develops early during this stage. This stage can last for several years. The level of protein excretion can be decreased, and the decline in GFR can be slowed with improved control of hyperglycemia and aggressive control of hypertension.

- Stage IV. This is the stage of overt nephropathy or dipstick-positive proteinuria and is characterized by fixed and repro-ducible proteinuria (more than 0.5 g/24 hr, detectable by dip-stick). Hypertension is invariably present, and the GFR gradu-ally declines. Histology reveals diffuse or nodular intercapillary glomerulosclerosis.

- Stage V. This is the stage of end-stage renal failure and on average occurs about 20 years from time of onset of diabetes in IDDM patients. In patients who progress to end stage, the time required to develop overt diabetic nephropathy (stage IV) is highly variable but averages 15 to 17 years. However, subsequent progression to end stage (stage V) is relatively predictable and averages 5 to 7 years. The histology is characterized by glomerular sclerosis and obsolescence. Evidence of other complications of diabetes such as retinopathy, neuropathy, cardiac disease, and vascular disease are usually present at this stage.

Non-Insulin-Dependent Diabetes Mellitus

Far less is known regarding the development of diabetic nephropathy in non-insulin-dependent or type II diabetes mellitus. At diagnosis, microalbuminuria is frequently present and is often reversible with proper metabolic control. In contrast to insulin-dependent or type I disease, hyperfiltration is detected only rarely, and there is no evidence of glomerular hypertrophy. It is clear, however, that in comparison with an age-matched population, the presence of microalbuminuria in NIDDM carries a worse prognosis.

Besides diabetic nephropathy, patients with diabetes mellitus are prone to an increased incidence of urinary tract infections (bacteriuria, cystitis, acute pyelonephritis), papillary necrosis, and neurogenic bladder with hydronephrosis. It is also important to consider other nondiabetic causes for renal disease in the diabetic patient because many diabetics with renal disease are incorrectly labeled as having diabetic nephropathy. Table 7.1 summarizes features that, if present, may raise the suspicion of a nondiabetic cause for renal disease.

PATHOLOGY

The histopathologic alterations observed in diabetic nephropathy typically affect the glomeruli, vasculature, and tubulointerstitial compartment (Table 7.2). Nodular intercapillary glomeruloscle-

TABLE 7.1 Features Suggestive of Nondiabetic Renal Disease in Diabetic Patients

Absence of diabetic retinopathy
Overt nephropathy with diabetes of less than 5 years' duration
Renal failure without significant proteinuria
Presence of RBC casts
Hypocomplementemia

TABLE 7.2   Histopathologic Features of Diabetic Renal Disease

Glomerular lesions
  Diffuse intercapillary glomerulosclerosis
  Nodular intercapillary glomerulosclerosis
  Capsular drop lesion
  Fibrin cap lesion
  Glomerular basement membrane thickening
Vascular lesions
  Subintimal hyalin arteriolosclerosis
  Benign arteriosclerosis
Tubular and interstitial lesions
  Hyalin droplets in proximal tubules
  Glycogen deposits (Armanni-Ebstein lesion)
  Tubular atrophy
  Interstitial fibrosis

rosis, although not pathognomonic of diabetic nephropathy, is the most characteristic of the renal lesions observed in this disease. However, a very similar lesion can be observed in light-chain deposition disease. Therefore, caution must be exercised when this lesion is found in patients with proteinuria in the absence of hyperglycemia or other signs and symptoms of diabetes mellitus.

PATHOGENESIS

The pathogenesis of diabetic nephropathy is undoubtedly multifactorial and includes hemodynamic alterations, level of glycemic control, genetic predisposition, and race.

Hemodynamic Alterations

Both systemic and renal hemodynamics are critical determinants in the pathogenesis of diabetic nephropathy. Hypertension usually occurs before the onset of a decline in GFR and is associated with a higher incidence of developing nephropathy. Glomerular hyperfiltration occurs early in the disease and, if persistent, is more likely to be associated with renal failure later. Hyperglycemia is thought to be one of the mechanisms responsible for glomerular hyperfiltration.

Glycemic Control

An abnormal metabolic milieu must also be present for development of the characteristic renal lesions. The Diabetes Control and

Complications Trial (DCCT) has clearly proven what many had long suspected, that glycemic control correlates with the appearance and progression of diabetic nephropathy. Improved control of hyperglycemia and reduction in intraglomerular and systemic hypertension can delay progression of the functional and histologic changes of diabetic nephropathy. Furthermore, normoglycemia following pancreas transplantation has recently been shown to reverse the lesions of diabetic nephropathy in native kidneys. Abnormal glycosylation of proteins that form the GBM and mesangial matrix, hyperperfusion of the glomerular capillaries with an associated increase in the transcapillary pressure gradient, and growth of the glomerular capillaries lead to progressive glomerulosclerosis.

Genetic Predisposition

Genetic susceptibility to diabetic nephropathy is supported by the association of a family history of hypertension and an increased incidence of nephropathy in siblings of affected individuals. Additionally, ongoing studies involving the renin–angiotensin system and its various components have provided further evidence for a genetic basis of diabetic nephropathy.

Race

Minority populations are more commonly affected with diabetic nephropathy. The incidence of diabetic nephropathy is two- to threefold higher in African-Americans and six times higher in Native Americans and Hispanics compared to Caucasians.

EVALUATION

The presence of proteinuria, with or without hypertension and renal insufficiency, in a patient with diabetes mellitus of several years' duration is diabetic nephropathy until proved otherwise. The presence of diabetic retinopathy, which is observed in more than 90% of patients with diabetic nephropathy, strengthens the diagnosis. However, only one-fourth to one-third of those patients with diabetic retinopathy have clinically detectable renal disease. There are situations in which renal disease other than diabetic nephropathy should be considered in the diabetic patient (see Table 7-1). These include the absence of diabetic retinopathy, overt nephropathy with diabetes of less than 5 years' duration, renal failure without significant proteinuria, presence of an active urinary sediment, and low serum complements. In these situations a percutaneous renal biopsy is often indicated to establish the diagnosis, determine the prognosis, and aid in management. A renal ultrasound should be obtained to exclude obstructive uropathy secondary to a neurogenic bladder.

MANAGEMENT

Management of the renal disease associated with IDDM depends on the point in the disease at which the patient is encountered.

Hypertension

One of the most important factors in the management of diabetic renal disease is control of hypertension. Lowering the blood pressure in the hypertensive diabetic patient can slow the rate of decline in GFR by 5 to 6 ml/min/year. Intraglomerular hypertension is thought by many to cause progressive glomerular destruction. Although lowering systemic blood pressure can lower intraglomerular pressures, angiotensin-converting enzyme (ACE) inhibitors lower intraglomerular hypertension more predictably by reducing postglomerular vascular resistance. This accounts for some of the evidence showing a delay in progression of diabetic nephropathy in type I patients with diabetic nephropathy. The ACE inhibitors are considered drugs of choice on the basis of these findings. By extension, it is reasonable to assume that the newer angiotensin type I receptor blockers (ARBs) would be reasonable alternatives to the use of ACE inhibitors, especially when patients develop intolerable side effects from the latter agents. Other useful agents to control hypertension include calcium channel blockers, α-receptor blockers, and cardioselective β-blockers.

Hyperglycemia

At the onset of diabetes mellitus, before insulin therapy is initiated (hyperfiltration–hypertrophy stage), the GFR is elevated and the kidneys are enlarged. With insulin therapy and proper diet, both the GFR and the size of the kidneys usually decrease. Evidence suggests that failure to correct the elevated GFR increases the likelihood of the development of progressive renal disease later; thus, proper control of blood glucose levels early in the disease is important. Normalization of blood glucose levels will reduce microalbuminuria, especially in patients in the so-called incipient nephropathy stage (stage III). Thus, proper control of blood glucose levels in any diabetic patient is an important treatment goal as demonstrated by the DCCT trial. With the development of progressive diabetic nephropathy and renal failure, close attention should be given to blood glucose levels because renal clearance of insulin is diminished and hypoglycemia is more common.

Urinary Tract Infection

In general, asymptomatic bacteriuria (more than 100,000 organisms/ml) should be treated in the diabetic patient. The development of acute pyelonephritis, especially if associated with obstruction, can result in papillary necrosis that can be life threatening.

Renal Insufficiency

Once it is established that renal insufficiency in a diabetic patient is secondary to the underlying disease and not to a superimposed or secondary problem that may be reversible, management is essentially the same as in any patient with renal insufficiency. Blood pressure control is essential, and ACE inhibitors have been established as the drugs of choice. Dietary protein restriction and a low-fat diet are important measures to slow progression of renal failure in diabetic nephropathy. Because of the high propensity for accelerated atherosclerosis in these patients, risk factors for coronary artery disease should be appropriately modified.

Dialysis and Transplantation

Hemodialysis and continuous ambulatory peritoneal dialysis offer a 3-year survival rate of approximately 50%. Patients should be educated to save one of their upper extremities for vascular access, which should be placed earlier in these patients than in nondiabetics. In the younger diabetic patient, and especially in the absence of severe peripheral vascular disease, renal transplantation offers the best chance for survival. The 3-year patient survival with a living related donor allograft is close to 85%. The disease does recur in the transplanted kidney and can cause destruction of the graft in 5 to 10 years or less. Unfortunately, the successful rehabilitation of the transplant patient often depends on the rate of progression of the disease in other organs. Because cardiovascular disease is the most common cause of death in the transplant patient, especially the diabetic transplant patient, attention needs to be given to the proper evaluation of these patients before transplantation. It has been clearly demonstrated that diabetics have a high incidence of asymptomatic coronary artery disease and that noninvasive stress tests in this group are not optimal. The appropriate cardiac evaluation, therefore, is somewhat controversial, though there is reasonable support for obtaining a coronary angiogram in all patients with IDDM over age 45, even if asymptomatic. In patients younger than 45 years, multiple cardiac risk factors, a heavy smoking history, or an abnormal electrocardiogram should prompt the cardiologist to perform an angiogram, even in the absence of classic symptoms. Whether these same findings can be extrapolated to include patients with NIDDM is unclear.

Suggested Readings

Brancati FL, Whelton PK, Randall BL, Neaton JD, Stamler J, Klag MJ. Risk of end-stage renal disease in diabetes mellitus: a prospective cohort study of men screened for MRFIT. Multiple Risk Factor Intervention Trial. *JAMA* 1997;278:2069–2074.

Diabetes Control and Complications Trial Research Group. The effect of intensive treatment of diabetes on the development of long-term complications in insulin-dependent diabetes mellitus. *N Engl J Med* 1993;329:977–986.

Ibrahim HN, Hostetter TH. Diabetic nephropathy. *J Am Soc Nephrol* 1997; 8:487–493.

Ismail N, Becker B, Strzelczyk P, Ritz E. Renal disease and hypertension in non-insulin dependent diabetes mellitus. *Kidney Int* 1999;55:1–28.

Lewis EJ, Hunsicker LG, Bain RP, Rhode RD. The effect of angiotensin-converting enzyme inhibition on diabetic nephropathy: the collaborative study group. *N Engl J Med* 1993;329:1456–1462.

Chapter 8

Glomerulonephritis

C. Craig Tisher

Glomerulonephritis results from stimulation of the immune system leading to inflammation of the glomerulus and other components of the renal parenchyma. When limited to the kidney parenchyma, it is termed a "primary" glomerulonephritis. If part of a widely disseminated immune process, it is classified as a "secondary" form of glomerulonephritis (see Chapters 9–11).

CLINICAL PRESENTATION

Typically, patients present with a "nephritic urinary sediment" characterized by hematuria, pyuria, cellular and granular casts, and varying degrees of proteinuria. However, many types of glomerulonephritis are associated with the nephrotic syndrome (e.g., membranous glomerulonephritis, minimal-change disease (MCD), or focal segmental glomerulosclerosis) (see Chapter 6) or with gross hematuria (e.g., IgA nephropathy). When glomerulonephritis is part of a multisystem disease, the clinical presentation will often be characteristic of that disease, and renal involvement may be clinically evident (e.g., Goodpasture's syndrome or systemic lupus erythematosus) (see Chapter 9). Patients who present with red blood cell casts in the urine sediment or with a rapidly rising serum creatinine deserve special consideration. Many will develop irreversible renal failure early in their disease and must be diagnosed and treated aggressively. The laboratory studies listed in the following section should be obtained, but a kidney biopsy should not be delayed while awaiting the results. Often institution of aggressive therapy, such as corticosteroids and a cytotoxic agent, is warranted even before the biopsy results are known.

LABORATORY EVALUATION

Careful examination of the urine sediment is the cornerstone of the evaluation of patients suspected of glomerulonephritis. A 24-hour urine collection for creatinine clearance and total protein should be obtained to quantify residual renal function and urine protein excretion. Renal ultrasound should be performed to exclude reversible causes of renal insufficiency, to measure kidney size, and to prepare for biopsy. Routine studies, such as electrolytes, liver function tests (especially albumin), and cholesterol, should be obtained early in the disease. Adults with significant proteinuria (>1 g/24 hr) need a serum immunoelectrophoresis and urine protein electrophoresis. To further characterize the etiology of glomerulonephritis, the following laboratory studies should be considered:

- Complement components (C_3, C_4, CH_{50})
- Antinuclear antibodies—rheumatoid factor—erythrocyte sedimentation rate
- Antiglomerular basement membrane (anti-GBM) antibody titer
- Hepatitis serologies
- Antineutrophilic cytoplasmic antibodies
- Streptococcal screen or antistreptolysin O titers
- Human immunodeficiency virus (HIV) titer

PATHOGENESIS

The etiology and pathogenesis of many forms of glomerulonephritis are poorly understood. Antigens, including DNA, viruses, bacteria, or proteins of other tissues, can stimulate immune activation and antibody formation in glomerulonephritis. This is followed by deposition of antibodies directed against glomerular tissues or antigen–antibody complexes in the nephron or invasion of the glomerulus by cellular elements of the immune system.

CLASSIFICATION AND MANAGEMENT

Minimal-Change Disease

Patients with minimal-change disease (MCD), also called "nil disease" or "lipoid nephrosis," usually present with the nephrotic syndrome. Ninety percent of children between the ages of 1 and 6 years with the nephrotic syndrome will have MCD, whereas approximately 20% of adults with the nephrotic syndrome have MCD. The onset may be acute and often follows an upper respiratory tract infection. Edema can be dramatic, and hypertension and hematuria occur in 20% to 30% of affected children. Creatinine clearance is usually near normal; however, renal failure can be seen that may be caused, at least in part, by volume contraction secondary to severe hypoalbuminemia, that is, "prerenal" azotemia.

The MCD kidney has normal glomeruli on light microscopy. Immunofluorescence microscopy is negative, but electron microscopy reveals fusion or effacement of the foot processes of the glomerular visceral epithelial cell.

Because MCD is by far the most common cause of childhood nephrotic syndrome, an empirical course of corticosteroids is usually administered, and biopsy withheld, unless a remission is not induced within 4 to 8 weeks. More than 90% of children with MCD will experience a complete remission, but fewer than 25% will be cured with one course of corticosteroids. The rest will relapse at varying intervals but are generally responsive to another course of corticosteroids. Cyclophosphamide and chlorambucil can decrease the frequency of relapse, but this therapy must be weighed against the risk of using a cytotoxic agent for a benign disease in childhood, especially because relapses usually end by adulthood. Those who fail to respond to corticosteroids require a kidney biopsy to establish the diagnosis.

Because more than two-thirds of adult patients with the nephrotic syndrome will have a lesion that does not respond to corticosteroids, most nephrologists obtain a kidney biopsy before initiating therapy. Prednisone is effective in inducing a remission in adults with MCD, albeit at a much lower rate than in children, and frequent relapses are the rule. Treatment failures will often respond to cyclophosphamide, but again, the risk of using this agent in a benign disease must be considered carefully.

Focal Segmental Glomerulosclerosis

Typically, patients with focal segmental glomerulosclerosis (FSGS) will have the nephrotic syndrome or nephrotic-range proteinuria. However, patients may also present with a "nephritic" urinary sediment or with isolated proteinuria. FSGS is a common cause of the nephrotic syndrome in adults, comprising 20% to 30% of all cases in some series. A light microscopic picture similar to FSGS can also be seen in IgA nephropathy, Alport's syndrome, reflux nephropathy, or human immunodeficiency virus nephropathy or in association with intravenous drug abuse.

There is segmental or total sclerosis of glomerular tufts, and increased mesangial matrix and cellularity are common. Diseased and normal glomeruli are interspersed, and there is a predisposition for involvement of juxtamedullary glomeruli. Both IgM and C_3 deposits are present in the sclerotic segments of the glomeruli.

In adults FSGS should be treated with prednisone at an average dose of 1 mg/kg body weight per day. A period of 5 to 8 months may be required to induce remission. A remission rate of 50% can be anticipated with this prolonged treatment. Favorable prognostic indicators include absence of tubulointerstitial disease on kidney biopsy, a normal or only modestly elevated serum creatinine, and nonnephrotic proteinuria. Failure to observe a decrease in urine protein excretion after 12 weeks of prednisone therapy in adults or 8 weeks in children raises the likelihood of steroid resistance. The use of angiotensin-converting enzyme inhibitors to reduce the level of proteinuria and control hypertension if the latter is present is recommended.

Membranous Glomerulonephritis

Patients with membranous glomerulonephritis usually present with the nephrotic syndrome, but many are asymptomatic, and proteinuria is discovered on routine urinalysis. This disease accounts for approximately 30% of all adults with the nephrotic syndrome. The peak age of incidence is 35 to 50 years, and men predominate by a ratio of 2:1. Patients can lose 10 to 20 g protein/day and experience severe disability. No specific laboratory or clinical features are pathognomonic, and kidney biopsy is required to make the diagnosis. Pathologically, the subepithelial surface of the glomerular capillary loops is irregular or "spike-like" as a result of extension of basement membrane material, which is best seen on silver stain of kidney tissue. On immunofluorescence microscopy of capillary loops, granular subepithelial immune deposits that stain for IgG and C_3 are present. Electron microscopy delineates the deposits from the spike-like deformities of the basement membrane.

Membranous glomerulonephritis is usually idiopathic, but up to 25% of patients can have an underlying disease such as systemic lupus erythematosus, hepatitis B and C, tumors, adverse drug reactions, or parasitic diseases. In addition to the laboratory tests mentioned earlier, antithyroid antibodies, serologic tests for syphilis, and anti-DNA antibodies should be obtained. Controversy exists regarding the likelihood of an underlying malignancy with idiopathic membranous glomerulonephritis; however, an evaluation for common malignancies should be undertaken, especially in older adults.

Approximately one-third of untreated patients require dialysis after 10 years, whereas another 20% to 30% have improvement in proteinuria or complete resolution of their disease. There are various therapies, but none has been proven superior. These include corticosteroids or cytotoxic agents or a combination of the two. Treatment should be tailored to the severity of symptoms, including proteinuria, as well as to the age and physical status of the patient. Prognosis is generally more favorable in women and in those with nonnephrotic proteinuria, a normal or mildly elevated serum creatinine, and an absence of tubulointerstitial scarring on renal biopsy.

Postinfectious Proliferative Glomerulonephritis

Postinfectious proliferative glomerulonephritis is usually observed after a streptococcal infection of either the upper respiratory tract or the skin. However, similar clinical and pathologic features can occur after any infectious process including subacute bacterial endocarditis, visceral abscesses, osteomyelitis, or bacterial sepsis. Poststreptococcal glomerulonephritis (PSGN) is discussed as a representative of this class of diseases.

Typically, PSGN presents with hematuria, hypertension, edema, proteinuria, and acute renal failure. In many patients, these signs may not be present or may be mild. Nephrotic-range proteinuria is uncommon in PSGN. Subclinical cases are common, especially in household contacts of the index case. PSGN is rare before the age of 2 years but is the most common glomerulonephritis in school-age children presenting with a nephritic urine sediment. It occurs at any age in adults and has a 2:1 male predominance. PSGN follows an infection with group A β-hemolytic *Streptococcus* of the throat, upper respiratory tract, or skin. There is typically an 8- to 14-day latent period after infection before the onset of glomerulonephritis. This period may last as long as 21 to 28 days after skin infections. Throat cultures are usually negative when active glomerulonephritis is detected, but the antistreptolysin O titer is positive in 90% of patients after upper respiratory tract infections and in 50% after skin infections.

Because PSGN is the most common etiology of an acute nephritic urinalysis in children, an antistreptolysin O titer and a complement profile are indicated initially. Kidney biopsy should be reserved for patients who present atypically or in whom the disease does not resolve spontaneously. In adults, postinfectious glomerulonephritis may mimic other types of glomerulonephritis. A kidney biopsy is indicated to establish the diagnosis.

In mild cases there is glomerular mesangial cell proliferation with an increase in mesangial matrix. Severe cases will also have diffuse endothelial cell proliferation with loss of glomerular capillary lumina, and crescents may be present. Electron microscopy reveals irregular subepithelial deposits or "humps" along the capillary loops.

Therapy is largely supportive, utilizing fluid and sodium restriction to control blood pressure and edema. Protein restriction is indicated in azotemic patients, and antihypertensive agents should be used to control blood pressure in those who fail to respond to conservative measures. Immunosuppressive agents are not indicated.

Family members of patients should have throat cultures, and those with streptococcal infection require antibiotic treatment. Children, even with severe disease, do well with supportive management; however, the presence of crescents on biopsy indicates a more guarded prognosis. Complete recovery is less certain in adults, particularly in those with a creatinine clearance of <40 ml/min/1.73 m^2, persistent proteinuria of >2 g/day, or increased age. Recurrence of PSGN is rare.

Rapidly Progressive Glomerulonephritis

Rapidly progressive glomerulonephritis presents clinically as acute renal failure and is associated with extensive glomerular crescent formation. It can be seen with an infectious etiology, vasculitis, or anti-GBM disease but is idiopathic in approximately 40% of patients. In half the patients it begins with a viral-like prodrome with myalgias, arthralgias, back pain, fever, and malaise. It may present with manifestations similar to a vasculitis. The urine often contains red blood cell casts.

The kidney reveals extensive cellular crescents with or without immune complex localization on immunofluorescence microscopy. Anti-GBM antibodies or antineutrophilic cytoplasmic antibodies may be present. In the absence of glomerular immune complexes or anti-GBM antibodies, a diagnosis of pauci-immune glomerulonephritis is likely. When glomerulosclerosis, crescents, or interstitial fibrosis is extensive, the lesion is usually irreversible.

Treatment for rapidly progressive glomerulonephritis is usually intravenous corticosteroids and cyclophosphamide. Plasmapheresis is useful only if the underlying disease, such as anti-GBM disease, is known to be responsive. Early diagnosis and treatment are key to a successful therapeutic response. The prognosis is poor when treatment is initiated after the serum creatinine is greater than 6 mg/dl or when oliguria is present. Red blood cell casts on urinalysis warrant aggressive diagnosis and treatment. Rapid loss of renal function may require empirical therapy with corticosteroids and cyclophosphamide until a specific diagnosis is obtained.

Goodpasture's Syndrome (Anti-GBM Disease)

Patients with Goodpasture's syndrome classically present with pulmonary hemorrhage and nephritis. Pulmonary involvement can range from frank hemoptysis to simple pulmonary infiltrates on chest x-ray and may not be concurrent with the presentation of nephritis. Most patients, however, will give some history of recent pulmonary complaints. Occasionally, patients present with pulmonary involvement in the absence of renal lesions. The peak incidence is in the third decade with a second peak in patients older than 60 years. The disease has a 2:1 male predominance.

The disease results from the formation of antibodies directed against an antigen in the GBM that cross-reacts with pulmonary tissue antigens. Linear deposits of IgG are found along the GBM, and circulating anti-GBM antibodies can be measured in the serum.

Treatment involves a 14-day course of plasma exchange with albumin, accompanied by the administration of corticosteroids and a cytotoxic agent such as cyclophosphamide. Unless patients present near end stage, they usually respond to therapy and eventually can be withdrawn from all agents. Recurrence is rare but is usually responsive to a second course of therapy. However, a significant number of patients eventually progress to end-stage renal failure. If renal transplantation is necessary, the procedure should be delayed until anti-GBM antibody titers are low or undetectable.

Membranoproliferative Glomerulonephritis

Membranoproliferative glomerulonephritis (MPGN) of the idiopathic variety frequently presents with a vague systemic illness (often described as similar to flu), accompanied by edema and gross hematuria. Edema and hematuria without systemic complaints are also commonly seen. Acute nephritis or rapidly progressive renal failure is less common. Complement levels are decreased in approximately 75% of patients. A serum IgG antiglobulin, C_3 nephritic factor, is present in some patients and may explain the decreased complement levels.

MPGN has been divided into three categories based on the histologic findings. Clinical differentiation of these subtypes is impossible. Type I is most common and is mediated by immune complexes with activation of the classical complement pathway. It is often associated with a chronic immunologic disease. Histologically there is an increase in mesangial cells with mesangial interposition in the capillary walls, which gives the appearance of reduplication of the GBM. Immune complex deposits are seen along peripheral capillary walls and in the mesangium. This form of MPGN has been reported with both hepatitis B virus (HBV) and hepatitis C virus (HCV) infection.

Type II MPGN, also known as dense-deposit disease, is characterized by activation of the alternate complement pathway. Most patients have C_3 nephritic factor in their serum. Histologically, there are intramembranous dense deposits in the basement membrane of the glomerulus, Bowman's capsule, and renal tubules as seen on electron microscopy. Type II MPGN is often associated with partial lipodystrophy but not with other immunologic diseases.

Type III MPGN has histologic lesions similar to those of type I, although less mesangial cell proliferation is seen. Electron microscopy usually reveals GBM spikes that are similar to those of membranous glomerulonephritis.

There is no definitive therapy for idiopathic MPGN. The natural history is one of acute deterioration in renal function and proteinuria followed by spontaneous improvement. Progressive loss of renal function or worsening proteinuria for more than 6 months is associated with a poor prognosis, as is diffuse glomerulosclerosis or the presence of large numbers of crescents on kidney biopsy. Focal and segmental involvement is associated with a more benign prognosis. In contrast, when MPGN is secondary to HBV or HCV infection, the glomerular lesions often improve or clear with control of the virus.

Immunoglobulin A Nephropathy (Berger's Disease)

Immunoglobulin A (IgA) nephropathy is the most common form of glomerulonephritis worldwide, comprising 20% to 40% of all biopsy-proven glomerulonephritides. It occurs most frequently in the second or third decade with a male predominance of 3:1. The IgA nephropathy typically presents with an episode of macroscopic hematuria, often after an upper respiratory tract infection and without other renal manifestations. It is often suspected on routine urinalysis because of microscopic hematuria. Proteinuria is usually mild, but the nephrotic syndrome is occasionally present. A kidney biopsy is required for diagnosis.

The IgA nephropathy is characterized by deposition of IgA, often accompanied by C_3, in the glomerular mesangium, as seen on immunofluorescence microscopy. There is less prominent localization of IgG and IgM in various combinations. This is usually accompanied by widening of the mesangium and cellular proliferation.

The IgA nephropathy typically progresses slowly to chronic renal failure; however, a significant number of patients do not have progressive disease. The 20-year kidney survival is about 75%. Aggressive therapy with corticosteroids or cytotoxic agents is indicated only for patients with acute renal failure or crescentic glomerulonephritis.

Fibrillary Glomerulonephritis

Fibrillary glomerulonephritis typically occurs in adults older than 50 who present with proteinuria in the nephrotic range, hematuria, elevations in serum creatinine, and hypertension. No specific laboratory finding or symptom is characteristic of this disease.

Histologically, there is mild to moderate hypercellularity of the mesangium with an increase in mesangial volume. There is infiltration of the mesangial matrix and capillary basement membrane that on electron microscopy represents an amorphous material that is distinct from amyloid. This material is composed of nonbranching, randomly arranged fibrils approximately twice the diameter of amyloid. Immunofluorescence microscopy reveals immunoglobulins and C_3 in the mesangium and capillary walls in a granular pattern along with κ and λ light chains. No effective therapy has yet been described. In a small series, 50% progressed to end-stage renal failure.

Suggested Readings

Banfi G, Moriggi M, Sabadini E, et al. The impact of prolonged immunosuppression on the outcome of focal-segmental glomerulosclerosis with nephrotic syndrome in adults: a collaborative retrospective study. *Clin Nephrol* 1991;36:53–59.

Couser WG. Mediation of immune glomerular injury. *J Am Soc Nephrol* 1990;1:13–29.

Falk RJ. ANCA-associated renal disease. Nephrology forum. *Kidney Int* 1990;38:998–1010.

Falk RJ, Hogan SL, Maller KE, Jennette C. Glomerular disease collaborative network: treatment of progressive membranous glomerulopathy. *Ann Intern Med* 1992;116:438–445.

Korbet SM, Schwartz MM, Lewis EJ. Primary focal segmental glomerulosclerosis: clinical course and response to therapy. *Am J Kidney Dis* 1994;23:773–783.

Madore F, Lazarus JM, Brady HR. Therapeutic plasma exchange in renal diseases. *J Am Soc Nephrol* 1996;7:367–386.

Ponticelli C, Altieri P, Scolani F, et al. A randomized study comparing methylprednisolone plus chlorambucil versus methylprednisolone plus cyclophosphamide in idiopathic membranous nephropathy. *J Am Soc Nephrol* 1998;9:444–450.

Reichert LJ, Koene RA, Wetzels JF. Prognostic factors in idiopathic membranous nephropathy. *Am J Kidney Dis* 1998;31:1–11.

Tisher CC, Brenner BM, eds. *Renal pathology with clinical and functional correlations, 2nd ed.* Philadelphia: JB Lippincott, 1994.

Chapter 9

Renal Involvement in Systemic Lupus Erythematosus

C. Craig Tisher

Systemic lupus erythematosus is an autoimmune disease chiefly affecting the skin, kidneys, joints, serous membranes, and blood vessels.

CLINICAL PICTURE

Systemic lupus erythematosus is more common in women aged 20 to 40 years (female-to-male ratio 9:1) and affects approximately 1 in 500 adult women in the United States. Fever, arthralgia, and a malar or butterfly rash are among the most common presenting symptoms. Photosensitivity, alopecia, serositis, cerebritis, and peripheral neuritis can occur.

Several drugs are associated with a systemic lupus erythematosus–like syndrome, including hydralazine, sulfonamides, procainamide, carbamazepine, and isoniazid, but renal involvement is rare.

Laboratory investigations may show a markedly elevated erythrocyte sedimentation rate, thrombocytopenia, anemia, and leukopenia. Antinuclear antibodies are positive in 90% to 95% of patients, but antibodies to double-stranded DNA are more specific. Hypocomplementemia is especially associated with certain types of lupus nephritis (LN).

RENAL INVOLVEMENT

Initial presentation may include mild proteinuria, microscopic hematuria, or hypertension or may be more severe with acute nephritis, nephrotic syndrome, rapidly progressive renal failure, chronic renal insufficiency, or even end-stage renal failure. Renal involvement is clinically apparent in 50% of patients at diagnosis, yet up to 95% have evidence of LN on kidney biopsy even in the absence of a clinical abnormality.

Lupus nephritis is extremely diverse in its presentation and pathology. Hematoxylin bodies, consisting of a basophilic amorphous substance found in areas of necrosis, are thought to be pathognomonic. The World Health Organization (WHO) classification (Table 9.1) is useful in determining prognosis and management. Transformation between classes may occur. In addition to glomerular involvement, tubulointerstitial disease with immunoglobulin and complement deposits in association with cellular infiltration may be seen in up to 50% of patients. Usually this accompanies glomerular disease, especially class IV LN, but it is occasionally seen alone. Certain clinical features are more closely associated with a particular pathologic class, but no clinical or laboratory parameters reliably predict findings on biopsy.

MANAGEMENT AND PROGNOSIS

Patients with WHO classes I (normal) and II (mesangial) disease and those who present with slowly progressive renal insufficiency or advanced renal failure are managed with blood pressure control and corticosteroids limited to the minimal dose that will control extrarenal disease. Class V (membranous) LN is also usually treated conservatively. Classes III (focal proliferative) and IV (diffuse proliferative) lesions, or patients presenting with a rapidly progressive renal failure, are treated aggressively with high-dose methylprednisolone followed by oral corticosteroids. Cytotoxic agents are often added, especially for the more active forms of class IV LN, which carry a worse prognosis. Pulse intravenous cyclophosphamide is often advocated for these patients.

WHO classes I, II, and III LN generally have a good prognosis. However, changes consistent with class IV disease may develop, especially in patients with class III disease. Thus, many nephrologists advocate aggressive treatment for class III lesions with features of highly active disease or if rapidly progressive renal failure supervenes. Also, the differentiation between "focal" (class III) and "diffuse" (class IV) proliferative glomerulonephritis is arbitrary (<50% glomeruli involved = focal). Class IV is the most ominous form of

TABLE 9.1 Lupus Nephritis According to WHO Classification

	Normal class I	Mesangial class II	Focal segmental proliferative class III	Diffuse proliferative class IV	Membranous class V
Overall incidence (%)	0–4	10–20	10–20	40–60	10–20
Light microscopy	Normal	Normal or diffuse mesangial proliferation	Focal segmental mesangial and endothelial proliferation ± segmental necrosis ± hyaline thrombi	Pronounced diffuse proliferation in mesangium and endothelium ± wire loops, crescents, and necrosis	Diffuse basement membrane thickening and mild mesangial proliferation
Immunofluorescence microscopy	Negative	Granular deposits of IgG and C_3 in mesangium ± subendothelium and capillary wall	Diffuse deposits of IgG, C_3, and C_4 in mesangium and subendothelium and capillary wall	Irregular diffuse granular deposits of IgG, IgM, IgA, C_3, C_4 throughout glomerulus	Diffuse granular deposits of IgG and C_3 in mesangium and along capillary walls
Electron microscopy	Normal	EDD in mesangium	Diffuse EDD in mesangium ± subendothelium	EDD throughout glomerulus	EDD in subepithelium and mesangium
Notes	Very rarely seen; complete absence of any structural abnormality or immune deposit	May have no detectable clinical abnormality or mild abnormality on urinalysis only; excellent prognosis	Hematuria or proteinuria on urinalysis; occasionally nephrotic; hypertension; renal insufficiency (usually indicates transformation)	Renal insufficiency, nephrotic syndrome; hypertension common; if untreated, progresses to end-stage within 2–4 years	Proteinuria is universal; 50% nephrotic initially; 90% eventually develop nephrotic syndrome; may slowly progress to end-stage

EDD, electron-dense deposits.

LN. This commonly progresses to end-stage renal failure (50% within 2 years if untreated), and, because it is often associated with severe extrarenal disease, up to 35% of patients die within 5 years. Membranous (class V) LN is generally associated with a good renal prognosis, with remissions occurring in one-third of patients. However, persistent nephrotic-range proteinuria or transformation to class IV LN is associated with a more rapid progression. Interestingly, recurrence of LN in the transplanted kidney is rare.

Suggested Readings

Appel GB, Cohen DJ, Pirani CL, et al. Long-term follow-up of lupus nephritis: a study based on the WHO classification. *Am J Med* 1987;83: 877–885.

Bansal VK, Beto JA. Treatment of lupus nephritis: a meta-analysis of clinical trials. *Am J Kidney Dis* 1997;29:193–199.

Cameron JS. Lupus nephritis. *J Am Soc Nephrol* 1999;10:413–424.

Kotzin BL, Achenbach GA, West SG. Renal involvement in systemic lupus erythematosus. In: Schrier RW, Gottschalk CW, eds. *Diseases of the kidney, 6th ed.* Boston: Little, Brown, 1997:1781–1800.

Ponticelli C. Treatment of lupus nephritis: the advantages of a flexible approach. *Nephrol Dial Transplant* 1997;12:2057–2059.

Chapter 10

Renal Vasculitis

C. Craig Tisher

Systemic necrotizing vasculitis is characterized by inflammation and necrosis of blood vessels. Virtually any size or type of blood vessel in any organ can be affected. Classification is difficult, and there is considerable overlap between diseases; however, certain general patterns can be recognized.

WEGENER'S GRANULOMATOSIS

Wegener's granulomatosis is a granulomatous systemic vasculitis affecting predominantly the small and medium-sized arteries of the respiratory tract and kidneys. It is uncommon.

Clinical Picture

Wegener's granulomatosis mostly affects middle-aged adults of either gender. The classic triad includes necrotizing granulomata of the upper and lower respiratory tract and a necrotizing glomerulonephritis. Clinical renal disease is almost always preceded by extrarenal manifestations, and patients commonly present with epistaxis or painful sinusitis and hemoptysis. Chest x-ray may show pulmonary nodules that may cavitate. Fever, rashes, digital infarction and arthritis, coronary artery disease, serositis, and mononeuritis multiplex occur. Antineutrophilic cytoplasmic antibodies (ANCA) are seen in many forms of vasculitis. "C" ANCA with a coarse, granular cytoplasmic staining pattern are highly specific for Wegener's granulomatosis. Moreover, titers of ANCA appear to correlate with disease activity and may be important in pathogenesis.

Renal Involvement

Renal disease is evident at presentation in about 85% of patients, with urinalysis revealing hematuria, red cell casts, and proteinuria. Only 10% of patients will have renal impairment initially, but characteristically there is progressive deterioration in function. Kidney biopsy usually shows a focal segmental or diffuse necrotizing glomerulonephritis. Rapidly progressive renal failure can occur and is associated with a large number of crescents. The pathognomonic granulomas as seen in the respiratory tract are typically absent. Immunofluorescence microscopy is usually negative, but there may be irregular granular deposits of IgG, IgM, and C_3 along glomerular capillary walls.

Management and Prognosis

Untreated, 80% of patients with Wegener's granulomatosis die within 1 year. Early, aggressive treatment is indicated in the presence of major organ disease because tissue necrosis is irreversible. The necessity of dialysis for acute renal failure should not preclude the use of aggressive therapy, because significant recovery of function can occur. The mainstay of treatment remains methylprednisolone (usually 500–1,000 mg, depending on body weight, on three successive days) followed by oral prednisone (1 mg/kg/day). This is tapered after 4 weeks and discontinued at 6 months. Cyclophosphamide is used in combination with corticosteroids either orally (starting at 2 mg/kg/day) or intravenously ($0.5–1.0$ mg/m²/ month). It is generally recommended that some form of immunosuppressive therapy be continued for at least 1 year because relapses are common. Plasma exchange is effective in controlling rapidly progressive renal failure or massive pulmonary hemorrhage. It is used in combination with prednisone and cyclophosphamide. With care and correct management, more than 90% of patients can be brought into remission.

POLYARTERITIS NODOSA

This is a vasculitis of small and medium-sized muscular arteries involving many organs, notably the kidneys, nervous system, and heart. The necrosed blood vessels heal by fibrosis, and the weakened wall develops aneurysms, hence the term "nodosa."

Clinical Picture

Polyarteritis nodosa (PAN) is most common in men aged 30 to 50 years. It presents with nonspecific symptoms of fever, weight loss, and arthralgia. Hypertension caused by hyperreninism secondary to glomerular ischemia is present in 50% of patients at presentation and will eventually occur in almost all. About 70% will develop cardiac manifestations including angina, infarction, and pericarditis. Mononeuritis multiplex occurs, and PAN is the principal cause of polyneuropathy in the United States after diabetes mellitus. Involvement of the central nervous system may cause strokes, seizures, and cerebellar dysfunction. Hepatitis B infection, intravenous drug use, and hairy cell leukemia can be associated with PAN.

Diagnosis is based on histology of a clinically affected organ such as a peripheral nerve or kidney. Alternatively, celiac and renal angiography may show characteristic aneurysms and segments of irregularly constricted larger vessels. ANCA are frequently detected, but the staining pattern is often perinuclear ("P" ANCA). Their significance is not as well established as that in Wegener's granulomatosis.

Renal Involvement

The kidneys are affected in 65% to 100% of patients, who may be asymptomatic, have minimal findings on urinalysis, or present with gross hematuria or renal failure. Lesions primarily affect the arcuate and interlobular arteries. Glomerular ischemia leads to fibrinoid necrosis, sclerosis, and patchy cortical infarction but little cellular proliferation. The fall in glomerular filtration rate results from reduced glomerular perfusion rather than direct inflammation. Although circulating immune complexes are suspected in the pathogenesis of these lesions, they are rarely found on biopsy. This has lead to the term "pauci-immune," which encompasses many ANCA-associated forms of vasculitis.

Necrotizing and crescentic glomerulonephritis are rare in classic PAN. Both are more common in the microscopic form of the disease. Resolving inflammation of the vessel walls leaves changes similar to those of chronic hypertensive vascular disease, but in the latter the elastic lamina is reduplicated, whereas it is destroyed in vasculitis.

Management and Prognosis

Rapid evaluation and initiation of treatment are important in PAN because the lesions are irreversible and the disease is potentially fatal. Treatment consists of cyclophosphamide and corticosteroids and has resulted in a 5-year survival rate as high as 80%.

MICROSCOPIC POLYARTERITIS

This disease may be considered a variant of PAN, but it tends to involve smaller vessels.

Clinical Picture and Renal Involvement

Microscopic polyarteritis may present with all features of classic PAN including multisystem involvement. However, hypertension is unusual, and glomerulonephritis is more common. There is inflammation of the glomerular capillaries, distal interlobular arteries, and afferent arterioles. Glomerular capillaries surrounding areas of fibrinoid necrosis collapse; the glomerular basement membrane is thickened; and there is cellular proliferation of the mesangium and endothelium. Crescent formation and a clinical picture of rapidly progressive glomerulonephritis may occur. The typical picture is one of focal, segmental glomerulonephritis with no immune deposits, although involvement may be diffuse. There is usually proteinuria and an active urinary sediment.

Management and Prognosis

Treatment guidelines are the same as those for PAN. Microscopic polyarteritis tends to have a better prognosis than classic PAN.

SCHÖNLEIN-HENOCH PURPURA

This is another vasculitis involving small vessels. Immune complexes containing IgA are deposited in vessels of the skin and kidneys.

Clinical Picture

Schönlein-Henoch purpura is a relatively common vasculitis that is most often seen in young children. Its incidence increases in winter and spring, when upper respiratory tract infections are epidemic, suggesting the possibility of an infectious etiology in some patients.

The skin is involved in all patients, and any rash from urticaria to the classic "palpable purpura" may be seen over the buttocks and the dependent extensor surfaces of the arms and legs. Skin biopsy reveals a leukocytoclastic vasculitis. Immunoglobulin A deposits are seen if new lesions are biopsied. Abdominal pain, arthralgia, and dorsopedal edema also occur.

Renal Involvement

The kidneys are commonly involved in Schönlein-Henoch purpura, and findings range from microscopic or macroscopic hematuria with proteinuria to acute nephritis with oliguria, a fall in glomerular filtration rate, and hypertension. Proteinuria in the nephrotic range may also be present.

Histologic changes are identical to those in IgA nephropathy, with IgA deposits located in the glomerular mesangium. Usually a mild glomerulonephritis with focal and segmental changes is present. In severe cases necrosis and crescents are seen. In addition to IgA, less intense IgG and C_3 deposition may be detected with immunofluorescence microscopy. Serum complement levels usually remain normal. The severity of glomerulonephritis does not correlate with the extent of extrarenal disease.

Management and Prognosis

Schönlein-Henoch purpura is usually self-limiting over weeks to months. However, relapses that are usually milder than the original presentation, with episodes of purpura and hematuria, may occur. Because the disease follows a benign course in most patients, specific treatment (corticosteroids) is limited to those with unusually debilitating or progressive disease. However, the value of corticosteroids is not proven.

Risk factors for developing progressive renal disease include the nephrotic syndrome, acute renal failure, and crescents on kidney biopsy. Methylprednisolone, cyclosphosphamide, and even plasma exchange have been used with varying success in patients with a picture of rapidly progressive glomerulonephritis.

The most important determinant of long-term prognosis is the extent of renal disease. For most patients the glomerulonephritis is self-limiting, and persistent hematuria does not necessarily indicate future renal insufficiency. Recurrence in the allograft after transplantation occurs in some 15% of patients.

Suggested Readings

Balow JE, Fauci AS. Vasculitic diseases of the kidney. In: Schrier RW, Gottschalk CW, eds. *Diseases of the kidney, 6th ed.* Boston: Little, Brown, 1997:1851–1878.

D'Agati VD, Appel GB. Polyarteritis nodosa, Wegener granulomatosis, Churg-Strauss syndrome, temporal arteritis, Takayasu arteritis, and lymphomatoid granulomatosis. In: Tisher CC, Brenner BM, eds. *Renal pathology with clinical and functional correlations, 2nd ed.* Philadelphia: JB Lippincott, 1994:1087–1153.

Feehally J. IgA nephropathy and Henoch-Schönlein purpura. In: Brady HR, Wilcox CS, eds. *Therapy in nephrology and hypertension.* Philadelphia: WB Saunders, 1999:138–144.

Nachman PH, Falk RJ. ANCA-associated small vessel vasculitis. In: Brady HR, Wilcox CS, eds. *Therapy in nephrology and hypertension.* Philadelphia: WB Saunders, 1999:158–164.

Chapter 11

Renal Involvement in Thrombotic Microangiopathy, Progressive Systemic Sclerosis, Multiple Myeloma, and Amyloidosis

C. Craig Tisher

THROMBOTIC MICROANGIOPATHY

This is a disease characterized by microangiopathic hemolytic anemia, thrombocytopenia, and variable renal and neurologic manifestations. Adult and childhood hemolytic-uremic syndrome (HUS) and thrombotic thrombocytopenic purpura (TTP) are included. Thrombotic microangiopathy may also be associated with preeclampsia, various malignancies, and the use of oral contraceptives.

Clinical Picture

Hemolytic-uremic syndrome and TTP occur with a female-to-male predominance of 10:1. Whether they should be regarded as separate diseases is still controversial. The syndrome tends to occur in childhood with an annual incidence of 2.65 per 100,000 children who are younger than 5 years in the United States, whereas most cases of TTP occur in the third to fourth decade with an incidence of 0.1 per 100,000 adults. However, patients of any age can be affected by either disease.

Hemolytic-uremic syndrome is frequently associated with infections, especially enteric involvement with *Escherichia coli* 0157:H7. Neurologic features including confusion, seizures, and paresis occur in both diseases but are much more common in TTP. These symptoms often wax and wane. More than 90% of patients in both groups present with purpura, variably associated with epistaxis, hematuria, and gastrointestinal hemorrhage. These problems are related to a thrombocytopenia that is present in virtually all patients, as is a Coombs-negative hemolytic anemia. One of the most helpful findings for diagnosis is evidence of erythrocyte fragmentation on a peripheral blood smear with schistocytes, burr cells, and helmet cells. Myalgia and arthralgia are not uncommon.

Renal Involvement

The kidneys are affected in both groups, but the process tends to be more common and more severe in HUS. About 90% of all patients will have proteinuria and microscopic or gross hematuria, and renal failure of varying severity occurs in 40% to 80%.

It is thought that the target organ damaged in TTP is the endothelium. In the acute stages, platelet and fibrin thrombi occlude the glomerular capillaries and arterioles, leading to ischemia and sometimes necrosis. Endothelial cell hypertrophy adds to the narrowing of the lumen. Immunofluorescence microscopy for immunoglobulins and complement is usually negative. The typical thrombotic angiopathy is also seen in the pancreas, adrenal glands, brain, and heart.

Management and Prognosis

Untreated TTP is almost invariably fatal within 3 months; HUS has a mortality of 50% if there is no intervention. Relapses are less common than in TTP and are usually mild.

Nearly all patients with TTP-HUS now receive corticosteroids, but this alone is usually inadequate to induce remission. The antiplatelet agents aspirin and Dextran 70 have been used in TTP but do not appear to be beneficial in HUS. Splenectomy, prostacyclins, and immunosuppressive agents have also been used with variable success. The most consistently useful form of management is plasma therapy, and sometimes plasma infusion alone is effective. More commonly, however, plasma exchange with fresh frozen plasma as a replacement fluid is required. A typical schedule consists of daily plasma exchanges for 7 days, followed by alternate-day exchanges until hematologic remission is achieved. Plasma therapy is successful in up to 90% of patients, although relapses occur.

Supportive therapy alone (including control of hypertension, blood transfusions, attention to fluid balance, and dialysis if indicated) is often sufficient for HUS, which may remit spontaneously.

Recurrence after renal transplantation occurs in up to 25% of patients and may be associated with the use of cyclosporine in some cases.

PROGRESSIVE SYSTEMIC SCLEROSIS

This is a systemic disease of collagen associated with obliterative vascular lesions. It mainly affects the skin, lungs, gastrointestinal tract, and kidneys.

Clinical Picture

Progressive systemic sclerosis (PSS) or scleroderma is a relatively rare disease that is most common in middle-aged women. Vessel walls are inflamed and thickened, with narrowed and eventually obliterated lumina. The skin is involved in 90% of patients: ischemic ulcers, subcutaneous calcinosis, Raynaud's phenomenon, telangiectasis, and sclerodactyly may occur. Esophageal dysmotility, pulmonary interstitial fibrosis, cardiomyopathy, polymyositis, and arthralgia are also seen.

Various immunologic abnormalities may be present. More than 90% of patients are antinuclear antibody positive (usually a speckled pattern on immunofluorescence microscopy). Highly specific for PSS and its variants are anticentromere antibodies and antibody to topoisomerase. These antibodies are found in 20% of the patients and correlate with the more severe, diffuse form of PSS.

Renal Involvement

The kidneys are involved in up to 50% of patients with PSS, and renal failure accounts for about 40% of deaths. Kidney biopsy characteristically reveals obliterative arterial lesions predominantly of the interlobular arteries. There is concentric proliferation of smooth muscle cells in the media that migrate into the intima to produce "onionskin" thickening. The glomerulus and tubulointerstitium may be affected by basement membrane thickening and areas of fibrinoid necrosis. There is interstitial edema and tubular atrophy. Immunofluorescence microscopy may show IgM or C_3 deposits, but they are rarely present in the glomerulus.

Because the disease is basically noninflammatory, the urinary sediment is often inactive. Ischemia-induced glomerulonecrosis may cause hematuria. Glomerular ischemia commonly leads to elevated renin levels and hypertension.

An important complication is the scleroderma renal crisis. This usually develops within 4 years after the onset of extrarenal disease, and hypertension is a prominent, but not absolute, feature. Scleroderma renal crisis is of abrupt onset and involves a rapid progression to renal failure over 1 to 2 months. Throughout this time the urinary sediment may remain inactive. Scleroderma renal crisis occurs in up to 25% of patients with PSS and is more common in the colder months. It is postulated that renal vasoconstriction caused by hypovolemia, cold-induced vasospasm, or heart failure superimposed on an already compromised circulation is the cause of this rapid deterioration. Renin levels are elevated.

Management and Prognosis

The general course of PSS depends on the distribution and severity of organ involvement. The overall mortality from renal, cardiac, or respiratory failure is about 65% at 7 years. Before the advent of angiotensin-converting enzyme inhibitor therapy, scleroderma renal crisis was almost invariably fatal.

The most important therapeutic step in the management of PSS is adequate control of blood pressure. Corticosteroids and cytotoxic agents do not affect the course of the disease. In scleroderma renal crisis, angiotensin-converting enzyme inhibitors successfully control hypertension in up to 90% of patients and, if instituted early, can stabilize or even improve deteriorating renal function. This improvement is often associated with a remission in extrarenal disease. Supportive therapy is also important and includes adequate nutrition, avoidance of cold, calcium antagonists for digital vasospasm, skin emollients, and dialysis. The 1-year survival has now increased to 75% with the use of angiotensin-converting enzyme inhibitors. Hemodialysis is often problematic because of the lack of good vascular access. Continuous ambulatory peritoneal dialysis is usually more successful, but impaired peritoneal blood flow sometimes reduces the efficiency of dialysis. After transplantation, the allograft may be involved in disease recurrence, but the incidence may be overestimated because the histologic features of chronic rejection are very similar to those seen in PSS.

MULTIPLE MYELOMA

This is a tumor of plasma cells in the bone marrow that produces excessive immunoglobulin (M protein). The light chains of this immunoglobulin are detected in the urine as Bence Jones protein.

Clinical Picture

Multiple myeloma usually affects adults older than 50 years. Many symptoms at presentation are caused by the abnormal protein, which may elevate the erythrocyte sedimentation rate, lead to renal failure, and cause the hyperviscosity syndrome. Bone involvement with pain, fractures, and hypercalcemia is common. Marrow infiltration causes anemia, thrombocytopenia, leukopenia, and immunoparesis, permitting opportunistic infections such as herpes zoster.

Renal Involvement

Renal dysfunction occurs in more than 50% of patients but does not dramatically alter prognosis. Proteinuria in the nephrotic range is quite common. The main pathology occurs in the tubules, where filtered proteins such as albumin and fibrinogen, along with Tamm-Horsfall mucoprotein, obstruct the lumen and form large glassy eosinophilic casts, which are accompanied by inflammation, interstitial fibrosis, and tubular atrophy. Free light chains spill into the urine and are in themselves nephrotoxic, causing tubular dysfunction. Amyloid deposition in the kidney can complicate the picture. Renal failure in multiple myeloma may be precipitated by hypercalcemia and dehydration, chemotherapy and hyperuricemia, and potential nephrotoxins such as nonsteroidal anti-inflammatory drugs prescribed for bone pain.

Management

One aim of treatment is to reduce production of the nephrotoxic light chains. Corticosteroids and melphalan are both effective. Advanced disease may be treated more aggressively with doxorubicin and vincristine and dialysis as indicated. Recently, plasma exchange has been recognized as an important part of treatment, although a small group of patients remain resistant. General measures such as avoiding dehydration, treating infections and hypercalcemia, and minimizing nephrotoxic drugs are important.

AMYLOID

Amyloid is a fibrous protein that produces a bright green birefringence with polarization of tissue sections stained with Congo red. Its deposition gradually destroys normal tissue and is seen in two basic patterns: primary amyloid and secondary amyloid (AA).

Clinical Picture

Primary amyloid mainly involves the kidneys, heart, gastrointestinal tract, nerves, and blood vessels. It is often associated with myeloma. In secondary amyloid, deposits are seen principally in the kidneys, spleen, and liver. Secondary amyloid is associated with chronic diseases such as rheumatoid arthritis, seronegative arthritis, tuberculosis, osteomyelitis, systemic lupus erythematosus, paraplegia, and Crohn's disease.

Renal Involvement

The kidneys are affected in more than 90% of patients in both primary and secondary amyloid, and up to 50% of patients have an elevated serum creatinine at presentation. Renal involvement may be the only clinically significant abnormality in secondary amyloid and usually manifests as proteinuria. Renal secondary amyloid tends to be a more slowly progressive entity than renal primary amyloid. Nephrotic syndrome caused by glomerular deposition of the abnormal protein is a common finding in both. If amyloid deposition is primarily tubular, nephrogenic diabetes insipidus, renal tubular acidosis, or hyperkalemia caused by diminished distal potassium secretion may be the predominant clinical picture. In primary amyloid, M protein is often detectable in the serum or urine, and malignant transformation to myeloma may occur.

Amyloid should be considered in any patient with nephrotic syndrome or renal insufficiency who has an associated chronic inflammatory disease or has evidence of multisystem involvement such as malabsorption, congestive heart failure, hepatomegaly, or neuropathy.

Management and Prognosis

Once suspected, amyloid may be confirmed by abdominal fat pad or bone marrow aspiration or by biopsy of the kidney, tongue, or rectum. Proteinuria may be relatively small in quantity for many years, especially in secondary amyloid. Once azotemia or the nephrotic syndrome appears, the prognosis is poor. Approximately 20% of the patients will die within 3 years.

Treatment of amyloidosis is difficult and usually centers on standard nephrotic syndrome therapy such as salt restriction and diuretics and dialysis when needed. Associated autonomic dysfunction or cardiac involvement may adversely affect hemodialysis. In secondary amyloid, treatment is directed toward control of the underlying disease, which also dictates the ultimate prognosis. In primary amyloid, melphalan and prednisone have been used with some success. Recurrence of disease can occur in up to 30% of renal allografts after transplantation, but the associated decline in function is often less severe than with native kidneys.

Suggested Readings

D'Agati VD, Cannon PJ. Scleroderma (systemic sclerosis). In: Tisher CC, Brenner BM, eds. *Renal pathology with clinical and functional correlations, 2nd ed.* Philadelphia: JB Lippincott, 1994:1059–1086.

Irish AB, Wineals CG, Littlewood T. Presentation and survival of patients with severe renal failure and myeloma. *Q J Med* 1997;90:773–780.

Kaplan BS, Meyers KE, Schulman SL. The pathogenesis and treatment of hemolytic uremic syndrome. *J Am Soc Nephrol* 1998;9:1126–1133.

Kyle RA, Gertz MA. Renal complications of amyloidosis. In: Glassock RJ, ed. *Current therapy in nephrology and hypertension, 3rd ed.* Philadelphia: Decker, 1992:188–195.

Rowe PC, Orrbine E, Lior H, et al. Risk of hemolytic uremic syndrome after sporadic *Escherichia coli* 0157:H7 infection: results of a Canadian collaborative study. *J Pediatr* 1998;132:777–782.

Ruggenenti P, Remuzzi G. Thrombotic microangiopathies. In: Brady HR, Wilcox CS, eds. *Therapy in nephrology and hypertension.* Philadelphia: WB Saunders, 1999:225–231.

Chapter 12

Tubulointerstitial Nephritis

Nicolas J. Guzman

Tubulointerstitial nephritis (TIN) is inflammation of the renal interstitium and tubules; TIN that accompanies glomerular diseases or allograft rejection is discussed in Chapters 8 and 30. Approximately half of the cases of acute TIN are drug related. The etiology is detailed in Table 12.1.

INCIDENCE

Tubulointerstitial nephritis accounts for 11% to 14% of acute renal failure (ARF) but few cases of end-stage renal disease (ESRD).

CLINICAL MANIFESTATIONS

Tubulointerstitial nephritis usually presents with a normal or mildly decreased glomerular filtration rate (GFR) and proteinuria of <2 g/24 hr. The urinary sediment usually contains white blood cells, red blood cells, and occasionally white blood cell casts. Eosinophils may be seen on Wright's or Hansel's stain of the urinary sediment in patients with drug-induced TIN. Peripheral eosinophilia is a more consistent finding. As inflammation progresses, the glomeruli may also be involved, resulting in progressive renal insufficiency, worsening proteinuria and hematuria, oliguria, and hypertension. At this time, the diagnosis may have to be made by kidney biopsy.

In its early stages, TIN can present as any combination of three patterns of renal dysfunction: proximal tubular dysfunction manifested as renal tubular acidosis:(type II) with or without Fanconi's

TABLE 12.1   Etiology of Tubulointerstitial Nephritis

Infections

Acute	Chronic
Bacterial	Bacterial
Acute pyelonephritis	Chronic obstructive pyelonephritis
Rocky Mountain spotted fever	Tuberculosis
Viral	Fungal
Cytomegalovirus	Histoplasmosis
	Parasitic infection
	Schistosomiasis
	Malaria (*Plasmodium* falciparum)
	Xanthogranulomatous pyelonephritis
	Malacoplakia

Drugs

Analgesic nephropathy	Lithium nephropathy

Metabolic causes

Hypokalemic nephropathy	Urate nephropathy
Hypercalcemic nephropathy	Oxalate nephropathy

Other causes

Heavy metals	Neoplastic diseases
Reflux nephropathy	Plasma cell dyscrasias
Sarcoid nephropathy	Myeloma kidney
Obstructive uropathy	Light-chain deposition disease
	Lymphoproliferative diseases
	Leukemia

syndrome (see Chapter 17); distal tubular dysfunction manifested as renal tubular acidosis (type I), salt wasting, or hyperkalemia; and renal medullary dysfunction resulting in decreased concentrating ability with polyuria and nocturia.

ACUTE TUBULOINTERSTITIAL NEPHRITIS

The two most common causes are bacterial pyelonephritis (see Chapter 20) and drug-induced hypersensitivity TIN.

Acute Drug-Induced Hypersensitivity TIN

Drugs implicated most frequently in TIN are the β-lactam antibiotics, particularly methicillin, and the nonsteroidal antiinflammatory drugs (NSAIDs), particularly propionic acid derivatives such as ibuprofen, fenoprofen, and naproxen (Table 12.2). Acute TIN can develop during prolonged therapy. The mean duration of therapy before the onset of methicillin-induced TIN is 15 days.

Pathophysiology

Drug-induced acute TIN occurs as a result of both humoral and cell-mediated hypersensitivity reactions mounted against a hapten (drug or drug metabolite)–protein complex. The response is not dose related and recurs rapidly after drug rechallenge. Within a class of related drugs, structural similarity can lead to immunologic cross-reactivity. For example, the presence of a sulfa group in both furosemide and bumetanide precludes their

TABLE 12.2   Drugs Commonly Associated with Acute Hypersensitivity TIN

Antibiotics
    β-Lactam antibiotics (e.g., penicillins, cephalosporins)
    Ethambutol
    Tetracyclines
    Sulfonamides
    Vancomycin
    Trimethoprim–sulfamethoxazole
    Erythromycin
    Rifampin
    Ciprofloxacin
Diuretics
    Furosemide
    Bumetanide
    Thiazides
Nonsteroidal antiinflammatory drugs
    Indomethacin
    Phenylbutazone
    Fenoprofen
    Mefenamic acid
    Ibuprofen
    Aspirin
    Naproxen
    Tolmetin
Others
    Cimetidine
    Phenytoin
    α-Methyldopa
    Carbamazepine
    Allopurinol

use in patients who have demonstrated hypersensitivity to either drug. Ethacrynic acid is a non-sulfhydryl-containing loop diuretic that can be selected in the circumstance (see Chapter 25).

Light microscopy reveals focal interstitial infiltrates of mononuclear cells, predominantly lymphocytes, accompanied by edema and some eosinophils. Acute tubular necrosis is common, but the medulla, glomeruli, and vessels are usually spared. Some patients have a granulomatous response (usually associated with allopurinol, thiazides, sulfonamides, oxacillin, and polymyxin); minimal-change nephrotic syndrome (associated with nonsteroidal antiinflammatory drugs); or a predominant tubular injury (rifampin-induced TIN).

Clinical Manifestations

This presents as an allergic reaction (Table 12.3). Blood eosinophilia is usually transient. Eosinophiluria is common but not specific. Drug-induced TIN should be suspected in all patients with ARF of unknown etiology.

Investigations

A detailed history of drug intake and previous allergic reactions and a careful examination of the urinary sediment are essential. Ultrasound may reveal kidney enlargement. Radioactive gallium scanning shows intense uptake of the isotope by the kidneys. It may differentiate acute TIN from acute tubular necrosis in which renal gallium uptake is not increased. A kidney biopsy should be performed when the diagnosis is unclear.

TABLE 12.3   Clinical Features of Acute Drug-induced TIN

Signs and symptoms
    Fever (85–100%)
    Maculopapular rash (25–50%)
    Arthralgias
    Uremic symptoms
Laboratory findings
    Hematuria (95%)
    Eosinophilia (80%)
    Sterile pyuria
    Low-grade proteinuria
    Eosinophiluria
    White blood cell casts

Treatment and Prognosis

The offending agent should be discontinued. Corticosteroids may be beneficial, but controlled clinical trials are not available. Most patients recover renal function fully within 1 year. Prolonged ARF lasting longer than 3 weeks and advanced age at onset are adverse prognostic indicators.

Nonsteroidal Antiinflammatory Drugs

Nonsteroidal antiinflammatory drugs (NSAIDs) can cause salt retention, hyporeninemic hypoaldosteronism with hyperkalemia, ARF, nephrotic syndrome, and acute TIN. Patients with TIN tend to be older and generally have taken the drugs for 1 to 2 years. Most patients with NSAID-induced minimal-change nephrotic syndrome do not have evidence of hypersensitivity. These syndromes are rapidly reversible.

Rifampin-Induced TIN

Rifampin causes three patterns of renal injury: classic acute TIN; direct proximal tubular injury with little interstitial involvement (probably because of a toxic mechanism); and minimal-change nephrotic syndrome. The clinical pattern of rifampin-induced TIN is unique, with abrupt onset of renal failure occurring on rechallenge with the drug. Most cases have occurred during intermittent therapy (two to three times per week) or after resumption of therapy following a drug-free interval. The patient presents with fever, chills, myalgias, arthralgias, skin rashes, eosinophilia, eosinophiluria, and oliguric ARF. The toxic form presents as a more gradual decline in renal function associated with granular casts. In either case, renal function improves over several weeks once the drug is discontinued.

CHRONIC DRUG-INDUCED TUBULOINTERSTITIAL NEPHRITIS

Analgesic nephropathy can lead to both chronic TIN and papillary necrosis.

Incidence

The incidence of analgesic nephropathy in patients with ESRD is generally 1% to 3%, but the incidence is 13% in patients in North Carolina where there is a high usage of over-the-counter phenacetin-containing powders.

Pathophysiology

Papillary necrosis occurs after ingestion of mixtures of aspirin and phenacetin. Tubulointerstitial nephritis occurs with prolonged use of various combinations of aspirin, phenacetin, acetaminophen, aminopyrine, phenazone, and salicylamide. Renal injury is dose dependent. A cumulative analgesic intake of more than 3 kg (1 g/ day for 3 years) is usually required. Phenacetin metabolites (e.g., acetaminophen) and aspirin are concentrated in the kidney, particularly in the papillae, where dehydration further increases their concentration. Acetaminophen is metabolized in the renal papillae to reactive metabolites that cause toxic injury by covalently binding to macromolecules or by lipid peroxidation.

The early stages of analgesic nephropathy are characterized by patchy necrosis of interstitial cells, loops of Henle, and capillaries of the inner medulla. Later, there is necrosis of the papillae and outer medulla and early focal atrophy of cortical tubules.

Clinical Manifestations

Analgesic nephropathy occurs most frequently in women with a history of chronic headaches, arthritis, or muscular pain. Nocturia, caused by an inability to concentrate urine, is common. Gross hematuria, sometimes associated with sloughed papillary fragments in the urine and renal colic, can occur. Patients commonly present with moderate hypertension and anemia. The latter is usually compounded by occult gastrointestinal blood loss from analgesic-induced gastritis or peptic ulcer. Both persistent sterile pyuria and bouts of bacterial pyelonephritis occur frequently. Proteinuria (<1 g/24 hr) and renal tubular acidosis are common. Occasionally, there is diminished citrate excretion leading to nephrocalcinosis.

Investigations

Most patients have an abnormal intravenous pyelogram. The calyces are widened, and there is leakage of contrast material into the renal parenchyma. Papillary necrosis results in cavity formation. Blunting of the calyces and reduction in kidney size occur in advanced disease. Computed tomography (CT) with contrast can be diagnostic.

Treatment

Cessation of analgesic abuse, control of hypertension, and treatment of urinary tract infections and obstruction can prevent progressive renal insufficiency. The prognosis in patients treated early is usually good, and renal function can stabilize or improve with time.

Suggested Readings

Cruz DN, Perazella MA. Drug-induced acute tubulointerstitial nephritis: the clinical spectrum. *Hosp Pract* 1998;33:151–152, 157–158,161–164.

Davison AM, Jones CH. Acute interstitial nephritis in the elderly: a report from the UK MRC Glomerulonephritis Register and a review of the literature. *Nephrol Dialysis Transplant* 1998;13 (Suppl 7):12–16.

Michel DM, Kelly CJ. Acute interstitial nephritis. *J Am Soc Nephrol* 1998;9:506–515.

Rastegar A, Kashgarian M. The clinical spectrum of tubulointerstitial nephritis. *Kidney Int* 1998;54:313–327.

Reddy S, Salant DJ. Treatment of acute interstitial nephritis. *Ren Fail* 1998;20:829–838.

Whelton A, Hamilton CW. Nonsteroidal anti-inflammatory drugs: effects on kidney function. *J Clin Pharmacol* 1998;31:588–598.

Chapter 13

Familial and Cystic Renal Diseases

Wen-Ting Ouyang
Thomas A. Rakowski

Renal cysts are fluid-filled cavities with epithelial linings. Simple renal cysts increase in frequency with age but are of little clinical importance. Ultrasound examination of simple renal cysts reveals a homogeneous pattern without internal echoes. Computed tomography (CT) scanning shows an attenuation value close to that of water, no enhancement with intravenous contrast, no enhanced thickness or irregularity of the cyst wall, and a smooth interface with the renal parenchyma. Cysts that lack these criteria are termed complex and require further evaluation.

Three adult cystic diseases cause significant complications: autosomal dominant polycystic kidney disease (adult-type ADPKD), medullary sponge kidney, and medullary cystic disease (Table 13.1). Additionally, an autosomal recessive polycystic kidney disease (ARPKD) is encountered predominantly in children. It presents with abdominal mass, liver involvement that can include portal hypertension, and renal failure. Not all congenital disorders are inherited.

ETIOLOGY

Renal cysts develop from tubules with which they may retain continuity. As they slowly enlarge by accumulation of glomerular filtrate, they lose their tubular connections and become isolated from the glomerulus. Further cyst expansion then depends on transepithelial transport of solutes and fluid. The etiology may involve tubular obstruction that elevates intraluminal pressure, increased elasticity of the tubular basement membrane, or prolif-

TABLE 13.1 Clinical Features of Major Renal Cystic Disease

	Autosomal dominant polycystic kidney disease	Simple renal cysts	Acquired cystic disease	Medullary sponge kidney	Medullary cystic kidney disease
Incidence	1:600	1:10	Common in patients on dialysis	1:5,000	Rare
Median age at presentation (yrs)	20–40	Variable	Variable	40–60	Variable
Inheritance	Autosomal dominant	None	None	None	Mainly autosomal dominant
Cyst location	Proximal and distal tubules	Variable	Variable	Collecting duct	Corticomedullary junction
Flank pain or hematuria	Frequent	Rare	Rare	With stones or infection	None
Major complications	Hypertension UTIs Renal stones Aneurysm	Rare	Renal cell carcinoma	UTIs Renal stones	Salt wasting Polyuria
Renal failure	Inevitable over time	Absent	Associated with pre-existing renal failure	Rare	Inevitable

eration of epithelial cells with production of excessive basement membrane.

AUTOSOMAL DOMINANT POLYCYSTIC KIDNEY DISEASE

Clinical Presentation and Diagnosis

Autosomal dominant polycystic kidney disease is one of the most common hereditary disorders. It affects 1:400 to 1:1,000 Americans. More than 500,000 persons in the United States are affected by this disorder. It accounts for 8% to 10% of the cases of end-stage renal disease (ESRD). About 85% of cases are caused by a dominant gene located on the short arm of chromosome 16 (the *ADPKD-1* gene). About 5% to 10% of cases result from an abnormal gene located on the long arm of chromosome 4 (the *ADPKD-2* gene). This gene defect causes a milder form of the disorder. A third genotype, *ADPKD-3,* has been identified, but the genomic locus has yet to be assigned. ADPKD is associated with hepatic cysts (approximately 50%; increasing with age), pancreatic cysts, and colonic diverticula. Cholangiocarcinoma, gonadal cysts, and cysts in the CNS occur rarely. Cardiac valvular abnormalities are present in 25% of patients. Renal tubular function shows impaired acidification and concentrating ability and diminished citrate excretion. Renal adenomas are present in 20% but are not normally malignant. Cystic calcification is observed commonly. Proteinuria is usually mild (<1 g/day). The plasma renin activity (PRA) is often elevated. Anemia is less common at any stage of renal failure because of persistent erythropoietin production. A positive family history is present in 60%.

Screening

The test of choice is renal ultrasound. The diagnosis is effectively secured if more than three cysts are detected in an individual with a family history of ADPKD. The number of cysts also depends on age of screening. Fewer than 25% of *ADPKD-1* gene carriers have detectable renal cysts before the age of 30 years. Gene linkage techniques can be used to diagnose presymptomatic individuals providing that at least two affected and related persons are also available for study. This test is useful for studying potential living related kidney donors among family members. Patients should be counseled about the risks and benefits of presymptomatic diagnosis. The identification of a gene-carrier state does not predict the clinical course.

Complications and Management

Activation of the renin–angiotensin pathway leads to hypertension in most patients. It usually responds to angiotensin-converting enzyme inhibitors (ACEIs) or angiotensin receptor blockers (ARBs), but they may precipitate renal failure.

Pain

Acute abdominal or flank pain may indicate hemorrhage into a cyst. This usually resolves with bed rest and analgesia. Cyst infection requires antibiotics. Drugs that penetrate into the cysts include trimethoprim-sulfamethoxazole or quinolones. Cyst infection should be differentiated from pyelonephritis, where patients often have WBC casts on urinalysis. Patients can develop calcium oxalate or uric acid stones. Patients with intractable pain from large cysts may respond to surgical decompression, percutaneous puncture and drainage, or laparoscopic unroofing.

Hematuria

Gross hematuria is usually self-limiting. It may be a sign of malignant transformation. Nephrolithiasis should be excluded.

Renal Insufficiency

About one-half of patients with the gene will have ESRD by the age of 60 years. Women have a less aggressive course than men. ESRD develops earlier in blacks. Nephrolithiasis should be excluded as a cause of rapid decline in renal function. Because of the limited peritoneal space as a result of enlarged kidneys, hemodialysis rather than peritoneal dialysis is preferred. Living related kidney donors must be screened carefully because some gene carriers may not show cysts until they are approximately 30 years old.

Cerebral Aneurysm

These affect 5% to 10% of patients with ADPKD. Routine screening is not recommended. Screening with magnetic resonance imaging or angiography (MRI/MRA) is reserved for patients with either a previous or family history of bleeding from a ruptured aneurysm or with uncontrolled hypertension. The diagnosis is confirmed by arteriogram. Aneurysms greater than 10 mm should be referred for surgery. Recommendations for screening and follow-up vary among centers.

Counseling

Family members should be counseled after the diagnosis of ADPKD.

Prognosis

Once real renal insufficiency is established, the creatinine clearance halves on average every 6 months. Not every carrier of an abnormal ADPKD gene progresses to ESRD.

ACQUIRED CYSTIC DISEASES

Simple renal cysts are common and increase with age. Usually these are single and unilateral and are nearly always benign.

Hypokalemia-related cystic disease develops in patients with hypokalemia and hyperaldosteronism. Multiple renal cysts can be visualized on ultrasound examination and regress after resection of the adrenal tumor.

Acquired cystic disease presents with benign or malignant cysts that develop in patients with ESRD. Ultrasound screening is recommended for patients on dialysis for more than 7 years. Patients with tumors greater than 2 cm should be referred for nephrectomy.

MEDULLARY SPONGE KIDNEY

Although medullary sponge kidney (MSK) is a congenital anomaly, it does not usually present until age 40 to 60 years. About one-quarter of patients have hemihypertrophy of the body. The syndrome is characterized by marked enlargement of the medullary and inner papillary portions of the collecting ducts.

Medullary sponge kidney is associated with recurrent gross or microscopic hematuria and urinary tract infections, nephrolithiasis, polyuria from an inability to concentrate the urine, and distal renal tubular acidosis. Diagnosis is made by intravenous pyelography, which shows striations in the papillae or cystic collections of contrast medium in ectatic collecting ducts. Patients with renal tubular acidosis require treatment with alkali. Those with renal calculi should drink enough fluid to maintain at least 2 L of urine output daily. Those with hypercalciuria should receive a thiazide diuretic.

MEDULLARY CYSTIC DISEASE

Juvenile nephronophthisis is an autosomal recessive defect in a gene on chromosome 2p. *Medullary cystic disease* is an autosomal dominant disease.

Renal–retinal dysplasia refers to medullary cystic disease associated with retinal degeneration, familial retinitis pigmentosa, and pigmentary optic atrophy.

The kidneys have small, thin-walled cysts at the corticomedullary junction. The childhood form presents with polydipsia, polyuria, anemia, lethargy, and growth retardation. It usually progresses to ESRD before the age of 20. The adult form presents with salt-wasting nephropathy that may require large amounts of salt and fluid to combat orthostasis.

VON HIPPEL-LINDAU DISEASE

This uncommon autosomal dominant disorder is associated with retinal angiomas, CNS hemangioblastomas, and pancreatic cysts. The development of renal cysts and bilateral or multicentric renal cell carcinomas mandates regular surveillance and early referral to surgery if detected. Pheochromocytomas occur in one-third of the patients.

TUBEROUS SCLEROSIS

This uncommon autosomal dominant disorder is characterized by epilepsy, mental retardation, adenoma sebaceum, ash-leaf skin pigmentation, angiomyolipomas of the kidneys, renal cysts, and pheochromocytomas.

SICKLE CELL NEPHROPATHY

Patients with sickle cell anemia can present with microscopic or gross hematuria from medullary congestion caused by sickling of erythrocytes at the low PO_2 values seen in the medulla or by papillary necrosis. Conservative treatment entails infusion of hypotonic fluid and diuretics. Patients may have tubular defects manifest as a concentrating defect, acidosis, hyperphosphatemia, hyperuricemia, or hyperkalemia. The development of focal segmental glomerulosclerosis (FSGS) with interstitial fibrosis is heralded by proteinuria and progresses to renal failure. Hypertension is infrequent in patients without nephropathy. Renal transplant can be successful, but nephropathy can recur.

ALPORT'S SYNDROME

This is usually an X-linked disorder presenting with microscopic hematuria. End-stage renal disease occurs early or after age 50. Men are more severely affected. Some families have high-frequency hearing loss. Anterior lenticonus, posterior polymorphous corneal dystrophy, and retinal flecks are rare diagnostic features. Leiomyomatosis of the female genitalia or esophagus occurs in some families. Anti–glomerular basement membrane disease occurs in 3% of transplant recipients.

FAMILIAL THIN MEMBRANE DISEASE

This benign condition presents with hematuria. The glomerular basement membrane is reduced to one-half of its normal thickness. Renal failure does not occur. Renal biopsy is diagnostic.

Suggested Readings

Chapman AB, Johnson AM, Gabow PA. Intracranial aneurysms in patients with autosomal dominant polycystic kidney disease: how to diagnose and who to screen. *Am J Kidney Dis* 1993;22:526–531.

Elzinga LW, Barry JM, Bennett WM. Surgical management of painful polycystic kidneys. *Am J Kidney Dis* 1993;22:532–537.

Fick GM, Gabow PA. Hereditary and acquired cystic disease of the kidney. *Kidney Int* 1994;46:951–964.

Greenberg A, ed. *Primer on kidney diseases, 2nd ed, Section 7.* New York: Academic Press, 1998:Section 7, 309–328.

Sarasin FP, Wong JB, Levey AS, Meyer KB. Screening for acquired cystic kidney disease: a decision analytic perspective. *Kidney Int* 1995; 48:207–219.

Chapter 14

AIDS and Kidney Disease

C. Craig Tisher

In most patients the kidney is not the major organ involved in acquired immune deficiency syndrome (AIDS). However, acute and chronic renal failure and significant fluid and electrolyte disturbances are observed in affected patients and often require intervention by a nephrologist. The magnitude of the problem is difficult to assess because detailed epidemiologic data are limited. However, it is clear that as the number of patients with HIV seropositivity, AIDS-related complex (ARC), and AIDS increases, the number of individuals who develop renal failure will increase in parallel.

Kidney involvement falls into three categories: (a) acute renal failure (ARF); (b) chronic renal failure, most often associated with proteinuria and histologic lesions of focal and segmental glomerulosclerosis, so-called HIV-associated nephropathy; and (c) patients with renal failure on maintenance hemodialysis who subsequently develop AIDS.

ACUTE RENAL FAILURE

Acute renal failure is a frequent complication in patients with HIV infection, especially those with the clinical picture of AIDS. Diagnosis is essentially the same as in any patient who manifests a rising blood urea nitrogen or serum creatinine (see Chapter 26). Sepsis with hypotension and drug nephrotoxicity secondary to pentamidine, antibiotics, foscarnet, and radiocontrast agents explain the ARF in most patients. Other potentially nephrotoxic agents commonly employed to treat many of the infectious complications in HIV-infected patients include rifampin, dapsone, trimethoprim-sulfamethoxazole, and amphotericin B. Occasionally, ARF may be secondary to a drug-induced allergic tubulointerstitial nephritis or to hyperuricemia resulting from the use of certain chemotherapeutic agents in the treatment of AIDS-related malignancies.

There is little doubt that ARF contributes to the mortality and morbidity in these patients, although sepsis remains the leading cause of death. If these patients are hemodynamically stable, hemodialysis can be beneficial, and the decision to treat should be made using the same clinical criteria as in non-HIV-infected patients.

CHRONIC RENAL FAILURE

Initially there was considerable controversy regarding the existence of a specific HIV-associated nephropathy. The clinicopathologic features that include proteinuria in the nephrotic range, rapidly advancing renal failure, and the histologic lesions of focal and segmental glomerulosclerosis (FSGS) are also observed in patients with prolonged heroin use in the absence of HIV infection. Because many HIV-positive patients are also intravenous heroin users, especially in large metropolitan areas where the disease is more prevalent, it was difficult to distinguish between these two potential etiologies. However, with more clinical experience gained by examining nonaddicted patients with HIV infection, it is now apparent that HIV-associated nephropathy should be considered a separate entity.

Although the histopathologic features of HIV-associated nephropathy resemble typical FSGS, certain distinguishing features can be seen in many patients. There is a greater tendency for collapse of the entire glomerular tuft, often in association with sclerosis. Tubulovesicular structures are observed in the endoplasmic reticulum of glomerular endothelial cells in virtually all patients. Tubular injury including microcyst formation is usually quite severe.

The early results of chronic dialysis treatment in patients with end-stage renal failure complicating AIDS generally were dismal. Many were too debilitated to be treated as outpatients and died of other complications of their illness within a few weeks. Often they became cachectic on hemodialysis despite intensive nutritional support and died of a combination of uremia, malnutrition, and infections. More recent reports suggest improved survival in this group of patients on both hemodialysis and peritoneal dialysis. The decision to treat must be individualized.

In contrast to the experience in patients with AIDS and end-stage renal failure, those individuals with chronic renal failure who have ARC or are seropositive for HIV appear to have a better prognosis on maintenance dialysis. Although the experience is limited to small numbers of patients, both continuous ambulatory peritoneal dialysis and hemodialysis, including self-dialysis at home, have met with some success. Again, treatment decisions must be individualized.

Another group of patients has been described who develop AIDS after becoming uremic and beginning dialysis. The typical patient has a history of intravenous drug use that often contributed to the chronic renal failure initially. Although intravenous drug addicts maintained on chronic hemodialysis exhibit a relatively stable course, the additional complications of AIDS are generally fatal within a few weeks.

FLUID AND ELECTROLYTE DISORDERS

Hyponatremia is the most common electrolyte disturbance observed in HIV-infected patients and has various causes. These include adrenal insufficiency with renal salt wasting, excessive vomiting and diarrhea often complicated by inappropriate fluid replacement with hypotonic solutions, and altered hormonal control of water excretion. Hypo- and hyperkalemia are also observed, the latter often in association with non-anion-gap hyperchloremic metabolic acidosis. Both hypo- and hypercalcemia can occur, although the latter entity is rare.

TRANSPLANTATION

Patients with AIDS and chronic renal failure are not candidates for renal transplantation in most transplant centers. The requirement for use of immunosuppressive drugs simply precludes serious consideration.

There are now several reported instances in which an organ donor has served as a source for transmission of an HIV infection. The recipients who have contracted AIDS via a graft or through contaminated blood products have generally experienced a rapid downhill course. Therefore, prospective donors with positive enzyme-linked immunosorbent assay screens are excluded in most transplant centers, regardless of the results of the Western blot. In addition, organ donation is avoided in certain high-risk groups for AIDS, including hemophiliacs, intravenous drug addicts, and homosexuals.

DIALYSIS PROCEDURES IN HIV-INFECTED PATIENTS

Because of the potential lethal nature of HIV infections, there has been great concern among health care workers regarding the establishment of necessary and proper precautions for dialysis of patients who are known to be HIV positive. At present, the Centers for Disease Control and Prevention recommends that those procedures currently employed in dialysis units to prevent hepatitis B transmission are adequate to prevent transmission of HIV. These include blood precautions, restriction of nondisposable supplies to a single patient unless the items are sterilized between uses, and cleaning and disinfection of dialysis machines and surrounding surfaces. It has also been suggested that to minimize blood spray from a dislodged needle, a transparent plastic bag should be placed over the patient's arm during dialysis.

In those patients being treated for end-stage renal failure with peritoneal dialysis, it is recommended that bleach be added to each bag of dialysate effluent before disposal of the bags.

Protection of the staff is critical. Even though the current experience with HIV-infected patients suggests that the risk of the infection to medical workers exposed to AIDS is extremely low, the lethal nature of the disease dictates extreme caution. Therefore, the policies developed by San Francisco General Hospital (see Humphreys and Schönfeld, 1987, under References) for their personnel remain quite appropriate (Table 14.1).

Some controversy exists regarding the value of routine screening for HIV antibodies in patients with end-stage renal failure, especially for those not in the high-risk categories. It is argued that the low transmission rate of HIV in dialysis units and the apparent success of current precautions to prevent transmission of viral infections render routine screening unnecessary. In many states, routine screening is not permitted without the consent of the patient. As noted under "Transplantation," where permitted, all prospective transplant donors should be tested. Otherwise, routine screening in patients who fall outside the high-risk categories is not advocated.

TABLE 14.1 Precautions When Caring for HIV-Infected Patients

Dispose of needles and syringes in puncture-resistant containers without breaking or recapping the needle

Dispose of needles immediately after use; do not throw needles into regular trash; home dialysis patients should be provided with containers that are brought to the hospital for disposal with other contaminated waste

Wear gloves for contact with blood or body substances

Wear gloves to cover cuts, abrasions, ulcers, rash, or skin infections on your hands while working

Wash hands as soon as possible after contact with blood or body substances or after touching objects that have been in contact with blood or body substances

Wear protective eyewear when performing procedures that may result in splashes to the face (e.g., operative procedures, venous catheter placement, dialyzer reuse, endoscopies)

Wear a mask when patient is coughing and diagnosis of tuberculosis has not been excluded or when performing a procedure that may result in splashes of blood or body fluids to the face and mucous membranes; wear a mask when specified for communicable diseases that require respiratory precautions

Wear a gown in anticipation of spills of blood or body fluids onto your clothing or when in contact with wounds or infected sites

Contact your supervisor when you have had a needle stick or other exposure or splash

---

Results of voluntary testing for HIV seropositivity in metropolitan chronic hemodialysis patients reveal that in high-risk patients, the prevalence of seropositivity is high (30–40%), whereas in patients without such risk factors (intravenous drug use, male homosexuality, Haitian background, blood transfusion), the risk is negligible. The findings provide additional evidence that transmission of HIV in chronic hemodialysis units must be a rare event. Another survey of voluntary testing involving several dialysis centers that included far fewer patients in high-risk categories for AIDS reported an HIV-seropositive rate of 0.77%, which is somewhat higher than that in blood donors.

Suggested Readings

Bourgoignie JJ. Renal complications of human immunodeficiency virus type I. *Kidney Int* 1990;37:1571–1584.

Chirgwin K, Rao TKS, Landesman SH, Friedman EA. Seroprevalence of antibody to human immunodeficiency virus (HIV) in patients treated by maintenance hemodialysis (MH). *Kidney Int* 1989;35:242.

D'Agati V, Appel GB. HIV infection and the kidney. *J Am Soc Nephrol* 1997;8:139–152.

D'Agati V, Suh JI, Carbone L, et al. Pathology of HIV-associated nephropathy: A detailed morphologic and comparative study. *Kidney Int* 1989;35:1358–1370.

Favero MS. Recommended precautions for patients undergoing hemodialysis who have AIDS or non-A, non-B hepatitis. *Infect Control* 1985;6:301–305.

Humphreys MH, Schönfeld PY. AIDS and renal disease. *Kidney* 1987; 20:7–12.

Ifudu O, Mayers JD, Matthew JJ, et al. Uremia therapy in patients with end-stage renal disease and human immunodeficiency virus: Has the outcome changed in the 1990s? *Am J Kidney Dis* 1997;29:549–552.

Kumar P, Pearson JE, Martin HD, et al. Transmission of human immunodeficiency virus by transplantation of a renal allograft, with development of the acquired immunodeficiency syndrome. *Ann Intern Med* 1987;106:244–245.

Stone HD, Appel RG. Human immunodeficiency virus associated nephropathy: current concepts. *Am J Med Sci* 1994;307:212–217.

Chapter 15

Disorders of Water Balance

Janet M. Crabtree
Charles S. Wingo

Under physiologic conditions, the osmolality of all body fluids is tightly regulated and maintained within a narrow range (285–295 mOsm/kg H_2O) by alterations in water intake and excretion. Water homeostasis is dependent on (a) access to water and an intact thirst mechanism, (b) appropriate renal regulation of solutes and water, (c) the magnitude of extrarenal solute and water losses, and (d) intact antidiuretic hormone (ADH) biosynthesis, release, and response to changes in serum osmolality. Derangements of water balance are reflected as changes in serum osmolality (S_{osm}), which are largely reflected as changes in serum sodium concentration (S_{Na}).

NORMAL WATER BALANCE

Total body water (TBW) constitutes 60% of lean body mass (LBM) in men and 50% in women. The TBW is distributed between the intracellular compartment (two-thirds) and the extracellular compartment (one-third). Three-fourths of the extracellular fluid volume is interstitial lymph fluid, and one-fourth is intravascular. Osmotic equilibrium is maintained between the intracellular and extracellular compartments by fluid shifts across cell membranes that are freely permeable to water.

Potassium salts are the predominant intracellular osmoles, and sodium salts are the major extracellular osmoles. Because cell membranes are freely permeable to water, S_{osm} is the same as extracellular fluid (ECF) osmolality and intracellular fluid (ICF) osmolality. Because S_{Na} is usually a major constituent of ECF osmolality, S_{Na} directly correlates with S_{osm}. Derangements in blood urea nitrogen (BUN) or glucose concentrations can also alter S_{osm} and are included in the formal calculation of S_{osm}:

$$S_{osm}(mOsm/kg\ H_2O) = 2\,S_{Na}(mEq/L) + [glucose\ (mg/dl)/18]$$
$$+ [BUN\ (mg/dl)/2.8]$$

This calculation should correlate to within 10 mOsm/kg H_2O of the measured S_{osm}. A greater disparity (an "osmolar gap") could result from an error of measurement, pseudohyponatremia, or the presence of another osmotically active solute such as mannitol or ethylene glycol. "Ineffective osmoles" such as urea and ethanol can alter S_{osm} but do not affect water distribution between the intracellular and extracellular compartments because they are membrane permeable. "Effective osmoles" such as sodium, mannitol, and glucose (in the absence of insulin) are distributed mainly extracellularly and can cause fluid shifts across the cell membrane.

Relatively small changes in S_{osm} are sensed by the hypothalamus, which stimulates thirst and ADH secretion. Hypotension and hypovolemia (>10% reduction of circulating plasma volume) can also stimulate thirst and ADH secretion through nonosmotic mechanisms. Thirst is the principal defense against hyperosmolality, whereas renal water excretion is the ultimate defense against hypoosmolality. ADH binds to specific receptors in the collecting duct to effect an increase in water permeability that promotes net water reabsorption into the interstitium. Maximal ADH action reduces urine volume to 500 ml/day and increases urine osmolality (U_{osm}) to 800 to 1,400 mOsm/kg H_2O. Complete absence of ADH results in a large diuresis (15–20 L/day) with a U_{osm} of 40 to 80 mOsm/kg H_2O. Any factor that impairs ADH release, tubular responsiveness to ADH, or medullary hypertonicity will also limit urinary concentrating ability.

S_{Na} is a measurement of concentration that reflects the balance of body sodium and water. Changes in total body sodium alter effective circulating volume, whereas changes in S_{Na} usually reflect changes in water balance. Therefore, S_{Na} does not necessarily correlate either with effective circulating volume or with renal sodium excretion.

HYPONATREMIA

Hyponatremia ($S_{Na} < 135$ mEq/L) is the most frequent electrolyte abnormality in hospitalized patients, with an incidence of 1% to 2%.

Pathophysiology

Hyponatremia occurs when water intake exceeds water excretion. This can occur by (a) excess water intake (water intoxication) with normal renal function or (b) a continued solute-free water intake with decreased renal diluting capacity. Appropriate excretion of a water load requires the following:

1. Adequate glomerular filtration without excessive proximal reabsorption to deliver tubular fluid to the diluting segments of the nephron (ascending limb of Henle and early distal convoluted tubule).
2. Normal function of diluting segments of the nephron.
3. Suppression of ADH to prevent reabsorption of solute-free water in the collecting ducts.

Classification

A diagnostic decision tree is presented in Fig. 15.1. Initial evaluation of hyponatremia includes measurement of S_{osm} and an assessment of the effective circulating volume (as an index of total body sodium). Accurate serial recordings of body weight and intake-output may be valuable. Signs of *hypovolemia* include poor skin turgor, dry mucous membranes, dry axillae, flat neck veins, tachycardia and postural changes in vital signs (hypotension or relative tachycardia). Hemoconcentration (increased hematocrit and serum protein), an increased BUN-to-creatinine ratio, and U_{Na} of <20 mEq/L are often seen. *Hypervolemia* is usually manifested by an elevated jugular venous pressure and peripheral or presacral edema. Hemodilution (decreased hematocrit and serum protein) and a decreased BUN-to-creatinine ratio are often observed, whereas the U_{Na} is less helpful.

ISOOSMOLAR HYPONATREMIA

Pseudohyponatremia (artifactual depression of the S_{Na}) can occur when the fraction of plasma that is water (normally 92%–94%) is decreased by excessive amounts of lipids or proteins. This may occur with severe hyperlipidemias (usually tri-

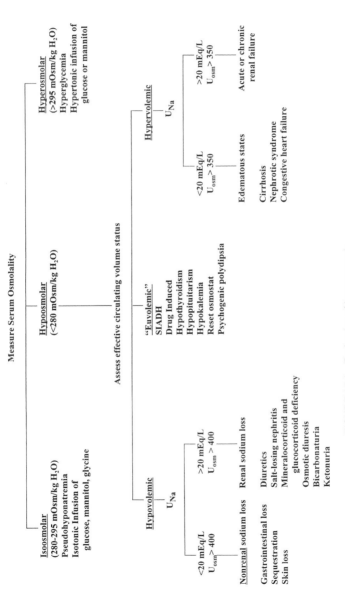

FIGURE 15.1 Evaluation of hyponatremia.

glyceridemia >1,500 mg/dL) or hyperproteinemias such as Waldenstrom's macroglobulinemia or multiple myeloma (serum protein >10 g/dL). In these instances, the measured S_{osm} will be normal, but the serum osmolar gap will be increased. Pseudohyponatremia must be distinguished from the true, potentially serious hyponatremia with normal S_{osm} that can occur with infusions of isosmotic, sodium-free solutions such as glycine in certain urologic procedures.

HYPOOSMOLAR HYPONATREMIA

Hypovolemic Hyponatremia

This condition implies a total body sodium deficit in excess of water losses and results primarily from renal or nonrenal sodium losses. The contracted effective circulating volume enhances isosmotic reabsorption of fluid in the proximal tubule and thereby limits fluid delivery to the distal diluting segments. With significant hypovolemia, nonosmotic stimulation of thirst and ADH also occur.

Nonrenal Sodium Loss
This results from loss (vomiting, diarrhea) or sequestration (pancreatitis, peritonitis) of gastrointestinal fluids.

Renal Sodium Loss

Diuretic Administration

This is most frequently seen in the elderly receiving thiazide diuretics, which can impair fluid delivery to the diluting segments (due to hypovolemia), inhibit NaCl reabsorption in the diluting segment, and potentiate ADH action and release.

Salt-Losing Nephritis

This can occur in patients with chronic renal failure given a sodium-deficient diet or in patients with relatively preserved glomerular filtration rate but significant interstitial disease such as polycystic kidney disease, medullary cystic disease, or chronic pyelonephritis.

Mineralocorticoid and Glucocorticoid Deficiency

A combination of volume depletion with enhanced proximal tubular reabsorption and nonosmotic stimulation of ADH may be implicated.

Osmotic Diuresis, Bicarbonaturia, Ketonuria

Excessive amounts of osmotically active solutes (glucose, bicarbonate, or ketones) in the urine can cause excessive renal sodium and water excretion.

EUVOLEMIC HYPONATREMIA

These patients generally have an increased TBW (by approximately 3–5 L) but normal total body sodium content and no edema. These disorders result primarily from nonphysiologic secretion, potentiation, or inappropriate action of ADH.

Syndrome of Inappropriate ADH Secretion

This syndrome (SIADH) is generally associated with:

1. *Malignancies.* Oat cell carcinoma of the lung, Hodgkin's and non-Hodgkin's lymphoma, thymoma, other carcinomas (duodenum, pancreas).
2. *Pulmonary disorders.* Tuberculosis, pneumonia, abscess, asthma, acute respiratory failure.
3. *Central nervous system disorders.* Tumors, head trauma, subarachnoid or subdural hemorrhage, meningitis, encephalitis, abscess, seizures, psychosis, delirium tremens.
4. *Postoperative period.*

SIADH is a diagnosis of exclusion and requires that the patient have no causes for nonosmotic ADH release (hypovolemia, nausea) and no other cause of decreased diluting capacity (thyroid, renal, adrenal, cardiac, or liver disease). The urine is less than maximally dilute (>100 mOsm/kg H_2O) despite low serum osmolality, and U_{Na} is usually >20 mEq/L. Hypouricemia (<4 mg/dl) is a useful diagnostic clue. Because hyponatremia itself implies impaired urinary dilution, the diagnosis is confirmed by an elevated ADH level and does not require a formal urine dilution test.

Reset Osmostat

This is most commonly seen in pregnant women and results from down-regulation of the central osmoreceptors. ADH release varies appropriately with changes in S_{osm}, but the S_{osm} threshold for ADH release is below normal. S_{Na}, although reduced, remains stable because water excretion is normal.

Psychogenic Polydipsia

Psychotic patients can drink sufficient volumes of fluid to exceed their capacity to excrete solute-free water. In addition, these patients may have a subtle impairment in diluting capacity.

Drugs

1. *May potentiate ADH action.* Clofibrate, cyclophosphamide, non-steroidal antiinflammatory agents, ADH analogs.
2. *May stimulate ADH release.* Vincristine, carbamazepine, narcotics, barbiturates, antidepressants.
3. *May potentiate ADH action and stimulate its release.* Thiazide diuretics, chlorpropamide, ADH analogs.

HYPERVOLEMIC HYPONATREMIA

Patients with edema (congestive heart failure, nephrotic syndrome, and cirrhosis with ascites) can have an increased TBW that exceeds the increase in total body sodium. In these patients, a reduced effective circulating volume (from reduced cardiac output or peripheral arterial vasodilation) decreases filtrate delivery to the diluting segment and stimulates ADH release. In the absence of concomitant diuretic use, U_{Na} is frequently <15 mEq/L, and U_{osm} is >350 mOsm/kg H_2O. In addition, acute or chronic renal failure can cause hyponatremia because renal diluting capacity is reduced.

CLINICAL PRESENTATION

Most patients with hyponatremia are asymptomatic. Symptoms generally occur when significant hyponatremia ($S_{Na} < 125$ mEq/L) has evolved in <24 hours (acute hyponatremia). Nausea, vomiting, and headache are common presenting symptoms, but the clinical course can rapidly deteriorate to seizures, coma, and respiratory arrest. Severe acute hyponatremia ($S_{Na} < 120$ mEq/L, developing over <24 hours) has a mortality of up to 50%, predominantly from complications of cerebral edema.

TREATMENT

Acute Versus Chronic Hyponatremia

Correction of hyponatremia in patients who are asymptomatic or who have only subtle neurologic dysfunction (and thus likely have chronic hyponatremia) should be gradual. Water restriction or the administration of a sodium chloride solution, if appropriate (described below), and frequent measurements of S_{Na} should be undertaken. *Overzealous correction of S_{Na} in patients with chronic hyponatremia has been associated with the cerebral demyelination syndrome (central pontine myelinolysis), which can result in flaccid paralysis and death.* Although the reasons are not clear, it appears that individual susceptibility to the osmotic demyelination syndrome may vary across patient populations, and specifically, premenopausal women appear to be at greater risk for residual neurologic injury. Caution should also be taken in treatment of the hypovolemic patient who is receiving isotonic saline, which will restore normovolemia and cause loss of the hypovolemic stimulus to ADH release. In this setting, rapid excretion of excess water can lead to overly rapid correction of hyponatremia. Suggested therapy for different clinical situations is described below.

Acute Symptomatic Hyponatremia

More rapid correction of hyponatremia is indicated if the risk of complications from cerebral edema outweighs the risk of aggressive treatment. The choice of 3% saline versus isotonic saline in the treatment of these patients remains controversial and should be guided by the severity of the clinical condition and the availability of intensive clinical monitoring. Symptoms attributable to acute severe hyponatremia may be subtle (lethargy, nausea, vomiting, agitation, hallucinations, weakness, headache) or severe (seizures, coma, Cheyne-Stokes respiration, pseudobulbar palsy). A well-designed treatment regimen should include:

1. Admission to an intensive care unit for monitoring of electrolytes, blood pressure, neurologic status, renal function, and frequent measurements of S_{Na} during its correction.
2. A loop diuretic (such as furosemide, 1 mg/kg lean body weight) should be given to initiate and maintain a salt and water diuresis.

3. Hourly urinary sodium and potassium losses should be measured and replaced with 3% NaCl (513 mEq sodium/L) and KCl until S_{Na} has increased by 10% or symptoms have stabilized.
4. Thereafter, aim for slower correction of S_{Na} by water restriction. The rate of S_{Na} correction should never exceed 1.5 to 2.0 mEq/L/hr or 20 mEq/L/day.

It is crucial to ensure that during treatment of hyponatremia the S_{Na} is raised only to the normal range. Central pontine myelinolysis has been correlated both with too-rapid correction of the S_{Na} and with over-correction.

Hypovolemic Hyponatremia

Initial therapy should include:

1. Discontinuation of diuretics.
2. Correction of nonrenal fluid losses.
3. Expansion of the effective circulating volume with 0.9% NaCl to replace one-third of the sodium deficit over 6 hours and the remainder over the next 24 to 48 hours.

A general estimate of the total body sodium deficit can be calculated as follows:

$$\text{Sodium deficit (mEq)} = 0.6 \times \text{LBM (kg)} \times (140 - S_{Na})$$

Euvolemic Hyponatremia

This type of hyponatremia can usually be treated by water restriction to 1 L/day. The volume of excess water that must be excreted to normalize S_{Na} can be calculated as:

$$\text{Excess water (L)} = \text{current TBW} - \text{normal TBW}$$

$$\text{Current TBW (men)} = 0.6 \times \text{current lean body mass}$$

$$\text{Current TBW (women)} = 0.5 \times \text{current lean body mass}$$

$$\text{Normal TBW} = (0.6 \times \text{current LBM} \times \text{current } S_{Na}/\text{normal } S_{Na})$$

A general estimate of lean body mass (LBM) can be obtained after measurement of 24-hour urinary creatinine and can be calculated as:

$$\text{Lean body mass (kg)} = 7.138 + 0.02908 \times \text{urine creatinine (mg)}$$

When the cause of SIADH is not reversible, medications may be used to create a state of drug-induced nephrogenic diabetes insipidus. These medications include (a) demeclocycline, 600 to 1,200 mg/day, or (b) lithium carbonate, 300 mg three times daily.

Hypervolemic Hyponatremia

Initial therapy should include salt and fluid restriction if the hyponatremia is caused by the primary disease. Therapy to improve the underlying disease should be undertaken (e.g., improve/optimize the cardiac output in patients with congestive heart failure).

HYPEROSMOLAR HYPONATREMIA

Hypertonic infusions of glucose, mannitol, or glycine can cause shifts of intracellular fluid to the extracellular compartment with corresponding reduction in S_{Na}. In the case of hyperglycemia, for every 100 mg/dl glucose greater than 100 mg/dl, S_{Na} will fall by approximately 1.6 mEq/L.

HYPERNATREMIA

Hypernatremia (S_{Na} > 145 mEq/L) is less frequent than hyponatremia and occurs in fewer than 1% of hospitalized elderly patients.

Pathophysiology

Hypernatremia implies a relative deficiency of TBW compared with total body sodium. In general, this results from excessive water loss or from excessive sodium retention such as administration of hypertonic NaCl or $NaHCO_3$. Normally, a small increase in S_{osm} stimulates ADH secretion and thereby increases renal water retention. Because hypertonicity also stimulates thirst, even patients who are ADH deficient (central diabetes insipidus) can maintain their S_{osm} if they can drink and have access to water.

Etiology

Hypernatremia can be classified according to the total body sodium content and the state of hydration.

Decreased Total Body Sodium

Loss of hypotonic body fluids results in effective circulating volume depletion and hypernatremia. The usual signs of hypovolemia are present: poor skin turgor, postural hypotension, tachycardia, dry mucous membranes, and flat neck veins. Hypotonic fluid losses can occur from:

1. *Extrarenal sources.* Skin or gastrointestinal losses (vomiting, nasogastric suction, osmotic diarrhea) are common. The renal response leads to a high U_{osm} (>800 mOsm/kg H_2O) and a low U_{Na} (<10 mEq/L).

2. *Renal sources.* Hypotonic polyuria can be produced by (a) diuretics; (b) osmotic diuresis caused by glucose, mannitol, or urea (postobstructive diuresis); or (c) nonoliguric acute tubular necrosis (ATN). The urine may be either hypotonic or isotonic, and the U_{Na} is usually >20 mEq/L. More commonly, osmotic agents shift fluid to the extracellular compartment, resulting in hyponatremia.

Normal Total Body Sodium

Losses of solute-free water can result in hypernatremia. Evidence of volume contraction is lacking unless the water losses are extreme. The usual causes include:

1. *Extrarenal water loss.* Both skin and pulmonary losses of water can result in hypernatremia. In addition, water can be drawn from the extracellular compartment into damaged cells (rhabdomyolysis) with similar consequences. The U_{osm} is high and U_{Na} reflects sodium intake.

2. *Renal water loss.* This more common cause of excess water loss is usually related to partial or complete failure to synthesize or secrete ADH (central diabetes insipidus) or to a diminished or absent renal response to its action (nephrogenic diabetes insipidus). These disorders are characterized by an inability to concentrate the urine maximally, the result of both ADH deficiency (or resistance) and washout of the medullary osmotic gradient by chronic polyuria. Approximately half of the cases of central diabetes insipidus are idiopathic and are usually diagnosed in childhood. The remainder are caused by head trauma, hypoxic or ischemic encephalopathy, and central nervous system neoplasms. Patients with nephrogenic diabetes insipidus have impaired urinary concentrating ability despite maximal synthesis and release of ADH. Nephrogenic

diabetes insipidus (DI) results from (a) a failure of the countercurrent mechanism to generate a hypertonic medullary and papillary interstitium and/or (b) a failure of ADH to increase the water permeability of the collecting duct. Nephrogenic DI may be congenital but more commonly is acquired. Chronic diseases of the renal medulla (medullary cystic disease, pyelonephritis), poor protein or salt intake, hypercalcemia, hypokalemia, various systemic diseases (amyloidosis, multiple myeloma), and numerous medications (demeclocycline, lithium, glyburide) have been implicated as causes of nephrogenic DI.

Increased Total Body Sodium

This is usually iatrogenic, resulting from administration of hypertonic sodium-containing solutions ($NaHCO_3$ given to patients with metabolic acidosis) or from inappropriate repletion of hypotonic insensible fluid losses with 0.9% saline in critically ill patients.

Clinical Presentation and Diagnosis

Signs and symptoms of hypernatremia include lethargy, restlessness, hyperreflexia, spasticity, and seizures, which may progress to coma and death. Patients with central or nephrogenic diabetes insipidus may have profound polyuria and polydipsia. Cerebral dehydration leads to capillary and venous congestion, cerebrovascular tears, venous sinus thrombosis, and subcortical–subarachnoid hemorrhages. Mortality in infants and children is 43% in acute and 7% to 29% in chronic hypernatremia, whereas adults with acute hypernatremia have mortality rates as high as 60%.

Central diabetes insipidus can be distinguished from nephrogenic diabetes insipidus by the fluid deprivation test (Table 15.1) followed by exogenous ADH administration. Patients with severe central diabetes insipidus have baseline S_{osm} and S_{Na} that are high normal, and their urinary concentrating ability improves after ADH administration but not after water deprivation. In patients with severe nephrogenic diabetes insipidus, baseline S_{osm} is also increased, but they fail to respond to either ADH treatment or water deprivation. A more direct approach to distinguish central diabetes insipidus is to measure plasma or urine ADH levels simultaneously with S_{osm} after either fluid restriction or hypertonic saline infusion. Patients with central diabetes insipidus will have

TABLE 15.1   Fluid Deprivation Test

During the test, urine output, weight, and vital signs must be strictly monitored to prevent severe volume contraction; weight loss should not exceed 3–5%.

Patients with mild polyuria (<10 L/day) should have fluids withheld the night preceding the test (e.g., 6 p.m.); patients with severe polyuria (>10 L/day) should be fluid deprived only during the day (e.g., 6 a.m.) to allow close observation; time to achieve a maximal U_{osm} varies from 4 to 18 hours.

S_{osm} should approach 295 mOsm/kg H_2O after fluid deprivation and before ADH administration.

U_{osm} is measured at baseline and hourly until two values vary by <30 mOsm/kg H_2O or 3–5% of body weight is lost.

Five units of subcutaneous aqueous vasopressin or 10 µg of intranasal DDAVP is administered, and 1 hour later, a final U_{osm} is measured.

DDAVP, deamino-8-D-arginine vasopressin.

subnormal levels of ADH for the level of S_{osm}, whereas patients with nephrogenic diabetes insipidus will exhibit normal or elevated ratios.

Treatment

Decreased Total Body Sodium

Initially patients should receive isotonic NaCl until the effective circulating volume has been restored. Thereafter, hypotonic solutions (D_5W or 0.45% NaCl) can be used.

Normal Total Body Sodium

Pure water loss should be replaced with D_5W. Free water deficit (FWD) can be calculated as follows:

$$FWD\ (L) = (0.6 \times current\ LBM) \times [(current\ S_{Na} \times 140)/140]$$

Normally the solute-free water deficit should be replaced over 48 hours with frequent monitoring of S_{Na} and S_{osm}. The S_{osm} should decrease by approximately 1 to 2 mOsm/kg H_2O/hr. Faster rates of correction can cause seizures.

The treatment of choice for central diabetes insipidus is intranasal deamino-8-D-arginine vasopressin (DDAVP), a synthetic analog of ADH, 10 to 20 µg twice daily. Therapy for acquired nephrogenic diabetes insipidus should be directed toward the primary disorder. Thiazide diuretics and a low salt intake will decrease the polyuria.

Increased Total Body Sodium

Hypertonic sodium-containing solutions should be discontinued and diuretics administered to promote excretion of the excess salt and water.

Suggested Readings

Anderson RJ. Hospital-associated hyponatremia. *Kidney Int* 1986;29: 1237–1247.

Arieff AI. Hyponatremia associated with permanent brain damage. *Adv Intern Med* 1987;32:325–344.

Ayus JC, Wheeler JM, Arieff AI. Postoperative hyponatremic encephalopathy in menstruating women. *Ann Intern Med* 1992;117:891.

Berl T. Treating hyponatremia: damned if we do and damned if we don't. *Kidney Int* 1990;37:1006–1018.

Marsden PA, Halperin ML. Pathophysiological approach to patients presenting with hypernatremia. *Am J Nephrol* 1985;5:29–235.

Robertson GL, Berl T. Pathophysiology of water metabolism. In: Brenner BM, ed. *The kidney, 5th ed.* Philadelphia: WB Saunders, 1996:873–928.

Schrier RW. Body fluid volume regulation in health and disease: a unifying hypothesis. *Ann Intern Med* 1990;13:155–159.

Chapter 16

Potassium Disorders

G. Edward Newman
Charles S. Wingo

Disorders of serum potassium concentration (S_K) are common, silent, and potentially lethal. Hypokalemia ($S_K < 3.5$ mEq/L) and hyperkalemia ($S_K > 5.0$ mEq/L) may result from dietary or hormonal imbalance, pharmacologic effects, or abnormalities of renal or gastrointestinal function.

PHYSIOLOGY

Approximately 90% of the daily potassium intake of 50 to 150 mEq is excreted in the urine, but with reduced renal function, up to 30% of daily potassium intake may be eliminated in the feces. When diarrhea is present, enteric losses of potassium can be substantial. Because only 2% of total body potassium is in the extracellular fluid and 98% is intracellular, factors causing transcellular potassium shifts can lead to large changes in S_K.

Key hormones closely regulate potassium balance through their effects on the ubiquitous Na^+/K^+-ATPase.

Insulin promotes cellular potassium uptake through stimulation of Na^+/K^+-ATPase. A feedback system exists whereby hyperkalemia stimulates insulin secretion, and hypokalemia inhibits its release.

Catecholamines have divergent effects on S_K. β-Agonists (particularly $β_2$-agonists, e.g., terbutaline) cause cellular potassium uptake, whereas β-blockers (e.g., propranolol) increase S_K. Pure α-agonists increase S_K by stimulating cellular K^+ release.

Aldosterone is the major regulator of total body potassium through its effects on the renal collecting duct, colon, sweat glands, and muscles. Its effects on transcellular potassium distribution are well documented, and its release is in part regulated by a feedback system based on S_K. Aldosterone deficiency can cause mild hyperkalemia, but hyponatremia is more common with adrenal insufficiency than hyperkalemia. With adrenal insufficiency, hyperkalemia may become severe if renal function is impaired or if sodium intake is restricted.

Thyroid hormone stimulates Na^+/K^+-ATPase activity, in part explaining the hypokalemia of hyperthyroidism. No known feedback system exists.

Dopamine and *parathyroid hormone* have been reported to affect S_K, but more studies are required to define the precise role of these hormones in potassium homeostasis.

Metabolic acidosis promotes hyperkalemia, whereas alkalosis promotes hypokalemia. Recent studies have confirmed the observation that alkali therapy has little effect on S_K in patients without endogenous renal function. These findings suggest that acid–base balance affects S_K primarily by altering renal potassium excretion. Specifically, exogenous mineral acid administration increases S_K, largely by reducing renal potassium clearance, whereas exogenous alkali decreases S_K, largely by increasing renal potassium clearance.

RENAL REGULATION OF POTASSIUM

The regulation of renal potassium excretion is primarily through active transport in the collecting duct. This segment has the capacity for active potassium secretion and active potassium absorption. Active potassium secretion occurs largely in the cortical collecting duct and its proximal extension, the initial collecting tubule. This secretory mechanism depends on sodium absorption and requires active cellular uptake of potassium from the peritubular or interstitial fluid. Cellular sodium uptake at the luminal membrane is necessary for basolateral sodium extrusion in exchange for potassium uptake by Na^+/K^+-ATPase. Potassium is secreted passively at the luminal membrane via potassium channels and coupled to chloride secretion. Potassium secretion is stimulated by hyperkalemia, a reduction in luminal chloride concentration, increased tubular fluid flow, and increased distal sodium delivery. Most diuretics (loop, osmotic, thiazides) enhance potassium secretion by increasing distal nephron luminal flow and sodium delivery.

Dietary potassium loading and chronic hyperaldosteronism each stimulate secretion by the cortical collecting duct.

The kidney conserves potassium when potassium intake is reduced by active potassium reabsorption, largely in the medullary collecting duct by a luminal proton-potassium pump, an H^+, K^+-ATPase.

HYPOKALEMIA

Evaluation

Hypokalemia is a common electrolyte abnormality, occurring in up to 20% of hospitalized patients. Symptoms are not common (<50% of cases), typically are present at concentrations <2.5 mEq/L, and correlate with the rapidity of the decrease in S_K (Table 16.1).

The evaluation should begin with a comprehensive history and physical examination and should particularly emphasize the drug history, volume status, and blood pressure. See Table 16.2 for a differential diagnosis. In particular, hypokalemia can lead to hypertension, which occurs as a result of the sodium retention promoted by potassium depletion.

Figure 16.1 provides a diagnostic approach to hypokalemia, and should include analysis of serum and urine electrolytes. Ini-

---

TABLE 16.1   Clinical Manifestations of Hypokalemia

Cardiac
    Predisposition to digitalis glycoside toxicity
    Ventricular irritability
    Abnormal ECG (flattened T Waves, U waves, and ST segment
      depression)
    Coronary artery spasm
Neuromuscular
    Skeletal (weakness, cramps, tetany, paralysis, and rhabdomyolysis)
    Gastrointestinal (constipation, ileus)
    Encephalopathy
Renal
    Polyuria
    Increased ammoniagenesis
    Decreased renal blood flow (increased renal vascular resistance)
Endocrine and metabolic
    Carbohydrate intolerance
    Decreased plasma aldosterone concentration

TABLE 16.2 Differential Diagnosis of Hypokalemia

Artifactual (high white blood cell count, leukemia)
Redistribution (cellular shift)
    β-Adrenergic agonists (epinephrine, terbutaline)
    Alkalosis
    Theophylline toxicity
    Refeeding (intravenous hyperalimentation)
    Insulin administration
    Periodic paralysis (familial, thyrotoxic)
    Barium poisoning
    Mineralocorticoid excess (both renal and extrarenal effects, see below)
Inadequate dietary intake
Gastrointestinal losses
    Diarrhea and chronic laxative abuse
    Ureterosigmoidostomy (urinary diversion)
    Villous adenoma
    Gastrointestinal fistulas
Renal losses
    Metabolic alkalosis (vomiting or nasogastric drainage)
    Diuretics
    Hypomagnesemia (frequently associated with diuretics)
    Antibiotic/antifungal/chemotherapeutic agents
        Penicillins (e.g., carbenicillin)
        Amphotericin B (renal tubular acidosis)
        Aminoglycosides
        cis-Platin
    Glucocorticoids (causes both increased cellular potassium loss and
        increased excretion)
    Cushing's syndrome
    Mineralocorticoid excess (enhanced renal potassium clearance)
        Adrenal adenoma or bilateral adrenal hyperplasia
        Glycyrrhizic acid intoxication (licorice ingestion)
        Adrenal enzyme deficiency syndromes
    Renal tubular acidosis (drug-induced, classic distal and proximal)
    Acute renal failure syndromes (typically observed with recovery of renal
        function)
        Diuretic phase of acute tubular necrosis
        Postobstructive diuresis
        Interstitial nephritis
    Bartter's syndrome
    Acute leukemia (lysozymuria)

tially, spurious values such as are seen in leukemia (white blood cell count >100–250,000) should be considered, and such pseudo-hypokalemia may require special laboratory procedures to avoid. In particular, questionable values should be rechecked, and additional samples should be measured after the plasma and cellular

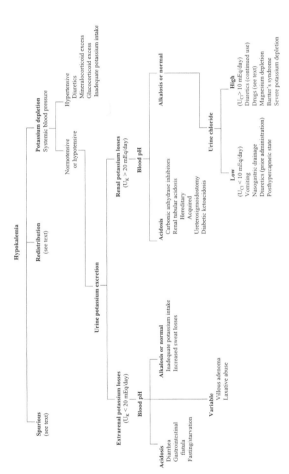

FIGURE 16.1   Diagnostic approach in hypokalemic patients.

components have been separated. Redistribution hypokalemia may result from drug (e.g., insulin, sympathomimetics) or non-drug (hyperthyroidism) causes.

True hypokalemia can be caused by either renal or extrarenal mechanisms. Renal conservation is present during extrarenal potassium losses when 24-hour urine potassium (U_K) excretion is <20 mEq. When U_K equals or exceeds potassium intake during a period of hypokalemia, a renal component is, at least in part, responsible for the hypokalemia.

Hypokalemia in the hypertensive patient can be caused by diuretics, potassium depletion, and primary mineralocorticoid excess (e.g., hyperaldosteronism). Cushing's syndrome is less frequently associated with hypokalemia. Thiazides and loop diuretics commonly cause hypokalemia, but rarely is it severe ($S_K < 3.0$ mEq/L) without other compounding factors such as increased sodium intake, reduced potassium intake, magnesium depletion, or hyperaldosteronism. Renin values may help distinguish the hypertensive patient with diuretic-induced hypokalemia (elevated renin activity) from those with mineralocorticoid excess (suppressed renin activity).

Other tests that aid in the evaluation of hypokalemia include serum magnesium, cortisol, simultaneous plasma renin and aldosterone, TSH, and arterial blood gasses.

Treatment

S_K is not an exact indicator of the total body potassium deficit but, excluding transcellular shifts the magnitude of hypokalemia, generally correlates with the degree of potassium depletion. For a typical adult, S_K decreases by an average of 0.3 mmol/L for each 100 mmol of potassium depletion. S_K levels below 3.0 mEq/L generally reflect potassium deficits of >300 mEq, whereas S_K levels of <2.0 mEq/L may reflect deficits of more than 1,000 mEq. Four factors should be considered in the correction of hypokalemia:

1. Acid–base status: correction of coexisting metabolic acidosis, particularly diabetic ketoacidosis, can cause the S_K to decrease further.
2. Intravenous glucose administration can cause potassium levels to decrease. In life-threatening hypokalemia, initial potassium replacement should be given in glucose-free solutions.
3. Overzealous administration of potassium, particularly intravenous administration, is the most common cause of hyper-

kalemia, especially with impaired renal function or with long-standing potassium depletion. In the latter case, aldosterone secretion is suppressed; hence, extrarenal potassium excretion is impaired. Urine output should be adequate before potassium replacement, and S_K should be checked periodically.

4. Coexisting hypomagnesemia can prevent correction of hypokalemia.

Potassium replacement is the mainstay of therapy for hypokalemia and may be administered orally or intravenously. Oral replacement over several days is safe and rarely causes hyperkalemia in patients with normal renal function when given in doses up to 120 mEq/day. KCl in liquid or tablet form is the therapy of choice when hypokalemia is associated with metabolic alkalosis and chloride depletion. The wax-matrix KCl tablets are preferred because of the gastrointestinal ulceration and bleeding associated with sustained-release tablets. Over-the-counter potassium salt substitutes contain 15 to 40 mEq/teaspoon of potassium and are well tolerated, especially if ingested with meals.

Intravenous replacement is more often associated with hyperkalemia and should be reserved for patients unable to take oral potassium or in life-threatening situations (e.g., paralysis, digitalis intoxication with arrhythmias, hypokalemia-induced hepatic coma) and those with ECG changes. Rates of up to 10 mEq/hr are safe without ECG monitoring, and concentrations of replacement solutions up to 30 mEq/L are safe and rarely produce pain or phlebitis. Doses up to 40 mEq/hr may be given through central venous catheters (with ECG monitoring) for $S_K < 2.5$ mEq/L when associated with ECG changes or symptoms; however, these doses are rarely necessary. S_K should be checked at least every 4 to 6 hours during high-dose replacement.

Treatment of ongoing potassium depletion, as observed with diuretic therapy, may require up to 40 to 120 mmol/day of potassium replacement. Combining potassium-sparing diuretics (e.g., spironolactone, amiloride, triamterene) with a loop or thiazide agent to minimize potassium loss is advocated by some but should not be combined with potassium supplementation in most cases. With intractable chronic hypokalemia (as seen in Gitelman's or Bartter's syndrome), these agents may be used in conjunction with a high-potassium diet or oral supplements.

HYPERKALEMIA

Evaluation

Hyperkalemia can develop when the balance between potassium intake and excretion or the distribution between intra- and extracellular compartments is disturbed. Clinical management requires exclusion of pseudohyperkalemia (Table 16.3), assessment of medications, and determination of adequate urine output. Drugs, diet history, and individual or family history of hereditary renal diseases are key points of the evaluation. Symptoms are not common but may include nonspecific complaints or neuromuscular weakness. *Life-threatening hyperkalemia can be silent,* so any of the classical ECG changes (Table 16.4) should be treated emergently, as progression to ventricular fibrillation may be rapid and unpredictable.

TABLE 16.3   Causes of Hyperkalemia

Spurious
  Hemolysis
  Thrombocytosis
  Leukocytosis
  Ischemic blood drawing
  Familial hyperkalemia
Redistribution
  Increased cellular release
    Exercise
    Tissue necrosis or trauma (rhabdomyolysis, hematoma, etc.)
    Hyperkalemic periodic paralysis, succinylcholine
    Hyperosmolality
  Decreased cellular potassium uptake
    Insulin deficiency (e.g., diabetic ketoacidosis)
    Aldosterone deficiency or blockade (spironolactone)
    β-Adrenergic blockers (e.g., propranolol)
    Digitalis poisoning
  Other
    Exogenous potassium administration (particularly intravenously)
    Arginine and lysine administration
    Fluoride intoxication
    Acidosis
Decreased renal clearance
  Acute or chronic renal failure
  Hyperkalemic renal tubular acidosis
  Drug-induced hyperkalemia (see Table 16-5)
  Mineralocorticoid deficiency (acquired and hereditary forms)
  Hyperkalemic hypertensive syndromes

TABLE 16.4   Electrocardiographic Findings in Hyperkalemia

Peaking or tenting of T waves
Flattening of P waves
Prolongation of PR interval
Widening of QRS complex (to sine wave)
Ventricular fibrillation, asystole, or both

Diagnosis

First, eliminate spurious hyperkalemia by drawing a fresh blood sample through a large-bore needle (to avoid hemolysis) without prolonged tourniquet time for a plasma potassium determination (heparinized tube). The white blood cell and platelet count also should be evaluated. If the clinical and initial laboratory findings suggest the need for urgent treatment, ECG confirmation of hyperkalemia may often be quicker than confirmation by measurement of plasma potassium. Moreover, this approach allows monitoring of the effectiveness of therapy.

Pseudohyperkalemia occurs from potassium released during clotting when the platelet count is >1,000,000/mm³ or the white blood cell count is >200,000/mm³. Even platelet counts between 500,000 and 1,000,000/mm³ are associated with a significant incidence of pseudohyperkalemia. In such cases the discrepancy between serum potassium and plasma potassium values may exceed 1.0 mEq/L. Rarely, pseudohyperkalemia may be caused by "leaky" erythrocytes of either acquired (infectious mononucleosis) or hereditary etiology.

In the absence of pseudohyperkalemia or potassium redistribution (Table 16.3), a S_K above 5.0 mEq/L reflects reduced renal potassium clearance. Diminished renal potassium clearance is frequently observed when kidney function is severely compromised (GFR < 20 ml/min) or with modest renal insufficiency (GFR, 20–60 ml/min) and impaired collecting duct function. In the latter case, patients may exhibit hyperkalemic renal tubular acidosis (HRTA). Conditions frequently present in patients with hyperkalemia include diabetic nephropathy, interstitial nephritis, and drug-induced hyperkalemia (Table 16.5). Most of these patients have some degree of intrinsic renal parenchymal disease. In contrast, less common causes of diminished renal potassium clearance such as defective adrenal mineralocorticoid production and the

TABLE 16.5   Drug-Induced Hyperkalemia

Common
  Potassium-sparing diuretics
  Nonsteroidal antiinflammatory drugs
  Cyclosporine and FK506 tricrolimus
  Heparin
  Angiotensin-converting enzyme inhibitors and receptor blockers
  Pentamidine
  Sulfamethoxazole–trimethoprim (high-dose therapy)
Uncommon
  β-Adrenergic antagonists
  Succinylcholine
  Digitalis poisoning

rare hyperkalemic hypertensive syndrome are not associated with intrinsic renal parenchymal disease.

HRTA may reflect either increased potassium reabsorption or diminished potassium secretion in the collecting duct. These patients usually have modest renal insufficiency, and both hypertension and edema are frequently present. Patients with true hyporeninemic hypoaldosteronism represent a subset of HRTA with impaired potassium secretion. In hyporeninemic hypoaldosteronism, plasma renin and plasma aldosterone values are decreased, but plasma cortisol values are normal. Mineralocorticoid replacement therapy should restore S_K to normal in patients with hyporeninemic hypoaldosteronism. However, this approach may aggravate fluid retention and hypertension that is present in most patients with HRTA. For this reason, HRTA is usually best managed with the combination of a loop diuretic and $NaHCO_3$ therapy.

Patients with adrenal cortical insufficiency (Addison's disease) may exhibit mild degrees of hyperkalemia, but impairment of renal sodium conservation is usually the predominant clinical finding. These individuals typically have hyperpigmentation, hypotension, hyponatremia, salt (NaCl) wasting, and acidosis. However, hyperkalemia can be severe during periods of volume depletion or in an Addisonian crisis. Treatment consists of saline administration and both glucocorticoid and mineralocorticoid replacement therapy.

Table 16.6 lists laboratory and diagnostic tests that are helpful in establishing the etiology of hyperkalemia. Frequent causes of hyperkalemia include drugs, intravenous potassium administration, and renal disease. The presence of "dirty-brown casts" in

TABLE 16.6   Laboratory and Diagnostic Tests to Evaluate Hyperkalemia

Urinalysis
Bladder catheterization
Renal ultrasound
ECG
Urine and serum electrolytes
Serum creatinine and blood urea nitrogen
Arterial blood gases and pH
White blood cell count
Platelet count
Hematocrit (if low, may indicate chronic renal failure)

the urine sediment may suggest the diagnosis of acute tubular necrosis. Bladder catheterization (to eliminate bladder neck obstruction) and renal ultrasonography (to eliminate hydronephrosis or small kidneys of end-stage renal disease) are important considerations.

Treatment

Hyperkalemia is life threatening because of its effects on cardiac conduction. Drug therapy for the acute treatment of hyperkalemia is listed in Table 16.7. Simultaneous use of several or all of these measures may be indicated if ECG abnormalities exist. With the exception of Na^+/K^+ exchange resins, none of the treatments removes potassium from the body, and they should be considered temporary measures. Severe hyperkalemia often requires emergent dialysis.

TABLE 16.7   Drug Therapy for Hyperkalemia

Drug	Dose	Onset of action (min)
Calcium gluconate or chloride	10–30 ml (10% solution) IV	1–3
Glucose/insulin	25–50 g glucose IV/5 units regular insulin (repeat every 60 min)	15–30
Albuterol	10 mg nebulized	30
NaHCO₃	50 mEq IV	See text
Kayexalate	Enema, 50–100 g, or oral, 40 g (see text)	60–120

Intravenous calcium is the most rapid way to treat hyperkalemia (onset of action within 1–3 minutes), but its specific potassium-antagonizing effects on cardiac muscle last only 30 to 60 minutes. A second dose may be given if no resolution of ECG changes is seen in 5 to 10 minutes, but additional doses are less effective. Slow infusions should be given over 20 to 30 minutes in patients on digitalis to prevent myocardial digitalis toxicity. Intravenous calcium should not be given in $NaHCO_3$-containing solutions to prevent precipitation.

Insulin acts to enhance cellular potassium uptake and is the second most rapid way to treat hyperkalemia (onset of action in 15–30 minutes). Ten units of regular insulin given intravenously will reliably decrease S_K in 10 to 20 minutes and should be accompanied by glucose ($D_{50}W$, 1 ampule) except in hyperglycemic patients. Effects of insulin and glucose last 4 to 6 hours and can be repeated every 20 minutes as needed to reverse ECG changes. Alternatively, 25 to 50 units of regular insulin may be mixed with 1L $D_{10}W$, and one-third may be infused over 20 minutes with the remainder infused as needed to maintain S_K.

β-Agonists also reduce S_K, though not as reliably as insulin. Nebulized albuterol, 10 to 20 mg (two to eight times the usual nebulized dose), has an onset of action in 30 minutes and can decrease S_K by up to 1 mEq/L. The major limitation of β-agonist therapy is tachycardia, but it may be given in combination with insulin.

The use of $NaHCO_3$ (one to two ampules intravenously) should be reserved for patients with frank acidosis, because its effect depends on residual renal function. Also, Blumberg et al. have shown that $NaHCO_3$, because of its hypertonicity, may precipitate volume overload and is therefore ineffective in chronic renal failure.

Definitive therapy of hyperkalemia requires potassium removal. This may be accomplished by loop or thiazide diuretics when renal function is adequate; otherwise, and in cases where more rapid elimination is needed, sodium polystyrene sulfate (Kayexalate) may be used. This Na^+/K^+ exchange resin binds approximately 1 mEq potassium/g resin when administered orally and approximately 0.5 mEq potassium/g resin when administered rectally. The full effect with oral or rectal administration is seen in 2 to 4 hours. Clinical volume overload is rare despite the 2 to 3 mEq Na^+/g resin load. Sorbitol, often given orally to improve intestinal transit, should not be given rectally because of the danger of possible colonic perforation. Retention enemas using Kayexalate only (with balloon inflation to ensure retention) are the preferred method of rectal administration. Dosing may be repeated every 4 to 6 hours until S_K is normal.

Hemodialysis is the most effective method of potassium removal when hyperkalemia is complicated by volume overload, acidosis, and renal failure. Potassium can be removed at a rate of 25 to 30 mEq/hr on hemodialysis, whereas peritoneal dialysis can remove 10 to 15 mEq/hr. Rapid removal can be problematic in cases of digitalis intoxication because the rapid reduction in S_K can accentuate the effects of digitalis toxicity. The use of a bath dialysate without potassium should be avoided in most cases because the rate of potassium removal is only marginally better than with 1 or 2 mEq/L K^+ baths and has the true risk of provoking life-threatening hypokalemia if not monitored closely.

Chronic hyperkalemia is rare unless renal function is impaired. In these cases, dietary potassium should be restricted to 40 to 60 mEq/day, and loop diuretics may be beneficial. Oral $NaHCO_3$ can be employed in an effort to maintain serum CO_2 in the 22 and 24 mEq/L range. Kayexalate, 15 to 60 g four times daily, is also an option. Finally, and particularly in patients with HRTA, fludrocortisone acetate (Florinef) can be given in initial doses of 0.1 to 0.3 mg daily when patients have no evidence of volume expansion, hypertension, or circulatory overload. Hypertension and sodium retention complicate its use.

Suggested Readings

Blumberg A, Weidmann P, Shaw S, Gnadinger MP. Effect of various therapeutic approaches on plasma potassium and major regulation factors in terminal renal failure. *Am J Med* 1988;85:507–512.

Genarri FJ. Hypokalemia. *N Engl J Med* 1998;339:451–458.

Greenberg A. Hyperkalemia: treatment options. *Semin Nephrol* 1998; 18:46–57.

Tannen RL. Potassium disorders. In: Kokko JP, Tannen RL, eds. *Fluids and electrolytes, 2nd ed.* Philadelphia: WB Saunders, 1990:195–256.

Weiner ID, Wingo CS. Hyperkalemia: a potential silent killer. *J Am Soc Nephrol* 1998;9:1535–1543.

Weiner ID, Wingo CS. Hypokalemia—consequences, causes, and correction. *J Am Soc Nephrol* 1997;8:1179–1188.

Wingo CS, Armitage FE. Potassium transport in the kidney: regulation and physiological relevance of H^+/K^+-ATPase. *Semin Nephrol* 1993;13: 213–224.

Chapter 17

Acid–Base Disorders

I. David Weiner
Charles S. Wingo

Acidosis is the manifestation of a disease process that, if left un-opposed, results in acidemia (blood pH < 7.35). *Alkalosis* is the man-ifestation of a disease process that, if left unopposed, results in alkalemia (blood pH > 7.45).

Acidosis can be subdivided into metabolic (a primary reduc-tion in plasma bicarbonate concentration) and respiratory (a pri-mary increase in the partial pressure of CO_2, PCO_2). Likewise, alkalosis can be divided into metabolic (a primary increase in plasma bicarbonate concentration) and respiratory (a primary decrease in PCO_2). Simple acid–base disorders are caused by a *sin-gle* primary change in either PCO_2 or bicarbonate concentration. In most cases, simple acid–base disorders result in an abnormal blood pH. Certain terms that are frequently confused are defined below.

- pH: a measure of acidity, equal to $-\log[H^+]$
- PCO_2: partial pressure (mm Hg or Torr) of CO_2 in a solution; concentration of CO_2 in blood, $[CO_2]$ (in mmol/L), is equal to $PCO_2 \times 0.03$, which is approximately 1.2 mM for a PCO_2 of 40 mm Hg
- Total CO_2: moles of CO_2 that can be released from a solution by adding a strong acid; plasma bicarbonate concentration approximates plasma total CO_2

The simple acid–base disorders are listed in Table 17.1 with the primary causes and compensatory changes.

TABLE 17.1 Simple Acid–Base Disturbances and Predicted Compensations

Disorder	Mechanism	Primary change	Compensatory change	Expected compensatory response[a]
Metabolic acidosis	Excessive acid production or retention	$\downarrow[HCO_3^-]$	$\downarrow P_{CO_2}$	$P_{CO_2} = 1.5 \times [HCO_3^-] + 8\ (\pm2)$ or
	Excessive base loss			$P_{CO_2} =$ last two digits of pH
Metabolic alkalosis	Excessive base intake or retention	$\uparrow[HCO_3^-]$	$\uparrow P_{CO_2}$	$P_{CO_2} = 0.9 \times [HCO_3^-] + 16\ (\pm5)$ or
	Excessive acid loss			$P_{CO_2} =$ last two digits of pH
Respiratory acidosis		$\uparrow P_{CO_2}$	$\uparrow[HCO_3^-]$	$[H^+] = 0.75 \times P_{CO_2} + 9\ (\pm4)$
Acute	Decreased CO_2 elimination			$\Delta[HCO_3^-] = 0.1 \times \Delta pCO_2$
Chronic	Decreased CO_2 elimination			$[H^+] = 0.3 \times pCO_2 + 28\ (\pm3)$
				$\Delta[HCO_3^-] = 0.4 \times \Delta pCO_2$
Respiratory alkalosis		$\downarrow P_{CO_2}$	$\downarrow[HCO_3^-]$	$[H^+] = 0.75 \times pCO_2 + 9\ (\pm4)$
Acute	Increased CO_2 elimination			$\Delta[HCO_3^-] = 0.2 \times \Delta pCO_2$
Chronic	Increased CO_2 elimination			$[H^+] = 0.3 \times pCO_2 + 28\ (\pm4)$
				$\Delta[HCO_3^-] = 0.5 \times \Delta pCO_2$

[a] These equations can predict expected steady-state relations between a primary and a compensatory change. For example, a decrease in $[HCO_3]$ to 15 mEq/L (metabolic acidosis) will produce a secondary change in P_{CO_2}. With 95% confidence P_{CO_2} will be $P_{CO_2} = 1.5 \times 15 + 8\ (\pm2) = 30.5 \pm 2$ or 28.5 to 32.5 mm Hg. By coincidence, the last two pH digits approximate the predicted P_{CO_2}.

PATHOPHYSIOLOGY

Acid–base homeostasis is maintained within a narrow range through a series of reversible chemical buffers and physiologic pulmonary and renal compensations. Intracellular and extracellular buffers that counteract changes in pH include CO_2/bicarbonate, phosphate, protein (particularly hemoglobin), and bone. Although all body buffers participate in acid–base regulation, it is convenient to think in terms of the bicarbonate buffer system because all extracellular buffers are essentially in equilibrium. This relationship may be expressed in terms of the Henderson-Hasselbalch equation as follows:

$$pH = 6.10 + \log\left\{[HCO_3^-]/(P_{CO_2} \times 0.03)\right\}$$

The normal blood pH of 7.40 ± 0.05 is equivalent to a hydrogen ion concentration of 40 ± 5 nM. Between pH 7.20 and 7.50, each 0.10 increase in pH is equivalent to a decrease in the hydrogen ion concentration of approximately 10 nM. Because the pH is the negative logarithm of the proton concentration, each 0.3 decrease in the pH is equal to a doubling of the proton concentration.

Compensation for Primary Acid–Base Disorders

Physiologic compensation for changes in systemic pH can involve changes in both alveolar ventilation (P_{CO_2}) and renal acid and alkali excretion. Respiratory compensation for metabolic acidosis begins within seconds and is predominantly completed within minutes. The kidney reacts more slowly to changes in systemic pH to alter net acid excretion. Renal excretion of an alkali load may require 24 to 48 hours, whereas full renal adaptation to an acid load may require 5 to 7 days or more.

Approach to Acid–Base Disorders

Evaluating a patient with an acid–base disturbance requires consideration of both the clinical presentation and the laboratory data. A carefully taken history can simplify a complex set of blood gas and electrolyte data. The arterial blood gas is the cornerstone of the diagnosis of most acid–base disturbances, but several caveats should be considered.

- Systemic pH, P_{CO_2}, bicarbonate, and electrolytes should be evaluated simultaneously, and the calculated bicarbonate from the blood gas should approximate the total CO_2.

- The pH should be independently calculated from the P_{CO_2} measured in the arterial blood gases (ABG) and the bicarbonate measured in the serum electrolytes using the Henderson-Hasselbalch equation. If the calculated pH differs from the measured pH by more than 0.04 pH units, then a laboratory error should be considered and all measurements repeated before corrective therapy is begun.
- A blood gas value represents a specific point in time; identical values can be obtained for different acid–base disturbances moving in opposite directions.
- Nomograms may lead to the wrong diagnosis if the clinical presentation is ignored.
- Physiologic compensation for a primary acid–base disorder seldom normalizes systemic pH. Metabolic acidosis represents a primary decrease in plasma bicarbonate concentration, which decreases blood pH.

METABOLIC ACIDOSIS

There are four mechanisms through which metabolic acidosis can develop:

1. Net acid production or net acid intake increases, thereby exceeding renal net acid excretion (e.g., ketoacidosis or lactic acidosis).
2. Renal net acid excretion fails to match endogenous net acid production [e.g., renal tubular acidosis (RTA) or administration of carbonic anhydrase inhibitors].
3. Bicarbonate loss via the gastrointestinal tract (e.g., diarrhea, fistula).
4. Extracellular fluid being diluted by a non-bicarbonate-containing solution (e.g., rapid saline administration).

The *compensatory response* to metabolic acidosis is an increase in ventilation that returns pH toward normal. When fully compensated, the P_{CO_2} closely approximates the last two digits of the serum pH. If this is not the case, a mixed acid–base disturbance should be considered.

Clinical Presentation

Metabolic acidosis can present with explosive, rapidly developing symptoms, or it can be very insidious in onset, avoiding detection for months or years before being recognized. Acute metabolic acidosis is typically associated with florid symptoms related to the underlying disease. For example, nausea, vomiting, and abdominal pain are frequent with diabetic ketoacidosis (DKA), while the patient with methanol or ethylene glycol poisoning may present with symptoms of alcohol abuse, nausea, and vomiting. In contrast, chronic metabolic acidosis is typically more insidious. Associated symptoms, such as recurrent renal stones, hypoalbuminemia, hypokalemia, osteomalacia or osteoporosis, or "failure to thrive" in pediatric patients will usually bring this condition to medical attention.

Respiratory compensation produces rapid, deep (Kussmaul) respirations. Severe acidosis can be associated with mildly decreased myocardial contractility, hypotension, pulmonary edema, and tissue hypoxia. The arterial blood gas reveals a reduced pH and plasma bicarbonate concentration and usually a reduced P_{CO_2}.

The anion gap helps in determining the etiology of metabolic acidosis. It is calculated from the following formula:

$$\text{Anion Gap} = \left[Na^+\right] - \left(\left[Cl^-\right] + \left[HCO_3^-\right]\right)$$

A normal anion gap ranges between 8 and 16 mM, provided that plasma albumin and globulin concentrations are normal. Table 17.2 provides the differential diagnosis of an elevated-anion-gap acidosis, key clinical features, supporting laboratory data, and a brief outline of treatment options. A non-anion-gap metabolic acidosis is generally caused by either gastrointestinal tract bicarbonate loss or renal tubular acidosis.

The primary therapy for these disorders is to treat the primary process. Alkali administration to correct the systemic pH should be undertaken only after the risks related to the acidosis are balanced against the risks of therapy.

For acute metabolic acidosis, there is limited to no benefit of alkali therapy of severe metabolic acidosis on either systemic hemodynamics or mortality. Furthermore, alkali therapy of acute metabolic acidosis is associated with a substantial cation load, which can lead to volume overload and pulmonary edema or to hypernatremia if the cation is sodium or to life-threatening hyperkalemia if the cation is potassium. However, if intravascular volume depletion is present, then administration of fluids using D_5W plus three ampules (150 mEq) of $NaHCO_3$ per liter can both increase intravascular volume and contribute to correction of the metabolic acidosis.

TABLE 17.2 Differential Diagnosis of Elevated Anion Gap Metabolic Acidosis

Etiology	Clinical features	Laboratory	Treatment
Diabetic ketoacidosis	Fruity breath	Increased glucose > 300 mg/dl; serum or urine ketones; increased BUN and creatinine; low urine output	Intravenous insulin and saline
Uremia	Oliguria, uremic breath; pericarditis		Consider dialysis
Salicylate intoxication	Tinnitus; hyperventilation	Positive urine ferric chloride test; increased serum salicylate	Diuresis and alkalinization of urine; hemodialysis
Starvation ketosis	None	Serum or urine ketones	Refeeding
Methanol	"Blind drunk"	Elevated osmolal gap	Ethanol infusion and dialysis
Alcohol ketoacidosis	Ethanol abuse, often with binge drinking	Increased alcohol level; serum lactate increased	Glucose and saline; phosphorus and potassium
Ethylene glycol	May have accompanying renal failure	Elevated osmolal gap; calcium oxalate crystals in urine	Consider ethanol infusion plus dialysis
Lactic acidosis	Shock, tissue hypoperfusion	Lactate level	Correct underlying cause

Chronic acidosis, in contrast to acute metabolic acidosis, leads to a wide variety of well-characterized sequelae. The best known are protein degradation, growth retardation, malnutrition, skeletal bone demineralization, and recurrent renal stone disease. In most cases of chronic metabolic acidosis, therapy can be administered with low doses of alkali (see below) with little risk of volume overload or hypertension from the sodium load. As a result, treatment of chronic metabolic acidosis with alkali, if the underlying condition cannot be treated, is generally beneficial.

If alkali therapy is initiated, then the dose should be estimated based on the period over which correction of the acidosis is desired. If rapid correction of acute metabolic acidosis is desired, then the base deficit should be calculated using the formula:

$$\text{Base deficit} \left(\text{mEq } HCO_3^-\right) = 0.6 \times \text{lean body weight} \left(\text{kg}\right)$$

$$\times \left(24 - \left[HCO_3^-\right]\right)$$

In severe metabolic acidosis, with plasma bicarbonate concentrations less than 5 mEq/L, the correction factor of 0.6 increases to 1.0 or more. For acute settings, 25% of the base deficit should be administered over the first 8 hours, with an additional 25% administered over the subsequent 16 hours, for a total dose of 50% over the first 24 hours. The response to therapy should be reevaluated after 24 hours, and dose adjustments made appropriately. In chronic settings, a replacement dose of 1 to 2 mEq/kg administered orally in two or three divided doses per day is frequently effective. However, in proximal RTA much larger doses are needed, e.g., 10 to 25 mEq/kg/24 hr (see below).

Non-Anion-Gap Metabolic Acidosis

The primary causes of a non-anion-gap metabolic acidosis are either bicarbonate loss in gastrointestinal fluids, such as diarrhea, or renal tubular acidosis. In theory the two can be easily differentiated based on the history and physical examination. However, some patients with chronic diarrhea may be receiving medications or have underlying conditions associated with RTA. Also, the patient may not admit to the diarrhea. The latter case is sometimes true in young adults self-inducing diarrhea through cathartic administration in order to control body weight.

Differentiating between these two conditions can be assisted by measuring the urine pH and the "urine anion gap" (UAG). If the urine pH is greater than 6 in the presence of systemic acidemia because of metabolic acidosis, then RTA can be diagnosed. If the urine pH is less than 6, then determining the urine anion gap is helpful. This is measured using the following formula:

$$\text{Urine anion gap} = U_{Na} + U_{K} - U_{Cl}$$

where U_{Na}, U_{K}, and U_{Cl} are the urinary concentrations of sodium, potassium, and chloride, respectively. If the UAG is either positive or between 0 and -5 to -10, then the patient is likely to have RTA. If the UAG is less than -20, then the patient is likely to have gastro-intestinal bicarbonate loss, and not an RTA.

Renal Tubular Acidosis

Renal tubular acidosis is a non-anion-gap metabolic acidosis caused by the kidney's inability to maintain a normal plasma bicar-bonate concentration in the absence of exogenous acid or alkali loads. Other causes of normal-anion-gap acidosis are listed in Table 17.3. The metabolism of a typical Western diet results in for-mation of ≈0.8 mEq/kg/24 hr of acid formation, predominantly in the form of hydrochloric, sulfuric, and phosphoric acid. This acid load is buffered by endogenous buffers, resulting in little effect over short periods on systemic pH. However, the buffers con-sumed in this process must be regenerated each day by the kid-neys, or progressive metabolic acidosis develops. When this occurs, it is termed an RTA. The RTAs can be divided into three types.

TABLE 17.3   Differential Diagnosis of Normal Anion Gap Metabolic Acidosis

Gastrointestinal tract bicarbonate loss from diarrhea, pancreatic or biliary fistulas, or an immature ileostomy yields fluid losses with a higher bicarbonate concentration than that of serum and produces potassium depletion
Ureterosigmoidostomy with urine retention in the colon causes chloride and water reabsorption with bicarbonate secretion
Ingestion of chloride salts or chloride-containing anion-exchange resins (i.e., $CaCl_2$, $MgCl_2$, or cholestyramine) causes chloride to exchange for bicarbonate across the gastrointestinal tract
Renal tubular acidosis may be associated with frank renal bicarbonate loss or failure to match net acid intake and production

Classic or distal (type I) RTA is characterized by hypokalemia and severe metabolic acidosis: [HCO_3^-] may be 5 to 10 mEq/L. Nephrocalcinosis or recurrent kidney stones may be present. It is caused by defective collecting duct acidification, resulting in an inability to normally acidify the urine (pH < 5.5), even when profound acidemia is present. This disorder can occur as either an autosomal dominant or an autosomal recessive inherited disease, or it can be acquired. Acquired forms are frequently associated with autoimmune diseases (e.g., systemic lupus erythematosus, pernicious anemia, or Sjögren's syndrome), nephrocalcinosis (e.g., hyperparathyroidism), or toxins (e.g., amphotericin B, lithium, or toluene).

Patients often present with musculoskeletal weakness or with nephrolithiasis. Severe distal RTA can present as a medical emergency with hypokalemic paralysis, coma, shock, or even death if the plasma bicarbonate concentration is below 5 mEq/L.

Some patients will have an incomplete distal RTA. These patients are typically not frankly acidemic, are generally asymptomatic, and may not be detected without a formal test of urine acidification. These patients fail to reduce urine pH below 5.5 following administration of an oral acid load with NH_4Cl.

Small amounts (1–2 mEq/kg/24 hr) of oral alkali are usually sufficient to correct the acidosis and will, given sufficient time, increase serum bicarbonate to normal levels. Alkali therapy may also improve the hypokalemia if given with potassium as the associated cation. Sources of alkali include the following:

- Sodium bicarbonate (325 mg = 4 mEq alkali)
- Shohl's solution (Bicitra) (1 ml = 1 mEq alkali and 1 mEq sodium)
- Polycitra (1 ml = 2 mEq alkali, 1 mEq potassium, and 1 mEq sodium)
- Polycitra-K (1 ml = 2 mEq alkali and 2 mEq potassium)

Other potassium citrate preparations include K-Lyte (25 mEq potassium and alkali), K-Lyte DS (50 mEq potassium and alkali), and Urocit-K (5 mEq potassium and alkali).

Proximal (type II) RTA is characterized by an acid urine pH in the presence of metabolic acidosis but excessive bicarbonaturia in the presence of a normal systemic pH, thereby differentiating it from distal RTA. Type II RTA is caused by a proximal tubular defect and can be observed with acetazolamide administration or with Fanconi's syndrome. In the latter case, glycosuria, phosphaturia, and aminoaciduria are present. Medullary cystic disease, multiple myeloma, nephrotic syndrome, and renal transplantation can also lead to proximal RTA.

Proximal RTA is the result of impaired reabsorption of bicarbonate in the proximal tubule. At normal plasma bicarbonate concentrations, the proximal tubule is unable to reabsorb sufficient filtered bicarbonate. This leads to bicarbonate delivery to the distal nephron, exceeding reabsorptive capacities in these segments and resulting in bicarbonaturia. Eventually the bicarbonaturia depletes total body bicarbonate stores, leading to metabolic acidosis. Eventually the plasma bicarbonate decreases sufficiently that the filtered bicarbonate load ($[HCO_3^-] \times GFR$) is within the reabsorptive capacity of the proximal tubule. This permits normal urine acidification by the distal nephron. As a result, patients with proximal RTA typically exhibit mild to moderate acidosis, with a plasma bicarbonate concentration of 15 to 18 mEq/L. The urine pH is generally below 6 in the absence of alkali therapy and increases above 6 when alkali is administered.

Proximal RTA usually occurs in children and presents as failure to thrive, growth retardation, vomiting, volume depletion, and lethargy. X-rays may reveal features suggestive of rickets in children and osteopenia in adults. Serum potassium is low or normal.

The fractional excretion of bicarbonate (FE_{HCO_3}) can be used to distinguish between proximal and distal RTA. It is calculated as: $FE_{HCO_3} = (U_{HCO_3}/P_{HCO_3})/(U_{Cr}/P_{Cr})$. It is important to emphasize that FE_{HCO_3} can be interpreted only when the plasma bicarbonate is normal. Under these conditions, FE_{HCO_3} is <5% in distal RTA but exceeds 15% in proximal RTA.

Proximal RTA can be difficult to treat, often requiring 10 to 25 mEq/kg/24 hr of oral alkali. Large doses of alkali are required because increasing the plasma bicarbonate causes increased bicarbonaturia as a result of the proximal tubular defect. Increased distal delivery of bicarbonate promotes secretion of potassium and can lead to severe hypokalemia. Thus, approximately 50% of the alkali therapy should be given as the potassium salt. Osteomalacia may require vitamin D and calcium supplements, whereas rickets can be corrected with vitamin D and 1.6 g/day of sodium phosphate.

Hyperkalemic (type IV) RTA is the most commonly encountered RTA. It is characterized by hyperkalemia and a mild, non-anion-gap metabolic acidosis; urine pH is frequently less than 6, indicating a retained ability to acidify the urine. Although type IV RTA frequently coexists with chronic renal insufficiency and diabetes mellitus, the hyperkalemia and metabolic acidosis are out of proportion to the degree of renal insufficiency. Occasionally this disorder occurs in the presence of normal renal function. In this case, a primary defect in aldosterone production or action is usually responsible for both the hyperkalemia and the acidosis.

Most cases of type IV RTA are related to an impairment in ammonium excretion that is the direct result of the hyperkalemia. The impairment in ammonium excretion leads to inadequate net acid excretion, resulting in the development of RTA. In these cases, the ability to acidify the urine is normal. The hyperkalemia reflects either impaired potassium secretion (primarily in the cortical collecting duct) or enhanced potassium reabsorption (primarily in the medullary collecting duct). Treating the hyperkalemia restores the normal ability to excrete ammonium and corrects the RTA and the metabolic acidosis.

Some cases of type IV RTA are secondary to impaired aldosterone production and respond well to mineralocorticoid replacement therapy (fludrocortisone acetate, Florinef, 0.1–0.2 mg/day). These cases are characterized by impaired urine acidification, intravascular volume depletion, and hypotension.

However, hyperkalemic RTA typically coexists with renal insufficiency, hypertension, and extracellular fluid volume expansion, features that are not typically associated with mineralocorticoid deficiency. In this latter group, mineralocorticoid therapy usually fails to restore serum potassium or plasma bicarbonate to normal and may worsen the hypertension and NaCl retention. Hyperkalemic RTA is especially common in diabetic nephropathy, interstitial nephritis, obstructive uropathy, and after renal transplantation. Most patients with hyperkalemia RTA are best treated with a loop diuretic (e.g., furosemide, 20–80 mg PO, two to three per day); sodium bicarbonate (0.5–1 mEq/kg/24 hr) can be generally reserved for refractory cases.

RESPIRATORY ACIDOSIS

Respiratory acidosis represents a primary increase in PCO_2, which decreases systemic pH. The increased PCO_2 is generally caused by failure of CO_2 excretion as a result of decreased alveolar ventilation and not increased CO_2 production. Respiratory acidosis frequently occurs with diseases involving the central nervous system, lungs, and heart. Chronic obstructive pulmonary disease (COPD) that results in loss of alveolar surface is the most common cause of respiratory acidosis. Sedatives and opiates that depress central nervous system centers of respiration are common iatrogenic causes of respiratory acidosis. Severe electrolyte abnormalities (hypokalemia or hypophosphatemia), impaired mechanical ventilation, and bronchopulmonary diseases are other common causes of respiratory acidosis (Table 17.4).

The retained CO_2 results in an increased carbonic acid concentration that is buffered, primarily, by intracellular buffers such as hemoglobin or phosphate, resulting in a small increase in plasma bicarbonate concentration. The kidneys compensate by increasing net acid excretion, which generates new bicarbonate that is returned to the blood. Enhanced urinary acidification also increases urinary chloride excretion, resulting in a decreased plasma chloride concentration. The renal response usually takes longer than 24 hours to develop fully.

Because the renal compensation to respiratory acidosis requires 1 to 3 days or more to become maximal, it is possible to differentiate between acute and chronic respiratory acidosis. In acute respiratory acidosis, less than 24 hours in duration, the serum bicarbonate can be calculated using the formula: $\Delta[HCO_3^-] = 0.1 \cdot \Delta P_{CO_2}$. In contrast, in chronic respiratory acidosis, the serum bicarbonate can be calculated using the formula: $\Delta[HCO_3^-] = 0.4 \cdot \Delta P_{CO_2}$.

TABLE 17.4   Causes of Respiratory Acidosis

Decreased alveolar ventilation and CO_2 removal
  Obstruction (e.g., bronchospasm, emphysema, or aspiration)
  Primary depression of respiratory center (e.g., drugs, trauma, neoplasm or infection)
  Mechanical or structural defect (e.g., pneumothorax, hemothorax, or adult respiratory distress syndrome)
  Mechanical or neuromuscular defect (e.g., primary muscular disease, neuromuscular diseases, drugs, botulism, or tetanus)
  Decreased stimulation of respiratory center (sleep apnea)
  Decreased capillary exchange of CO_2
    Cardiac arrest
    Circulatory shock
    Severe pulmonary edema
    Massive pulmonary embolus

Patients with respiratory acidosis may present with respiratory distress, dyspnea, or obtundation if the disease is acute in onset. They may complain of headaches or show signs of increased intracranial pressure caused by cerebral vasodilation produced by CO_2. The P_{CO_2} is increased, and the blood pH is decreased. In contrast, chronic respiratory acidosis typically produces few symptoms. The treatment for both acute and chronic respiratory acidosis is restoration of adequate ventilation.

METABOLIC ALKALOSIS

Metabolic alkalosis is due to a primary increase in plasma bicarbonate concentration, resulting in an increase in blood pH. This increase in plasma bicarbonate concentration can result from addition of bicarbonate or its precursors to the extracellular fluid or loss of fluid with a chloride-to-bicarbonate ratio greater than that of serum.

The administration of either bicarbonate or compounds that, when metabolized, cause bicarbonate formation, such as citrate, lactate, or acetate, increases the plasma bicarbonate concentration, but if the glomerular filtration rate is normal, most of the bicarbonate load is excreted. The kidney's ability to rapidly excrete an alkali load depends on several factors, including aldosterone and total body chloride stores. Hyperaldosteronism, whether primary or secondary, directly increases renal net acid excretion, thereby impairing the ability to excrete bicarbonate. When total body chloride stores are normal, the kidney is able to rapidly excrete bicarbonate, whereas when chloride depletion is present, the kidneys are unable to excrete bicarbonate.

Metabolic alkalosis is frequently related to a loss of either chloride salts or acid. Certain diuretics and gastrointestinal diseases, e.g., vomiting or nasogastric suction, induce a greater loss of chloride than bicarbonate. This leads to extracellular fluid volume contraction and to an increase in bicarbonate concentration. Alveolar hypoventilation leading to an increased P_{CO_2} is the compensatory respiratory response to this primary disturbance; however, this compensation is usually limited to a rise in P_{CO_2} to 55 to 60 mm Hg because hypoxia stimulates ventilation. Volume depletion, if present, increases renal bicarbonate retention by decreasing the glomerular filtration rate, thereby decreasing the filtered bicarbonate load. Volume depletion also reduces luminal chloride delivery to the collecting duct, thereby inhibiting bicarbonate excretion via chloride–bicarbonate exchange. Hyperaldosteronism, whether primary or secondary, further contributes to metabolic alkalosis by stimulating renal bicarbonate generation. In this condition the increase in plasma bicarbonate reflects the generation and retention of bicarbonate by the kidney as a consequence of increased net acid excretion.

Clinical Presentation

The clinical presentation of most common causes of metabolic alkalosis can be divided into those with and those without volume depletion. Metabolic alkalosis associated with volume depletion is invariably related to chloride depletion. Such individuals may exhibit orthostatic hypotension, tachycardia, azotemia, and other features of reduced effective circulating volume. Unless a renal mechanism is responsible for the volume and chloride depletion (e.g., diuretics), these patients will exhibit intense chloride conservation, and the urinary chloride concentration will be <10 mEq/L. Table 17.5 lists some common causes of chloride-responsive metabolic alkalosis.

TABLE 17.5   Causes of Metabolic Alkalosis

Chloride-responsive metabolic alkalosis: frequently observed with extracellular fluid contraction (urine [Cl⁻] < 10 mEq/L without diuretics)

  Vomiting/nasogastric suction
  Villous adenoma
  Diuretic therapy (urine [Cl⁻] < 10 mEq/L)
  Posthypercapnia state

Chloride-resistant metabolic alkalosis: frequently observed with excessive mineralocorticoid effect and hypokalemia (urine [Cl⁻] > 20 mEq/L and typically reflects intake)

  Primary hyperaldosteronism (Conn's syndrome)
  Bilateral adrenal hyperplasia
  Other causes of excessive mineralocorticoid effect
    Glycyrrhizic acid (licorice)
    Cushing's syndrome or disease
    Congenital adrenocorticoid excess or ectopic ACTH
    Diseases associated with high plasma renin activity
  Potassium depletion
  Bartter's syndrome

Milk-alkali syndrome
Acute alkali load

In contrast, the most common cause of chloride-resistant metabolic alkalosis is excessive mineralocorticoid action. Blood pressure is usually increased, and volume depletion is not present. Urinary chloride excretion typically reflects intake and is usually >20 mEq/L.

Hypokalemia is a common feature of metabolic alkalosis unless frank renal insufficiency is present. The hypokalemia and decreased ionized calcium may contribute to muscle cramps, weakness, and hyperreflexia. Plasma bicarbonate concentration and pH are increased, and the compensatory alveolar hypoventilation increases PCO_2 but decreases O_2 partial pressure that can lead to signs of hypoxia. Severe alkalemia can lead to cardiac arrhythmias.

Therapy

Chloride-responsive metabolic alkalosis will correct with administration of chloride, usually provided as 0.9% NaCl (saline), but coexisting depletion of potassium, magnesium, and phosphate must also be sought and corrected if detected. Chloride-resistant alkalosis is usually caused by mineralocorticoid excess and coexisting hypokalemia. Both of these disorders must be corrected for acid–base balance to be restored. Spironolactone can be used to treat some causes of primary hyperaldosteronism; otherwise, the underlying causes of secondary hyperaldosteronism should be identified and treated. In particular, angiotensin-converting enzyme inhibitor administration to patients with congestive heart failure may be helpful.

RESPIRATORY ALKALOSIS

Respiratory alkalosis results from a primary decrease in PCO_2 caused by alveolar hyperventilation. Pain, anxiety, hypoxia, severe anemia, progesterone and other drugs, endotoxin, and primary pulmonary disease can increase ventilation and lead to hypocapnia (Table 17.6). The initial response to alkalemia is buffering with intracellular protons. The renal compensation, which occurs over several days, is decreased net acid excretion, thereby decreasing plasma bicarbonate concentration and restoring pH toward normal. Patients often present with hyperventilation, perioral and extremity paresthesias, muscle cramps, hyperreflexia, seizures, or cardiac arrhythmias.

TABLE 17.6   Causes of Respiratory Alkalosis

Increased central nervous system drive for respiration
    Anxiety
    Central nervous system infection, infarction, trauma
    Drugs: salicylates, nicotine, aminophylline
    Fever, sepsis, especially gram-negative sepsis
    Pregnancy, progesterone
    Liver disease
Increased stimulation of chemoreceptors
    Anemia
    Carbon monoxide toxicity
    Pulmonary edema, pneumonia
    Pulmonary emboli
    Reduced inspired O_2 tension: high altitude
Increased mechanical ventilation
    Iatrogenic

The arterial blood gas measurement reveals a decreased P_{CO_2} and an increased pH. Plasma bicarbonate concentration will be decreased, and serum chloride concentration is usually increased. Some electrolyte changes of chronic respiratory alkalosis may mimic a non-anion-gap acidosis. The only effective therapy is to eliminate the cause of the hyperventilation.

MIXED ACID–BASE DISORDERS

Patients may present with two or even three primary acid–base disorders. The first step in diagnosis is to define the primary disorder and the pulmonary or renal compensation (Table 17.1). Identification of the primary disturbance can be made from the pH. A pH below 7.35 indicates a primary acidosis, whereas a pH above 7.45 indicates a primary alkalosis. "Overcompensation" does not occur for primary acid–base disturbances.

A reduced plasma bicarbonate concentration indicates a metabolic acidosis or respiratory alkalosis. A bicarbonate concentration below 15 mEq/L is typically a result of metabolic acidosis. A bicarbonate concentration over 45 mEq/L occurs most commonly with metabolic alkalosis. Use of the formulas in Table 17.1 assumes adequate time for compensation.

The most common clinical settings for mixed acid–base disorders appear in Table 17.7. Severe acidemia can result from combined metabolic and respiratory acidosis. Even though the P_{CO_2}

and bicarbonate concentration may be only moderately abnormal, the resulting acidemia is quite severe because of the lack of compensatory processes.

A mixed *metabolic acidosis* and *metabolic alkalosis* can be difficult to diagnose because both disorders affect the plasma bicarbonate concentration. The pH and bicarbonate concentration can be increased, decreased, or normal. An elevated anion gap with an increased or normal bicarbonate concentration is the key to recognizing this diagnosis, as an elevated anion gap only rarely occurs except in the presence of an anion-gap metabolic acidosis. Many causes of metabolic acidosis are accompanied by vomiting, so this mixed disorder is not uncommon.

A *combined metabolic alkalosis* and *respiratory acidosis* is characterized by an increased bicarbonate concentration and increased Pco_2. Based on the formulas in Table 17.1, the elevation in bicarbonate concentration will be greater than predicted for compensation caused by respiratory acidosis.

Severe alkalemia can result from a *combined metabolic* and *respiratory alkalosis*. A mixed disorder is present if a respiratory alkalosis is not accompanied by the appropriate decrease in bicarbonate concentration or if metabolic alkalosis is not accompanied by the appropriate increase in Pco_2. This combination occurs frequently in critically ill patients because of excessive mechanical ventilation and diuretic use.

Finally, a triple acid–base disturbance can exist. This is *combined metabolic acidosis* and *metabolic alkalosis* accompanied by either respiratory acidosis or respiratory alkalosis. It frequently occurs in an alcoholic or diabetic patient with vomiting (metabolic alkalosis), lactic or ketoacidosis (metabolic acidosis), and a respiratory alkalosis caused by sepsis or liver disease. As with mixed metabolic acidosis and metabolic alkalosis, this diagnosis should be considered whenever an elevated anion gap is present and the serum bicarbonate is either normal or elevated. Alternatively, knowledge of previous laboratory values showing a chronic metabolic alkalosis, frequently as compensation for chronic respiratory acidosis, that is now apparently normalized should raise the consideration of a triple acid–base disorder.

Suggested Readings

Adrogué HJ, Madias NE. Medical progress: management of life-threatening acid–base disorders. *N Engl J Med* 1998;338:26–34, 107–111.

DuBose TD Jr, Good DW, Hamm LL, Wall SM. Ammonium transport in the kidney: new physiological concepts and their clinical implications. *J Am Soc Nephrol* 1991;1:1193–1203.

Gluck SL, Iyori M, Holliday LS, Kostrominova T, Lee BS. Distal urinary acidification from Homer Smith to the present. *Kidney Int* 1996; 49:1660–1664.

Perazella MA, Brown E. Electrolyte and acid–base disorders associated with AIDS: an etiologic review. *J Gen Intern Med* 1994;9:232–236.

Chapter 18

Calcium, Phosphorus, and Magnesium Disorders

Marnie J. Marker
R. Tyler Miller

DISORDERS OF CALCIUM HOMEOSTASIS

Regulation of Serum Calcium

The parathyroid gland is the principal sensor of extracellular calcium (Ca), and parathyroid hormone (PTH) is the principal hormone that regulates Ca metabolism. Hypercalcemia suppresses PTH secretion through activation of a membrane-bound Ca receptor. Lower PTH levels reduce bone osteoblast activity (reduced Ca resorption from bone) and reduce vitamin D synthesis, which in turn reduces vitamin D–dependent Ca absorption in the GI tract and bone resorption. The same Ca receptor that is found in the parathyroid glands is also expressed in other tissues, including the kidney. Elevated Ca levels stimulate the renal Ca receptor located in the medullary thick ascending limb of Henle (MTAL) and distal convoluted tubule (DCT), which leads to a Na and H_2O diuresis and loss of Ca in the urine. In response to hypocalcemia, PTH secretion increases, leading to increased osteoblast activity with increased Ca resorption from bone, increased renal reabsorption of Ca, and increased renal production of vitamin D. The increased vitamin D levels cause increased vitamin D–dependent Ca reabsorption from the GI tract and increased osteoblast activity. Elevated levels of vitamin D reduce Ca-stimulated PTH secretion, whereas low vitamin D levels have the opposite effect. Although administration of calcitonin reduces serum Ca levels, its role in normal Ca homeostasis is not clear. Ninety-nine percent of total body Ca is in bone, while the remainder is in the extracellular and intracellular fluids. The normal serum Ca concentration is 8.5 to 10.5 mg/dl, and the ionized Ca (physiologically relevant form) ranges from 1.17–1.33 mmol/L.

Factors Affecting Calcium Concentration or Measurement

Changes in the serum albumin level alter the total Ca concentration without affecting ionized Ca. The total serum Ca concentration is corrected for hypoalbuminemia by adding 0.8 mg/dl for every 1 g/dl of albumin below 4 g/dl. A change in 0.1 pH units causes a reciprocal change of 0.12 mg/dl in ionized Ca because of increased protein binding with increased pH.

Hypercalcemia

Hypercalcemia is diagnosed with a total serum Ca over 10.5 mg/dl or ionized Ca over 1.33 mmol/L. The common presenting symptoms or findings of hypercalcemia are shown in Table 18.1.

Etiology and Differential Diagnosis
- Primary hyperparathyroidism—elevated PTH, adenoma (85%), hyperplasia (15%), parathyroid malignancy (1%)

TABLE 18.1   Presentation of Hyper- and Hypocalcemia

Hypercalcemia	Hypocalcemia
Asymptomatic	Asymptomatic
Confusion or obtundation	Tetany
Polyuria, polydypsia, and dehydration	Muscle spasm
Constipation	Laryngospasm
Weakness	Chvostek's sign: facial twitch in response to tapping on the facial nerve, present in 25% of normal individuals
Hypertension	
Renal insufficiency or acute renal failure (decreased GFR)	
Metastatic calcification	Trousseau's sign: carpal spasm 3 minutes after inflation of BP cuff above systolic pressure
Peptic ulcer disease	
Reduced cardiac conduction times	
Nephrolithiasis	Seizures
Digitalis toxicity—enhances effects of digoxin	Prolonged QT interval
	Hypotension

- Malignancy—three mechanisms: (a) cytokine-induced destruction of bone; (b) parathyroid hormone-related peptide (PTHrp) production by epithelial tumors (squamous cell cancers) or carcinomas of the kidney, ovary, or bladder; and (c) vitamin D production by hematopoietic tumors such as B-cell lymphomas
- Granulomatous conditions—e.g., sarcoidosis or mycobacterial infections (production of vitamin D by macrophages)
- Thyroid disease—increased bone turnover because of elevated T_3 or reduced renal Ca excretion in hypothyroidism
- Vitamin D intoxication—exogenous vitamin D (dialysis patients) or treatment for osteoporosis
- Immobilization—usually patients with Paget's disease, malignancy, or conditions of rapid growth (adolescents)
- End-stage renal disease—vitamin D intoxication (iatrogenic), secondary hyperparathyoidism or aluminum toxicity, post renal transplant (preexisting parathyroid hyperplasia)
- Milk-alkali syndrome—ingestion of large amounts of Ca (>5 g/day) and alkali (e.g., antacids)
- Recovery from acute renal failure—mobilization of the Ca and PO_4 deposited in soft tissues during the oliguric phase
- Thiazide diuretics—enhanced calcium reabsorption
- Lithium—alters the parathyroid setpoint for Ca so that PTH secretion is increased for a given level of serum Ca (10%)

Evaluation

Hypercalcemia may represent evidence of a relatively benign disease, hyperparathyroidism, a paraneoplastic syndrome, or a clue that a granulomatous disease is present. Figure 18.1 summarizes the evaluation of hypercalcemia.

Treatment

Patients with mild, asymptomatic hypercalcemia usually require no treatment but do warrant appropriate evaluation. Patients with moderate to severe symptomatic hypercalcemia (altered CNS function or Ca > 13 mg/dl) or a Ca: PO_4 product over 80 require treatment. Initial therapy is induction of a saline diuresis. Most patients present with some degree of volume depletion and require replacement of NaCl and water before induction of a diuresis. If a patient is hypovolemic, diuretic therapy exacerbates volume depletion and contributes to further Ca reabsorption, thus worsening the hypercalcemia. In patients with adequate renal function (those who respond to diuretics), treatment with furosemide allows the infusion of large volumes of saline without the risk of pulmonary edema. Usually, normal saline is infused at 100 to 200 cc/hr with the addition of furosemide, 40 to 160 mg/day, once intravascular volume is restored. With saline diuresis, the calcium concentration should decrease by 2 to 3 mg/dl within 24 hours.

If the serum Ca remains elevated, treatment with hypocalcemic agents or dialysis should be considered. The bisphosphonate drugs, etidronate, pamidronate, and clotidronate, inhibit osteoblast activity. Pamidronate and clotidronate are more potent than etidronate. The dose of pamidronate is 15 to 45 mg IV daily or as a single 24-hour infusion of up to 90 mg. Most patients with hypercalcemia of malignancy respond within 6 days, and the effect lasts 1 to 2 weeks. Side effects include fever and leukopenia. Mithramycin acts within 12 hours (peak 48 to 92 hours) to lower Ca via interference with osteoclast activity. The recommended dose is 25 μg/kg IV over 3 hours, which can be repeated every 3 to 4 days. Side effects are hepatotoxicity, nephrotoxicity, and thrombocytopenia. Mithramycin is used primarily for refractory hypercalcemia of malignancy and only for 2 to 3 weeks. Calcitonin inhibits bone resorption and can lower Ca 1 to 3 mg/dl in hours. Tachyphylaxis develops within days. The recommended dose is 4 to 8 IU/kg IM or SQ every 6 to 8 hours. Side effects include flushing, nausea and allergic reactions. For elevated Ca levels caused by vitamin D intoxication and granulomatous diseases, steroids are used. Prednisone impairs intestinal absorption of calcium when given in doses of 40 to 50 mg/day. In oliguric patients, hemodialysis is substituted for saline diuresis and lowers Ca temporarily.

Hypocalcemia

Hypocalcemia is defined as a low serum Ca concentration, <8.5 mg/dl when corrected for serum albumin. If the serum albumin is <4 g/dl, the total serum Ca is reduced by 0.8 mg/dl Ca for each 1 g/dl reduction in the serum albumin below 4 g/dl. Hypocalcemia is also defined as a low ionized Ca (<1.17 mmol/L). The common presenting symptoms or findings of hypocalcemia are shown in Table 18-1.

Etiology and Differential Diagnosis

- Hypoparathyroidism—idiopathic or from thyroid, parathyroid, or neck surgery.
- Hypomagnesemia—low Mg inhibits PTH synthesis and secretion, so hypocalcemia is refractory to treatment with calcium, vitamin D, and PTH and requires Mg therapy.
- Vitamin D deficiency—(a) sunlight deprivation, (b) malabsorption (gastric surgery, intestinal resection, celiac disease, steatorrhea), (c) liver disease (impaired 25-hydroxylation, bile salt formation, reduced synthesis of vitamin D binding protein), (d) nephrotic syndrome (urinary losses of vitamin D and vitamin D binding protein); and e) chronic renal failure (impaired production of vitamin D, hyperphosphatemia, chronic metabolic acidosis).
- Acute pancreatitis—precipitation of calcium salts in the pancreas.
- Enhanced bone turnover or hungry bone syndrome—occurs after surgical treatment of hyperparathyroidism, increase in bone formation.
- Miscellaneous—critically ill patients associated with sepsis, tumor lysis syndrome, rhabdomyolysis, albumin infusion and use of foscarnet.

Treatment

Treatment depends on the severity and the presence of symptoms. Mild hypocalcemia may require no treatment or the use of oral Ca supplements (250 to 500 mg of elemental Ca every 6 to 8 hours). Hypocalcemia associated with symptoms requires parenteral Ca. Calcium gluconate (9 mg of Ca per 10-cc ampule) is less irritating to veins than $CaCl_2$ (272 mg of Ca per ampule). Calcium gluconate can be given in 5 to 10 cc of 5% dextrose over 5 to 10 minutes and repeated as necessary. A continuous Ca infusion for persistent hypocalcemia can be given as 10 ampules/L of 5% dextrose at 50 cc/hr (45 mg/hr). Typically a dose of 15 mg/kg of calcium over 4 to 6 hours raises the serum Ca by 2 to 3 mg/dl.

PHOSPHORUS

The normal serum concentration of PO_4 is 3 to 4.5 mg/dl. Approximately 80% of the total body PO_4 is contained in bone, 9% in skeletal muscle and the remainder in other tissues and the extracellular fluid. Serum PO_4 levels are dependent on PO_4 intake (800 to $1,600$ mg/day), vitamin D, and PTH levels. The jejunum is the primary site of gastrointestinal absorption, and absorption is stimulated by vitamin D. In the absence of vitamin D, more than 60% of dietary phosphorus is still absorbed. Phosphorus is excreted primarily by the kidney, and 200 to 300 mg/day is excreted in sweat, saliva, and stool. Approximately 80% of the filtered PO_4 is reabsorbed in the proximal tubule (stimulated by vitamin D). The PTH inhibits renal reabsorption of PO_4, and increased PO_4 levels stimulate PTH secretion.

Hypophosphatemia

Hypophosphatemia is defined as a serum phosphorus below 2.5 mg/dl. Pseudohypophosphatemia can occur with the use of mannitol or with high bilirubin levels, which interfere with the laboratory measurement of phosphorus. Common clinical presentations or findings in hypophosphatemia are shown in Table 18.2.

Etiology and Differential Diagnosis
- Decreased GI absorption—(a) starvation (combined with vitamin D deficiency, e.g., alcoholism), (b) corticosteroids, (c) Al-, Mg-, and Ca-containing antacids
- Increased renal excretion—primary and secondary hyperparathyroidism (including postrenal transplant)
- Malignancies—production of PTH-related protein (PTHrp) by tumors

TABLE 18.2 Presentation of Hypophosphatemia or Hyperphosphatemia

Hypophosphatemia	Hyperphosphatemia
Asymptomatic (<2.5, >1.0 mg/dl)	Metastatic calcification (Ca × PO_4 > 70)
Muscle weakness (respiratory failure and left ventricular dysfunction)	
Encephalopathy	Secondary hyperparathyroidism (renal failure)
Increased erythrocyte fragility	
Decreased oxygen delivery by RBCs (depletion of 2,3-DPG)	
Impaired leukocyte chemotaxis Reduced platelet survival Chronic defective bone mineralization	

- Fanconi syndrome—associated with multiple myeloma
- Diuresis—(a) diuretics, mainly acetazolamide, (b) postobstruction, (c) recovery from ATN; and (d) recovery from diabetic ketoacidosis
- Intracellular shift—respiratory alkalosis

Treatment

Oral or intravenous therapy may be used, depending on the severity of hyposphosphatemia. Oral phosphorus can be given in various forms to provide 1,000 to 2,000 mg of elemental phosphorus per day to replete body stores in 7 to 10 days. If IV therapy is required, the usual dose is 2 mg/kg every 6 hours.

Hyperphosphatemia

Hyperphosphatemia is defined as a serum phosphorus over 4.5 mg/dl. Common clinical presentations or findings in hyperphosphatemia are listed in Table 18.2.

Etiology and Differential Diagnosis

- Pseudohyperphosphatemia: in vitro hemolysis or interference with the PO_4 assay in multiple myeloma (increased PO_4 binding by globulins)
- Increased PO_4 intake (GI absorption): (a) vitamin D intoxication; (b) iatrogenic (phosphorus repletion or Fleet enemas, which are rich in PO_4), especially in patients with renal insufficiency
- Rapid release of PO_4 from tissues: tumor lysis syndrome, rhabdomyolysis
- Transcellular shifts: acidosis shifts PO_4 into the extracellular space
- Decreased renal excretion: decreased GFR (<25 ml/min) or increased tubular reabsorption (hypoparathyroidism, acromegaly, thyrotoxicosis)

Treatment

Prevention of PO_4 absorption by the GI tract with oral PO_4 binders is the principal therapy for hyperphosphatemia. Calcium-containing binders such as $CaCO_3$ or Ca acetate are given with meals to decrease PO_4 absorption. However, when the PO_4 level exceeds 6.5 mg/dl, or the Ca to PO_4 product exceeds 70, aluminum binders are preferable. In acute severe hyperphosphatemia, saline infusion can increase renal PO_4 clearance. For patients with reduced renal function and Ca to PO_4 products above 70 to 80, dialysis may be required, although the clearance of PO_4 by dialysis is not efficient.

MAGNESIUM

The normal serum Mg level is 1.7 to 2.3 mg/dl. Soft tissue and bone contain 50% of the total body Mg, and 50% remains in the ECF and ICF. Average daily intake is 300 to 360 mg, of which 25% to 60% is absorbed primarily in the small intestine. Fecal losses account for 12 to 24 mg/day, and the kidney is responsible for the remainder of Mg excretion. Regulation of Mg metabolism is not well understood.

Hypermagnesemia

Hypermagnesemia is defined as a serum magnesium level over 2.3 mg/dl. Common clinical presentations or findings in hypermagnesemia are shown in Table 18.3.

Etiology and Differential Diagnosis

Hypermagnesemia usually results from renal failure or massive intake (e.g., Mg therapy for treatment of preeclampsia).

TABLE 18.3   Presentation of Hypermagnesemia and Hypomagnesemia

Hypermagnesemia	Hypomagensemia
Asymptomatic (Mg ≤ 5 mg/dl)	Asymptomatic
Nausea, vomiting, lethargy	Apathy, depression, confusion
Depressed neuromuscular function; decreased DTRs, muscle weakness, paralysis, hypoventilation (blocks acetylcholine release)	Hypocalcemia (hypoparathyroidism) Seizures Tetany and tremor Chvostek's sign
Bradycardia, heart block, cardiac arrest	Ventricular tachycardia, ventricular fibrillation, asystole
Effects exacerbated by hypocalcemia	

Treatment

In severe hypermagnesemia (neuromuscular depression), IV calcium (100 to 200 mg) can be given to antagonize the effects of the Mg. A saline diuresis should be induced, or hemodialysis can also be used, especially in patients with renal failure.

Hypomagnesemia

Hypomagnesemia is defined as a serum magnesium level below 1.7 mg/dl and is relatively common, with a reported frequency of 7% to 20% in hospitalized patients. Common clinical presentations and findings in hypomagnesemia are listed in Table 18-3.

Etiology and Differential Diagnosis
- Decreased intake: malnutrition, malabsorption (short bowel, chronic diarrhea)
- Increased renal excretion: diuresis (diuretics, especially loop diuretics; diuretic phase of ATN; postobstruction, previous renal transplant; hyperglycemia)
- Drugs: cisplatin, aminoglycosides, cyclosporine, amphotericin B, foscarnet, ethanol
- Congenital defects of Mg absorption: Bartter's and Gitelman's syndromes

Treatment

Mild asymptomatic hypomagnesemia can be treated with oral Mg supplements in the form of MgO (1 g, which contains 600 mg of Mg). If hypomagnesemia is severe, intravenous therapy is required. With normal renal function, 2 g of $MgSO_4$ administered IV over 15 minutes is the usual dose.

Suggested Readings

Auerbach GD, Marx SJ, Spiegel AM. Parathyroid hormone, calcitonin, and the calciferols. In: Wilson JD, Foster DW, eds. *Williams textbook of endocrinology, 8th ed.* Philadelphia: WB Saunders, 1992:1397–1476.

Bilzekian JP. Management of acute hypercalcemia. *N Engl J Med* 1992; 326:1196–1203.

Hruska KA, Slatopolsky E. Disorders of phosphorus, calcium, and magnesium metabolism. In: Schrier RW, Gottschalk, eds. *Diseases of the kidney, 6th ed.* Boston: Little, Brown, 1996:2477–2526.

Hruska KA, Teitlebaum SL. Renal osteodystrophy. *N Engl J Med* 1995; 333:166–174.

Knochel JP, Agarwal R. Hypophosphatemia and hyperphosphatemia. In: Brenner BM, ed. *The kidney, 5th ed.* Philadelphia: WB Saunders, 1996: 1086–1136.

Singer FR, Ritch PS, Lad TE, et al, and the Hypercalcemia Study Group. Treatment of hypercalcemia of malignancy with intravenous etidronate: a controlled multicenter trial. *Arch Intern Med* 1991;151:471–476.

Sutton RA, Dirks JH. Disorders of calcium and magnesium metabolism. In: Brenner BM, ed. *The kidney, 5th ed.* Philadelphia: WB Saunders, 1996:1038–1085.

Chapter 19

Renal Stone Disease

I. David Weiner

Renal stone disease is a common condition that affects wide ranges of the population and causes significant morbidity. Therapeutic advances including extracorporeal shock wave lithotripsy (ESWL), percutaneous lithotripsy, and ureteroscopic laser treatment have improved our ability to treat the acute manifestations of renal stone disease. However, in many individuals renal stone disease is chronic, with high rates of recurrence.

EPIDEMIOLOGY

Renal stone disease affects approximately one in every 500 individuals in the United States each year. Over a lifetime about 1 of 14 men and 1 of 30 women will develop this disease. The disease is frequently recurrent. In the absence of preventive treatment, recurrence rates are ≈5% to 10% at 1 year, 15% to 20% at 5 years, and 30% to 40% after 25 years. The decrease in the recurrence rate with time suggests a gradual waning of the disease.

In the southeastern United States, the rate of kidney stone disease is approximately twice as high as in the rest of the country. The increased incidence is possibly related to the hotter climate, with increased insensible fluid losses and reduced urine output leading to increased concentration of stone-forming molecules in the urine.

PHYSIOLOGY AND PATHOPHYSIOLOGY

Most renal stones contain calcium in the form of calcium oxalate (35–70% of all stones), calcium phosphate (6–20%), or a mixture of both (10–30%). Pure uric acid stones account for 10% of all stones. Struvite stones, composed of magnesium ammonium phosphate, account for 15% to 20% of stones, and rare stones consist primarily of cystine. Figure 19.1 summarizes the typical distribution of renal stones.

Kidney stones form when stone-forming crystalloids normally present in urine come out of solution. The most common stone-forming crystalloids are calcium phosphate, calcium oxalate, uric acid, magnesium ammonium phosphate, and cystine.

Several factors interact to cause these stone-forming crystalloids to come out of solutions. The most important factors are (a) supersaturation of the crystalloids in the urine; (b) the presence of physical or chemical stimuli that promote stone formation; and (c) inadequate amounts of inhibitors of stone formation. Therefore, stone formation can result from any combination of:

- Low urinary volume (e.g., hot climates)
- High urinary excretion of calcium, uric acid, or oxalate (the most common components of renal stones)
- Abnormal urinary pH (e.g., uric acid and cystine are less soluble in acid urine, whereas struvite and calcium phosphate are less soluble in alkaline urine)
- A nidus for crystal precipitation (e.g., sodium urate crystallization promotes calcium oxalate deposition on the sodium urate crystals and speeds the rate of stone formation)

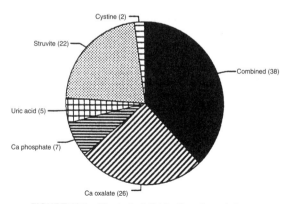

FIGURE 19.1 The typical distribution of renal stones.

- A deficiency of inhibitors of stone formation such as citrate and Mg^{2+}

Most patients with renal stones will have one or more identifiable causes of stone formation. The most common include hypercalciuria, hyperoxaluria, hypocitraturia, hyperuricosuria, and infection.

Hypercalciuria is the most commonly identified cause of renal stone disease. Excessive urinary calcium excretion leads to supersaturation of urine with calcium and the subsequent development of calcium oxalate (acid urine) or calcium phosphate (alkaline urine) stones. Hypercalciuria has several causes. Primary absorptive hypercalciuria leads to subclinical increases in serum calcium, mild suppression of parathyroid hormone, increased renal calcium filtration, and decreased calcium reabsorption leading to an increase in urinary calcium excretion. A second cause is a primary renal calcium "leak," whereby a primary decrease in renal calcium reabsorption leads to increased urinary calcium excretion. A rarer but easily treatable cause is a primary renal phosphate "leak" that leads to hypophosphatemia, stimulation of PTH release, a secondary increase in gastrointestinal calcium absorption, a subclinical increase in the serum calcium, and a subsequent increase in urinary calcium excretion. Finally, excessive dietary sodium intake can increase urinary calcium excretion.

Most patients with calcium oxalate stones excrete normal amounts of urinary oxalate. However, increased gastrointestinal oxalate absorption can occur either from a primary increase in gastrointestinal uptake or from enhanced endogenous production. Gastrointestinal oxalate absorption can be increased by conditions that cause fat malabsorption, such as Crohn's disease, celiac sprue, or intestinal bypass surgery. Increased endogenous production occurs from either increased intake of foods rich in oxalate such as spinach, peanuts, and cocoa, or excessive intake of vitamin C, which is metabolized to oxalate.

Citrate plays an important role in the defense against stone development because of its ability to complex urinary calcium, thereby preventing its incorporation into either calcium oxalate or calcium phosphate stones. Hypocitraturia may result from conditions that increase endogenous acid production, such as excessive dietary protein intake, or increase base loss, as in chronic diarrhea.

Hyperuricosuria can cause renal stone formation in either of two ways. First, uric acid crystals may serve as a nidus on which calcium oxalate crystals deposit, leading to increased rates of calcium oxalate stone growth. Second, pure uric acid stones can form in persistently acid urine. The solubility of uric acid is strongly pH dependent, with markedly lower solubility at acid pH. For example, at pH 5, the normal rate of uric acid excretion for men, 800 mg/day, can lead to uric acid supersaturation and stone formation if urine volume is 1 L per day or less.

Infection with urea-splitting bacteria, such as *Proteus* and some species of *Klebsiella pneumoniae,* can lead to increased formation of specific stones. Bacterial urease hydrolyzes urinary urea to ammonia in a reaction that consumes a proton, thereby increasing both urinary ammonia and pH. At high urine pH, magnesium, phosphate, and ammonium form struvite, which is insoluble and can rapidly grow in size until it fills the collecting system, forming the classic "staghorn" calculi. The bacteria are frequently incorporated into the growing struvite stone, leading to difficulty in sterilizing the urine.

CLINICAL PRESENTATION

There are several clinical presentations of stone disease:

- *Severe, intense pain* is the most common presentation of renal stone disease. It typically has a sudden onset, although it may increase over a period of hours to a peak in some individuals. It may be either steady or colicky. An obstructing or partially obstructing stone in the renal pelvis or upper ureter is characteristically associated with flank and abdominal pain. Stones present in the middle and lower thirds of the ureter typically cause pain that radiates downward to the inguinal ligament and into the urethra or testicle and penis. When stones are present in the portion of the ureter within the bladder wall, they may cause dysuria and frequency. Nausea and vomiting frequently accompany the pain and may contribute to the development of dehydration. Many affected individuals characterize the pain as the worst they have ever experienced. For unclear reasons, recurrent stones are typically less painful than on initial presentation.
- *Hematuria* may occur as a result of local trauma to the renal pelvis or bladder from the stones.
- *Infection* of the stone may lead to either recurrent symptomatic urinary tract infections or asymptomatic infections, which lead to progressive renal dysfunction.

- *Obstruction* of the renal pelvis or the ureter may occur. Untreated obstruction, even if partial, can lead to irreversible loss of renal function.
- *Asymptomatic* stones may be discovered on an abdominal radiograph or ultrasound obtained for other reasons.

DIAGNOSIS

- *History* should emphasize diet, drug ingestion, familial disorders, and the presence or absence of previous renal stones.
- *Urinalysis* usually reveals either gross or microscopic hematuria. If pyuria is present, then infection should be excluded by urine culture. Crystalluria may permit a presumptive identification of stone type (see Fig. 19.2). However, only freshly voided, warm urine should be used for examination; when urine is cooled the solubility of dissolved crystalloids decreases, possibly leading to their precipitation and an incorrect diagnosis.
- *Radiologic studies* play an important role in the evaluation of renal stone disease. A plain abdominal radiograph may show radiodense stones (85–90% of all stones) containing either calcium, struvite, or cystine but may miss radiolucent uric acid stones. An ultrasound or an intravenous urogram is needed to identify radiolucent stones or to confirm that a radiodensity seen on plain radiograph is in fact within the renal

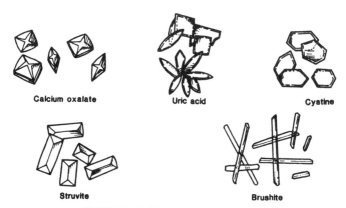

Calcium oxalate   Uric acid   Cystine

Struvite   Brushite

FIGURE 19.2   Urinary crystal morphology.

pelvis or the ureter, and to determine whether partial or complete ureteral obstruction is present.

- *Crystallographic stone analysis* is critical for establishing the chemical nature of a stone and guiding therapy. Patients should strain their urine through a filter until the stone is passed in order to obtain the stone for crystallographic analysis of its composition.

MANAGEMENT

The management of renal stone disease should be divided into two components, the acute presentation, in the patient with acute renal colic, and the chronic management, after the pain, obstruction, and/or infection is treated.

Acute Management

Patients presenting with acute renal colic caused by renal stone disease are frequently in great discomfort and require aggressive treatment. Once other conditions such as appendicitis, cholecystitis, or pyelonephritis are shown not to be the cause of the patient's symptoms, pain control is essential. Most pain can be controlled with intravenous ketorolac or parenteral narcotics. Oral analgesics should generally be avoided because of the nausea and vomiting or abdominal ileus that is frequently present. In addition, rapid pain control is generally desired and is best accomplished with parenteral analgesics.

Second, these patients are frequently intravascularly volume-depleted by nausea and vomiting or an avoidance of oral intake because of the pain they are experiencing. Intravenous rehydration will assist both in decreasing symptoms related to dehydration and by increasing urine output, which may aid in the passage of the renal stone.

If infection is suspected, either because of the presence of fever and leukocytosis or pyuria and bacteriuria on urinalysis, empirical antibiotics should be started. In general, all patients should have their urine cultured appropriately for bacteria.

In most patients the acute renal colic can be managed in an outpatient setting. An exception to this rule is the patient in whom nausea and vomiting cannot be controlled, who thus requires hospitalization for continued hydration. A second exception is the patient with a fever or urinary tract infection and ureteral obstruction. This patient is at high risk for severe, rapidly progressive urosepsis and should have emergent relief of the obstruction. Ureteral obstruction in the absence of infection is not an indication for emergent hospitalization unless the patient has a solitary functional kidney. Otherwise, the stone can be observed for spontaneous passage over a period of days.

Most renal stones pass spontaneously. The patient with acute renal colic should filter their urine until the stone passes in order to retrieve the stone for accurate identification of the composition, to gain insight into the factors that caused the problem. However, stones greater than 7 mm in size are less likely to pass spontaneously.

Stones that do not pass spontaneously or require urgent intervention for the reasons detailed above can be approached with a variety of techniques including basket extraction, cystoscopy with laser lithotripsy, extracorporeal shock wave lithotripsy (ESWL), and percutaneous extraction or shock wave lithotripsy. Usually stones in the distal third of the ureter can be treated with cystoscopic techniques. Stones in other locations can be treated with ESWL, leading to the formation of multiple small fragments that will usually pass with few symptoms.

Chronic Management

The chronic management of renal stone disease is based on two observations. First, renal stone disease may be the initial presentation of an underlying, systemic disease that may cause morbidity or mortality unrelated to the renal stone disease if not identified. Second, approximately 40% of patients with renal stone disease will develop at least one recurrence, and of those some will develop frequent recurrences that can lead to a substantial impact on the quality of life.

The first goal of the chronic management of renal stone disease is to exclude an underlying systemic disease that caused the renal stone disease. Table 19.1 lists the likely systemic diseases and their recommended screening tests. Patients with hypercalcemia, whether overt or borderline, should have an ionized calcium and a parathyroid hormone level measured to identify whether they have primary hyperparathyroidism. Patients with hypokalemic, non-anion-gap metabolic acidosis should have the urine pH and urine

TABLE 19.1 Systemic Diseases Causing Renal Stone Disease

Disease	Screening tests
Primary hyperparathyroidism	Serum calcium
Distal renal tubular acidosis	Serum electrolytes
Inflammatory bowel disease	History
Gout	History, uric acid
Inborn error of metabolism	Onset in childhood

anion gap measured to determine whether they have distal renal tubular acidosis. Inflammatory bowel disease and gout are generally suspected based on a typical history, although the presence of hyperuricemia may be helpful in the diagnosis of gout. Inborn errors of metabolism that cause renal stones are frequent causes of renal stones in children. These include cystine stones in cystinosis, glycine stones in hyperglycinuria, uric acid stones in Lesch-Nyhan syndrome, and oxalate stones in oxalosis. Congenital distal renal tubular acidosis may also present in children; it is frequently associated with impaired growth or failure to thrive or both.

The second component of the chronic management of renal stone disease is prevention of recurrence. As many as 40% to 50% of individuals with an initial stone will develop one or more recurrences. Measures to prevent recurrence can be helpful in many individuals. The simplest measure to prevent recurrence is to increase the urine volume to decrease the concentration of crystalloids, leading to a decreased rate of stone formation and even, in some patients, to dissolution of existing stones. Increasing urine volume by 1 L per day can decrease the risk of recurrence by 50%.

Other measures to decrease recurrence are based on treating the common causes of stone formation. Automated analysis of calcium, oxalate, uric acid, citrate, pH, total volume, and sodium in a 24-hour urine specimen (e.g., StoneRisk Profile, Mission Pharmacal, San Antonio, TX) can be helpful. Those abnormalities found can be treated as described below.

Hypercalciuria should be treated by measures that decrease urinary calcium excretion. First, primary hyperparathyroidism or other causes of hypercalcemia should be investigated and treated if present. If hypercalcemia is not present, then thiazide diuretics are effective at decreasing urinary calcium excretion. Because thiazide diuretics decrease urinary citrate excretion, they should be combined with administration of potassium citrate. Sodium citrate is usually avoided because the sodium content can increase urinary calcium excretion.

Hyperoxaluria is treated by addressing the underlying cause whenever possible. Fat malabsorption should be treated aggressively. If marked hyperoxaluria, greater than five to ten times the upper limit of normal, is identified, then evaluation for primary hyperoxaluria related to genetic defects in oxalate metabolism should be initiated.

Hyperuricosuria can be treated by measures that either increase the solubility of uric acid or decrease the production of uric acid. Alkalinizing the urine markedly increases the solubility of uric acid. Potassium citrate is effective because oral citrate intake can cause mild metabolic alkalosis and subsequent alkalinization of the urine. Allopurinol, 300 mg per day, decreases the production of uric acid and is also beneficial in patients with documented hyperuricosuria, particularly if uric acid stones have been documented.

Hypocitraturia is easily treated with oral potassium citrate. As noted above, citrate ingestion leads to mild metabolic alkalosis, which increases urinary citrate excretion. Potassium citrate, 40 to 60 mEq a day in divided doses, should be used; sodium citrate should be avoided as noted previously.

Struvite stones require treatment of the underlying infection. Appropriate antibiotics should be administered based on the results of urine culture and sensitivity and should be continued for 4 to 6 months. Because the offending bacteria can become incorporated into the stone matrix, prolonged antibiotic treatment, even in the presence of apparently negative urine cultures, is necessary. Acetohydroxamic acid, a urease inhibitor, may be helpful.

Suggested Readings

Ackermann DK. Prospective therapeutic studies in nephrolithiasis. *World J Urol* 1997;15:172–175.

Borghi L, Meschi T, Amato F, Briganti A, Novarini A, Giannini A. Urinary volume, water and recurrences in idiopathic calcium nephrolithiasis: a 5-year randomized prospective study. *J Urol* 1996;155:839–843.

Bushinsky DA. Nephrolithiasis. *J Am Soc Nephrol* 1998;9:917–924.

Coe FL, Parks JH. New insights into the pathophysiology and treatment of nephrolithiasis: new research venues. *J Bone Miner Res* 1997;12:522–533.

Pak CY. Nephrolithiasis. *Curr Ther Endocrinol Metab* 1997;6:572–576.

Pak CY. Southwestern Internal Medicine Conference: medical management of nephrolithiasis—a new, simplified approach for general practice. *Am J Med Sci* 1997;313:215–219.

Ruml LA, Pearle MS, Pak CY. Medical therapy, calcium oxalate urolithiasis. *Urol Clin North Am* 1997;24:117–133.

Saklayen MG. Medical management of nephrolithiasis. *Med Clin North Am* 1997;81:785–799.

Wasserstein AG. Nephrolithiasis: acute management and prevention. *Dis Month* 1998;44:196–213.

Chapter 20

Urinary Tract Infection

R. Tyler Miller

Urinary tract infections can be separated into three categories: (a) lower tract infections that involve the bladder (cystitis) or urethra (urethritis); (b) upper tract infections that involve primarily the kidneys (pyelonephritis); and (c) complicated urinary tract infections in which structural abnormalities such as strictures, stones, obstruction, or foreign bodies predispose to infection and may interfere with effective treatment. Urinary tract infections are common in both inpatient and outpatient populations, and they range in severity from causing discomfort and annoyance to being life threatening. Upper tract and complicated infections are generally the most severe, are often the most difficult to treat, often require radiologic evaluation, and frequently require treatment beyond antibiotics. Usually lower tract infections are not life threatening and respond readily to standard treatment. The reasons for infection, and consequently the approach to treatment, depend on the age, gender, and underlying conditions in the patient and must be considered in the evaluation and management of patients with urinary tract infections.

ETIOLOGY

Urinary tract infections occur as a consequence of impaired host defenses and bacterial virulence factors. Factors that impair bacterial invasion and colonization include periodic voiding, which dilutes bacteria and flushes them out of the bladder and urethra; urine composition, where extremes of pH and osmolality impair bacterial growth; presence of Tamm Horsfall protein, which competes with bacterial adhesion molecules; and prostatic secretions in men, which are bacteriostatic. Factors that promote urinary tract infections include bacterial colonization of the distal urethra, alteration of the normal host flora with antibiotics, the short urethra in female patients, stones or other foreign bodies (catheters, stents) that are difficult or impossible to sterilize, obstruction, strictures, diverticuli, reflux, or abnormal neural function (neurogenic bladder) that impairs emptying of the bladder, contraception (diaphragms, spermicide) that may alter the structure or chemical composition of the urinary tract, and estrogen status, which may alter bacterial binding to uroepithelium. Depending on the patient's gender or age, certain factors are more common in predisposing to urinary tract infections (Table 20.1). Bacterial virulence factors include fimbriae and pili that recognize specific host carbohydrate molecules (mannose or galactose) and are responsible for specific adhesion of pathogenic bacteria to the uroepithelium; K antigen, which confers resistance of bacteria to phagocytosis by host cells; and production of extracellular proteins and toxins such as hemolysin that make bacteria resistant to the bactericidal activity of serum and increase their invasiveness.

Table 20.2 depicts the various types of bacteria that are found characteristically in different types of urinary tract infections. In general, the bacteria are enteric organisms that gain access to the

TABLE 20.1   Epidemiology of UTI by Age Group

Age	Female Prev %	Female Risk factor	Male Prev %	Male Risk factor
<1	1	Structural/functional abnormalities	1	Structural/functional abnormalities
1–5	4–5	Congenital abnormalities/reflux	0.5	Congenital abnormalities/ uncircumcised men
6–15	4–5	Reflux	0.5	None
16–35	20	Sexual activity/ diaphragm	0.5	Homosexuality
36–65	35	Gynecologic surgery/prolapse	20	Prostatism/catheters/ obstruction/surgery
>65	40	As above/ incontinence	35	As above/ incontinence

TABLE 20.2   Bacteriology of Urinary Tract Infections

Organism	Cystitis	Pyelonephritis	Complicated	Catheter-associated
E. coli	79	89	32	24
S. saprophiticus	11	0	1	0
Proteus	2	4	4	6
Klebsiella	3	4	5	8
Enterococcus	2	0	22	7
Pseudomonas	0	0	20	9
Mixed	3	5	10	11
Other[a]	0	0	1	10
Yeast	0	0	1	28
S. epidermidis	0	0	15	8

[a] *S. aureus* suggests hematogenous spread from another source.

urinary tract through local contamination. As noted in the table, *S. aureus* is an unusual pathogen in urinary tract infections, and finding it in a urine culture suggests that the urinary tract has been infected secondarily, either through a communicating wound or by hematogenous spread. In most patients, infecting bacteria are the same species that colonize the colon and urogenital areas. In community-acquired infections, the predominant organism is *E. coli,* and the pattern of antibiotic resistance will reflect that found in the community, whereas in infections in hospitalized or institutionalized patients (nursing homes), the patterns of anti-biotic resistance will reflect those of the institution. Complicated and catheter-associated infections are often associated with patients who have been hospitalized. Although *E. coli* is still a common cause of infection, other enteric gram-negative rods (*Klebsiella* and *Enterobacter*) and enterococcus are found with a similar frequency as *E. coli*. Antibiotic-resistant (vancomycin-resistant) enterococcus is becoming an increasing problem in institutions.

DIAGNOSIS OF URINARY TRACT INFECTIONS

Patients with infections limited to the urethra usually complain of dysuria and urethral discomfort. Patients with lower urinary tract infections (cystitis) usually present with a history of dysuria, frequency, urgency, or suprapubic pain. Upper tract infections (pyelonephritis) are usually characterized by signs of lower tract infection in association with back pain, flank pain, fever, and chills.

In all cases of suspected urinary tract infections, a history of instrumentation, sexual activity, trauma, or structural abnormalities of
the urinary tract should be sought. Physical findings may include
urethral discharge in cases of urethritis, suprapubic tenderness in
cystitis, and flank and back tenderness (costovertebral angle tenderness) with upper tract infections. Fever is usually absent in
lower tract infections. Evidence of past urinary tract surgery (flank
or lower abdominal surgical scars) should also be sought.

Laboratory analysis should include a urinalysis, microscopic
examination of the sediment, urine culture, CBC, and electrolytes
if an upper tract or complicated infection is suspected or if warranted because of other medical conditions. Urine should be
obtained with a clean-catch or catheter technique to minimize
contamination. If a bacterial infection is present, the dipstick may
be positive for heme (50%) and should be positive for leukocyte
esterase and nitrite. False-negative leukocyte esterase results may
occur with high glucose levels, a high urine specific gravity, and
with some antibiotics (cephalexin, cephalothin, tetracycline) or
oxalic acid. False-negative nitrite results may arise from urine with
a high specific gravity or high levels of ascorbic acid. Microscopic
examination should reveal white blood cells (neutrophils) with
rare epithelial or squamous cells and may reveal bacteria or yeast.
Red blood cells are also seen in 50% of patients. A urine culture
that is diagnostic of a urinary tract infection should contain
$>10^5$ bacteria/ml of a single type, although infection can be diagnosed with pure cultures of fewer organisms. Mixed cultures when
other findings point to infection suggest bowel communication.
Electrolytes and renal excretory function are rarely abnormal in
uncomplicated infections.

If new electrolyte abnormalities are found, particularly elevations of the BUN and creatinine, urinary obstruction should
be suspected, and the diagnosis pursued with catheterization or
radiographic tests. Ultrasound is the best initial test to identify
obstruction. A type IV RTA pattern (elevated K and Cl levels and
a reduced HCO_3^- level) may be an early clue to a urinary tract
obstruction. Obstruction should be pursued aggressively if suspected because infection behind an obstruction will not respond
satisfactorily to antibiotics.

The value of radiographic studies and the studies chosen will
depend on the type of suspected infection (see Table 20.3). In
general, uncomplicated lower tract infections and uncomplicated

TABLE 20.3   Radiologic Studies in Urinary Tract Infections

Condition	IVP	Ultrasound	CT
Uncomplicated pyelonephritis	75% Nl, ↑ renal size, prolonged nephrogram	↑ Renal size, variable echo-genicity, no hydronephrosis	↑ renal size, ↓ cort.-med. def. ↓ function
Chronic pyelonephritis	↓Cortex, ↓ function, focal scarring caliectasis	↓ Renal size, lobular hyper-trophy, pseudo-tumor	↓renal size, ↓ function, pseudotumor
Renal/peri-nephric abscess	Mass effect, distortion of renal contour/calices	Thick-walled cystic mass with external echoes	Thick-walled cystic mass, ↓ attenuation
Obstruction	↓ Function, mass effect	Dilated collect-ing system	Dilated collect-ing system

pyelonephritis require only the diagnostic studies described above. However, if a complicated infection is suspected (newly elevated BUN and creatinine, abnormal urinary tract, urinary tract surgery, stones, pelvic tumors, neurogenic bladder, etc.), radiologic studies may be warranted to look for obstruction or localized foci of infection that do not have free drainage to the urinary space (e.g., perinephric abscess). Table 20-3 shows the characteristic findings with IVP, ultrasound, and CT in several types of urinary tract infections. Ultrasound is the best initial test for suspected obstruction in most cases, because it is possible to visualize the bladder, ureters, and collecting systems of both kidneys. A false-negative ultrasound examination can result from processes that infiltrate or encase the ureter such as retroperitoneal fibrosis or metastatic tumors.

DIAGNOSIS AND TREATMENT OF THE ACUTE URETHRAL SYNDROME

Patients with this syndrome usually present with symptoms of burning on urination, urethral discomfort, frequently a urethral discharge, and a history compatible with a sexually transmitted infection. The physical and laboratory findings are a purulent urethral discharge or no discharge and, if present, bacteriuria less than 10^4 CFU/ml. The organisms responsible for the acute urethral syndrome are *Chlamydia trachomatis, N. gonorrheae, Trichomonas,* or often undefined organisms. Treatment is based on culture of the discharge for *N. gonorrheae* and will depend on the current local guidelines for *N. gonorrheae:* flagyl or tetracycline. The outcome depends on the organism, the ability to make a diagnosis, and patient compliance.

DIAGNOSIS AND TREATMENT OF UNCOMPLICATED CYSTITIS

Patients with uncomplicated cystitis usually present with complaints of burning on urination, frequent urination, and suprapubic pain. Urinary tract instrumentation and sexual activity are common inciting events. Back pain, fever, chills, and other systemic symptoms suggest pyelonephritis. The findings that support a diagnosis of cystitis are pyuria, which is required for diagnosis, and bacteriuria (10^5 CFU/ml, single organism). In community-acquired infections, *E. coli* (>90%) and *S. saprophyticus* are the most frequently isolated organisms. Appropriate treatment includes TMP-SMX, TMP, norfloxacin, ciprofloxacin, sulfa, or nitrofurantoin for a period of 1, 3, or 7 days. The shorter courses of therapy are reserved for young patients without underlying disease and a normal urinary tract. More than 95% of patients with cystitis are cured. True relapses are rare, but reinfection occurs with some frequency. Unsuspected upper tract infections frequently do not respond to short-duration therapy. With recurrent and prolonged symptoms of cystitis, interstitial cystitis, an inflammatory condition of the bladder, should be considered.

DIAGNOSIS AND TREATMENT OF UNCOMPLICATED PYELONEPHRITIS

In pyelonephritis, the symptoms include burning on urination, urinary frequency, suprapubic pain, back pain, fever, chills, and other systemic symptoms. Physical examination may reveal fever, suprapubic tenderness, flank tenderness, and costovertebral angle tenderness. Laboratory findings include pyuria (usually required for diagnosis but occasionally not present with complete obstruction). The urine culture should be positive for bacteria (10^5 CFU/ml, single organism). *E. coli* is the causative organism in more than 90% of patients. A urine culture with antibiotic sensitivity testing is important to guide antibiotic therapy. A leukocytosis is frequently found.

Appropriate treatment involves antibiotics including TMP-SMX, TMP, norfloxacin, ciprofloxacin, sulfa, nitrofurantoin, or a β-lactam and an aminoglycoside. Patients with pyelonephritis are treated for 14 days. Initial treatment may be with IV antibiotics for 3 days or until a clinical response is achieved (resolution of fever, pain), and then with oral antibiotics. Uncomplicated pyelonephritis is usually cured in more than 90% of patients, and relapses are rare. However, a relapse or a poor initial response to therapy should lead to suspicion of a urinary tract abnormality, and appropriate evaluation is necessary. Recurrent infections should suggest reflux and prompt an evaluation.

DIAGNOSIS AND TREATMENT OF PYELONEPHRITIS WITH SEPSIS OR PROSTRATION

The symptoms and physical findings in pyelonephritis with sepsis and prostration are similar to those with uncomplicated pyelonephritis but may also include systemic symptoms such as hypotension and the sepsis syndrome. This manifestation of pyelonephritis is more common in older and debilitated patients such as nursing home residents, where a history may be unreliable. The physical findings are also similar to uncomplicated pyelonephritis but in addition include positive blood cultures and may include laboratory evidence of the sepsis syndrome (leukocytosis, leukopenia, acidosis, DIC). In these patients, *E. coli* is still the most frequently found organism, but other gram-negative rods such as *Klebsiella* and *Proteus* are also found. Treatment is with IV antibiotics such as a third- or fourth-generation cephalosporin or an aminoglycoside and a β-lactam, pending determination of bacterial sensitivities. In these patients the outcome remains relatively good with a >80% cure rate. As described above, with a relapse or a poor initial response, urinary tract abnormalities should be suspected, and their identification pursued.

DIAGNOSIS AND TREATMENT OF COMPLICATED URINARY TRACT INFECTION: STONES OR ANATOMIC ABNORMALITIES

In complicated urinary tract infections, the symptoms of burning on urination, frequency, suprapubic pain, back pain, fever, and chills are similar to those found in other urinary tract infections but may be modified by the urinary tract abnormality. Patients with kidney stones may have chronic pain and low-grade infection, patients with urinary diversion procedures may have no symptoms referable to the bladder, or patients with new-onset abnormalities (diabetics with neurogenic bladders or patients with urinary obstruction from tumors) may simply have a poor response to initial treatment. Complicated infections are likely to have systemic sequelae and symptoms including hypotension, nausea and vomiting, and sepsis. The physical and laboratory findings include pyuria, obstruction, stones, strictures, an enlarged prostate, evidence of malignancy, gynecologic pathology, retroperitoneal tumors or fibrosis, and abnormal bladder function. Pyuria and bacteriuria (10^5 CFU/ml, single organism *E. coli,* klebsiella, proteus, enterococcus) are the common laboratory findings in addition to the urinary tract abnormality. Treatment depends on the nature and severity of the infection and the goals of therapy (suppression vs. cure) and may involve either IV or PO antibiotics with a standard 14-day course or long-term suppression. The outcome depends on the nature of the urinary tract abnormality and the ability to correct it.

SPECIAL SITUATIONS

Several special situations are worthy of note because they either fall outside the definitions of urinary tract infections described above, or they represent patient groups where special care is warranted. Asymptomatic bacteriuria is defined as $\geq 10^5$ bacterial CFU/ml in the absence of urinary tract symptoms. Treatment is indicated for this condition in children, patients who are immune-suppressed (transplant recipients or those receiving chemotherapy), patients with diabetes mellitus, and pregnant women. Treatment usually involves a short course of antibiotics. Patients with diabetes mellitus are at risk for complications including atonic bladder (functional obstruction), neuropathy, and abnormal WBC function. Consequently, if they show systemic symptoms including deterioration in glucose control, altered mental status, and certainly urinary tract symptoms, their urine should be examined for infection. Asymptomatic bacteriuria should be treated in this population. Enlarged prostates can cause partial or complete obstruction, and chronic prostatitis may be a source of recurrent bacteriuria. A high index of suspicion should be maintained for urinary tract obstruction in elderly men. Pregnant women have decreased smooth muscle tone, dilated ureters, increased hydronephrosis, and an increased incidence of urinary tract infections, especially pyelonephritis. In these patients, the urine should be examined for evidence of infection and asymptomatic bacteriuria. In pregnancy, asymptomatic bacteriuria is associated with an increased incidence of premature labor. Lower urinary tract infections are treated with a 3-day course of sulfonamides, β-lactams, or nalidixic acid. TMP-SMZ should be avoided in the third trimester. Immune-suppressed patients, patients with primary diseases that result in immune suppression (e.g., lymphoma, leukemia, myeloma) or patients who are treated with immune-suppressive drugs (kidney transplant, chemotherapy for cancer, steroids for inflammatory diseases) should be evaluated carefully for urinary tract infections, even when presenting with nonspecific symptoms, because their reduced inflammatory responses may mask classic urinary tract symptoms, and early treatment may avoid systemic infections. Asymptomatic bacteriuria should be treated in this group of patients as well.

Suggested Readings

Schaefer AJ. Urinary tract infections. In: Jacobsen MR, Striker GE, Klahr S, eds. *The principles and practice of nephrology, 2nd ed.* St Louis: CV Mosby, 1995:480–509.

Sobel JD, Kaye D. Urinary tract infections. In: Mandell GL, Bennett JE, Dolin R, eds. *Principles and practice of infectious diseases, 4th ed.* New York: Churchill Livingstone, 1995:662–689.

Stamm WE. Urinary tract infections. In: Gorbach SL, Bartlett JG, Blacklow NR, eds. *Infectious diseases.* Philadelphia: WB Saunders, 1992:788–797.

Chapter 21

Approach to the Hypertensive Patient

Christopher S. Wilcox

Hypertension is a level of blood pressure (BP) sufficiently high to increase the risk of stroke or renal or cardiovascular system (CVS) disease. Blood pressure above 140/90 mm Hg in an adult is usually considered abnormal.

INCIDENCE

The incidence of hypertension is about 5% in young adults, 20% by age 50 to 60 years, and 50% by age 80. The incidence increases in those with diabetes mellitus or renal insufficiency.

ISOLATED SYSTOLIC HYPERTENSION

Systolic hypertension in the young implies a high cardiac output and rapid left ventricular ejection. This responds well to β-blockade. Systolic hypertension in the elderly results from the loss of elasticity in the large arteries or aortic atherosclerosis. Thus, it carries an unfavorable prognosis for stroke and myocardial infarction. It responds well to diuretics.

RISKS

Hypertension increases the risk of the following:

- Myocardial infarction (MI)
- Cerebrovascular accident (CVA)
- Chronic renal failure (notably nephrosclerosis)

- Congestive cardiac failure (CHF)
- Aortic aneurysm
- Peripheral vascular disease

The risk of vascular complications is increased by the following:

- Smoking
- Age (elderly have worse prognosis)
- Previous organ injury (e.g., stroke)
- Coincident arterial disease (e.g., atherosclerosis, aneurysm, diabetes mellitus)
- Race (African-Americans have a worse prognosis)
- Left ventricular hypertrophy (LVH)
- Hypercholesterolemia
- Obesity/underactivity
- Family history of death below age 50 from MI or vascular disease

Hypertension accelerates damage caused by other diseases affecting the heart, kidneys, and brain. The decline in renal function in azotemic patients with diabetic nephropathy and those with other renal diseases who are excreting more than 1 g daily of protein is enhanced by hypertension. In these patients, the target BP should be 120/70 mm Hg. Hypertension accelerates the decline in cognitive function in patients with dementia and in cardiac function in those with CHF.

CLASSIFICATION

Each patient with hypertension should be classified according to the severity, the pathologic type (benign, accelerated, or malignant), and the cause (essential or secondary).

Severity of Hypertension

- Borderline: 130 to 139/85 to 89 mm Hg
- Mild: 140 to 159/90 to 99 mm Hg
- Moderate: 160 to 179/100 to 109 mm Hg
- Severe: above 180/110 mm Hg

Treatment of mild hypertension is not urgent. Moderate hypertension requires treatment within weeks, and severe hypertension within hours.

Pathogenic Type

Benign hypertension is usually asymptomatic and progresses slowly. Pathologic changes in large and small arteries include concentric medial hypertrophy without necrosis. There is hypertrophy of the heart and fibrosis and sclerosis of the kidneys.

Accelerated hypertension implies a recent sharp increase in BP associated with vascular damage but without papilledema.

Malignant hypertension accounts for less than 1% of all hypertension. The hallmarks are grade IV funduscopic changes of papilledema, retinal hemorrhages, and exudates. The BP is severe and accompanied by headache and often by fluctuating neurologic signs caused by increased intracranial pressure and patchy ischemia. This can progress to seizures, fixed neurologic deficits, coma, and death. Patients have proteinuria and may progress rapidly to renal failure. Some have a microangiopathic hemolytic anemia. Further details appear in Chapter 24.

Cause

Essential hypertension encompasses the majority (85–95%), with no discernible cause. Most (60%) have a family history of hypertension that usually presents between 20 and 55 years of age.

Secondary hypertension encompasses the 5% to 15% who have an identifiable cause (see Chapter 22).

ETIOLOGIC FACTORS IN ESSENTIAL HYPERTENSION

Genetic

The probability of hypertension is increased sixfold if one parent is hypertensive and tenfold if an identical twin is hypertensive. The genes responsible are unknown.

Diet

Excessive intake of the following dietary constituents is associated with increased BP: sodium chloride, fat, caffeine, and alcohol (more than two drinks per day). Lower BP is associated with high intakes of calcium, potassium, and fish oil.

Renin–Angiotensin–Aldosterone Axis

There is an abnormal spread of renin values in hypertensive patients. About 40% are in the low-renin category, which includes many African-Americans, elderly, and hypertensives with renal insufficiency, who often have salt-sensitive hypertension. About 10% are in the high-renin category but do not have renovascular hypertension; they are often young, white patients.

Sympathetic Nervous System

Plasma levels of norepinephrine and epinephrine are normal or mildly elevated in most hypertensives. However, a subgroup has increased sympathetic tone (hyperdynamic circulation, raised heart rate, elevated catecholamine levels). Baroreceptor function is impaired in elderly hypertensives and predisposes to fluctuations of BP.

Renal Function

Early in the development of hypertension, the renal blood flow is reduced while the glomerular filtration rate is maintained. The ensuing rise in the filtration fraction promotes renal salt retention. In many hypertensives, renal function deteriorates, creating a vicious cycle whereby a decline in renal function impairs salt excretion, which raises BP and perpetuates further renal damage.

Life Style

The BP is increased by emotional stress, anxiety, obesity, and smoking but reduced by regular exercise.

CLINICAL PRESENTATION OF HYPERTENSION

There are no specific symptoms. Headaches occur in severe hypertension; they are usually occipital, throbbing, and present on awakening. Initial examination of all hypertensive patients should include measurement of BP and pulse by the physician while the patient is lying down and after 2 minutes of standing. An orthostatic fall in BP implies blocked cardiovascular reflexes (e.g., drugs, such as α-receptor blockers, autonomic neuropathy, pheochromocytoma) or volume depletion (heart rate rises more than 20 beats/min with standing). Initially, measure the BP in both arms and examine the timing of femoral and radial pulses (marked differences in pulse pressure or a delayed femoral pulse suggests aortic atherosclerosis or coarctation). In children or adolescents, measure the BP in the leg to exclude coarctation of the aorta. Examine the fundi (see Table 21.1) for hypertensive or atherosclerotic changes. More severe changes imply prolonged duration of disease and a poor prognosis.

The following questions should be answered in the routine history and examination of each patient suspected of hypertension.

Does the Patient Have Hypertension?

Several measurements of BP are necessary because patients are often anxious at the first visit. Patients should take their BP regularly at home, record the values, and bring them to clinic visits. The self-recorded BP should be checked against a clinic measurement to ensure accuracy. "White coat" or "office" hypertension is defined as elevated BPs in the clinic but not in the home setting. It is seen in 20% to 30% of patients with mild hypertension. It probably does not need treatment but should prompt arrangement for regular BP checks. A more precise diagnosis of white coat hypertension can be achieved with an ambulatory 24-hour BP monitor. The following can overestimate BP: fear, pain, anxiety, a rigid arterial wall (checked by palpation at wrist during BP measurement), or a large arm (use a large cuff).

Is the Blood Pressure Stable, Labile, or Accelerated?

Labile hypertension is seen in the prehypertensive phase and in the elderly. An accelerated rise in BP or drug requirements suggests malignant hypertension or a secondary cause (e.g., renovascular hypertension).

Has There Been Organ Damage?

Assess the impact on the heart (heart failure, hypertrophy, extra heart sounds, pulmonary rales, a raised jugular venous pressure), kidney (proteinuria, hematuria, azotemia, reduced creatinine clearance), vessels (peripheral pulses and bruits, abdominal aneurysms), and fundi (Table 21.1).

Is There a Secondary Cause?

Most patients with essential hypertension present between age 20 and 55 years. For further discussion see Chapter 22.

TABLE 21.1 Classification of Hypertension Retinopathy

Class	Arterial-to-venous ratio[a]	Focal arteriolar spasm[b]	Hemorrhages and exudates	Papilledema	Arteriolar light reflex
Normal	3:4	1:1	0	0	Fine yellow line, blood column seen
Grade I	1:2	1:1	0	0	Broad yellow line, blood column seen
Grade II	1:3	2:3	0	0	Broad "copper wiring" line, no blood column seen
Grade III	1:4	1:3	+	0	Broad "silver wire" line, no blood column seen
Grade IV	Fine	Obliteration	+	+	Fibrous cords, no blood column seen

[a] Ratio of arterial to venous diameters.

[b] Ratio of diameter of regions of spasm to more proximal segments.

Are There Dietary Factors Contributing to Hypertension?

Assess the level of sodium intake from measurements of 24-hour renal sodium excretion. (Measure creatinine excretion to assess the adequacy of collection, which should be 15–25 mg/kg). Patients on a "no added salt" diet should achieve a daily sodium excretion of 120 mmol (equals 120 mEq) or less. More than two alcoholic drinks per day raises BP.

What Are the Coincident Risk Factors for Vascular Disease?

These include dyslipidemia, smoking, glucose intolerance, electrocardiogram evidence of LVH, obesity/underactivity, hyperhomocysteinemia, and death of a parent from MI before age 50.

ROUTINE LABORATORY TESTS

The following are ordered routinely in the author's clinic in patients with hypertension to assess the effect on end organs and to screen for some secondary causes:

- Urinalysis (protein, glucose, and blood; microscopy if dip is abnormal)
- Electrolytes, calcium, blood urea nitrogen, and serum creatinine
- Fasting blood sugar and lipid profile
- Electrocardiogram
- Twenty-four-hour urine for sodium excretion, creatinine clearance, and total protein excretion (important where proteinuria is detected on dipstick or serum creatinine concentration is increased). A more sensitive index of renal damage is microalbuminuria, which is also a risk factor for cardiovascular disease.

Additional tests that are often helpful, especially in severe hypertension, include:

- Plasma renin activity and plasma aldosterone concentration (a guide to treatment or a secondary cause)
- Echocardiogram. This is more sensitive for LVH than is an EEG but is considerably more expensive. It documents ventricular wall thickness and ejection fraction and also reveals diastolic dysfunction in patients with LVH and severe hypertension.
- Plasma homocysteine. This is an important risk factor for vascular disease. It is treated by increased intakes of folic acid and

vitamins B_6 and B_{12}, which should also be measured in patients with elevated plasma total homocysteine levels.

These tests will not identify renovascular hypertension or pheochromocytoma.

SPECIAL INVESTIGATIONS

The following have value in selected patients.

Intravenous Pyelogram, Computed Tomography, or Renal Ultrasound

These are indicated where the kidneys are palpated on examination (suggesting polycystic kidney disease or tumor) or anatomical abnormalities of the collecting system are suspected (patients with recurrent urinary tract infection, unexplained pyuria or hematuria, symptoms of prostatism, or previous renal stone disease). Renal ultrasound assesses renal size (decreased in unilateral renal artery stenosis or parenchymal disease) and structure.

Radionuclide Scanning

These tests are described in Chapters 3 and 22.

Renal Arteriography

Aortography and selective renal arteriography are the definitive procedures for visualizing renal artery stenosis. They are also valuable in the workup of polyarteritis nodosa (classic type for demonstration of renal aneurysms) and in the diagnosis of renal infarction or tumor. A digital-subtraction arteriogram decreases the dye load and the risk of contrast-induced nephropathy in patients with impaired renal function or diabetes mellitus.

Suggested Readings

Joint National Committee on Detection, Evaluation, and Treatment of High Blood Pressure. *Sixth report.* Bethesda, MD: National Institutes of Health, 1998.

Krakoff LR. Treatment decision for hypertension. In: Brady HR, Wilcox CS, eds. *Therapy in nephrology and hypertension.* Philadelphia: WB Saunders, 1998:387–391.

Laragh JH, Brenner BM, eds. *Hypertension: pathophysiology, diagnosis and management.* New York: Raven Press, 1998.

Chapter 22

Secondary Forms of Hypertension

Christopher S. Wilcox

Some 10% of patients with hypertension have a secondary cause. The low prevalence mandates a discrete screening program to limit expensive testing (Table 22.1). The prevalence of secondary hypertension increases substantially among patients with severe and drug-resistant hypertension. It should be considered in all whose BP is not controlled on three or more medications. Specific clinical and laboratory findings should prompt appropriate screening tests, which must be highly sensitive (few false negatives) to avoid missing these patients.

RENAL PARENCHYMAL DISEASE

Any decrease in renal function may cause hypertension. Conversely, hypertension itself may cause nephrosclerosis, especially in African-Americans. Hypertension accounts for 24% of cases of end-stage renal disease. It accelerates the progression of renal injury in patients with diabetes mellitus or those with more than 1 g daily of proteinuria. Renal parenchymal hypertension is caused predominantly by excessive salt and water retention, but inappropriate secretion of renin and angiotensin contribute. Consequently, the mainstays of therapy are salt-depleting therapy with salt restriction and a diuretic and therapy to reduce angiotensin II generation with an angiotensin-converting enzyme inhibitor (ACEI) and/or an angiotensin receptor blocker (ARB). Calcium antagonists are effective in most patients. For details of drug treatment, see Chapter 23.

179

TABLE 22.1   Secondary Causes of Hypertension

Cause	Prevalence (%)
Renal parenchymal disease	5
Renovascular disease	0.5–5
Primary aldosteronism	0.5–1
Thyroid disease	0.5–1
Pheochromocytoma	<0.2
Cushing's syndrome	<0.2
Drug-related	0.1–1

RENOVASCULAR HYPERTENSION

Renal artery stenosis is a narrowing (usually greater than 65% to be functionally significant) of one or both renal arteries or their branches. Renovascular hypertension is that which is improved or cured by correction of a renal artery stenosis. Renovascular disease encompasses both diagnoses. Ischemic nephropathy is chronic renal failure caused by renal artery stenosis that is often bilateral. If unilateral, it is accompanied by renal functional impairment in the contralateral kidney, usually nephrosclerosis (Table 22.2).

Pathophysiology

Renal hypoperfusion releases renin from the myoepithelial cells of the afferent arteriole. Renin catalyzes the transformation of angiotensinogen to angiotensin I (Ang I), which is itself inert. Angiotensin-converting enzyme (ACE), located predominantly on the vascular endothelium, catalyzes the formation of Ang II from Ang I. Ang II is a potent vasoconstrictor and causes renal sodium and water retention both by a direct action on the kidney and by stimulating aldosterone secretion. If only one kidney is hypoperfused, the sodium-retaining effects of the reduced renal

TABLE 22.2   Renal Lesions Causing Renovascular Hypertension

Intrinsic renal lesions	Extrinsic lesions
Atherosclerosis	Urinary tract obstruction
Fibromuscular dysplasia	Abdominal aortic aneurysm
Vasculitis	Emboli
Renal cysts	Renal capsular hematoma

perfusion pressure and the increased Ang II and aldosterone secretion are counterbalanced by a pressure natriuresis in the contralateral kidney. Therefore, there is little salt and water retention. However, where there is no normal kidney (e.g., patients with bilateral renal artery stenosis or stenosis of a transplanted, solitary, or dominant kidney), there is retention of salt and water, and hypertension becomes volume dependent. Such patients may have episodes of "flash" pulmonary edema caused by inappropriate renal salt retention. Acute or recurrent pulmonary edema in a hypertensive and azotemic patient with a preserved left ventricular (LV) ejection fraction suggests this diagnosis. The natural history of atherosclerotic renovascular disease is a presentation in middle or late life leading to a progressive decrease in renal blood flow, which ultimately results in complete loss of renal function ("ischemic nephropathy"). In contrast, fibromuscular dysplasia occurs in women, usually presents earlier in life, is not progressive, and rarely ends in ischemic nephropathy.

Clinical Features

Clinical features suggestive of renovascular hypertension follow:

- Hypertension resistant to two or more drugs and a diuretic
- Onset of hypertension before 20 in women or after 55 years
- Accelerated or malignant hypertension
- Arteriosclerosic disease elsewhere
- Smoking history
- Azotemia, especially developing with ACEIs or ARBs
- Abdominal bruit (especially diastolic or flank)
- Recurrent pulmonary edema with preserved LV ejection fraction
- Kidneys with a size differential greater than 1.5 cm
- Hypokalemic alkalosis (suggesting hyperaldosteronism)

Screening Tests

The rapid sequence of intravenous pyelogram, renogram, unstimulated plasma renin activity (PRA), intravenous digital subtraction angiogram, and renal vein renins are not sufficiently accurate for routine use. Currently, three tests with sensitivities above 90% in clinical trials are available for screening.

The *captopril-PRA* or *captopril challenge test* is detailed in Table 22.3.

TABLE 22.3   Captopril Challenge or Captopril–PRA Test

Patients must have a moderate or high probability of renovascular hypertension

Exclude those with serum creatinine > 2.5 mg/dl, CVS instability, or edema
No special requirement for regulation of dietary salt intake

Antihypertensives and diuretics are discontinued over 10 days or replaced with labetalol and/or calcium antagonists

Antihypertensives are withheld on the test day
Administer 50 mg of crushed captopril with water while the patient is seated
Monitor BP
Blood for PRA is drawn 60 minutes after captopril
Check standing BP to ensure patient is not orthostatic before discharge
A postcaptopril PRA >5.7 ng/ml/hr is positive

The preferred tracer for the *ACEI-renogram* presently is [^{99m}Tc]mercaptotriglycine (MAG$_3$). This is filtered at the glomerulus and by the proximal tubule.

The glomerular filtration rate (GFR) of a hypoperfused, poststenotic kidney is dependent on the contractile effects of Ang II on the efferent arterioles. Therefore, ACEIs reduce the GFR in such a kidney. This test detects a selective reduction in single-kidney GFR after ACEI in patients with renovascular hypertension. The ACEIs maintain the renal blood flow and, therefore, the delivery of MAG$_3$ to the nephron, yet retard the elimination of MAG$_3$ because of the fall in GFR. Captopril is given, and, after 1 hour, the kidneys are scanned for 20 to 30 minutes after IV MAG$_3$. If the test is abnormal, it is repeated without captopril to detect an ACEI-induced change in the renogram. Such changes imply functional renovascular hypertension, whereas fixed abnormalities imply renal parenchymal disease or outflow obstruction. Diagnostic criteria for renovascular hypertension include an ACEI-induced delay in the time to peak or in the washout. In extreme cases, there is a progressive renal accumulation of the tracer after ACEI.

The captopril-PRA and ACEI-renogram tests are functional indices of renovascular hypertension. In contrast, *renal ultrasound with duplex Doppler velocimetry* is a test of renal artery stenosis. First, the lengths of the kidneys are measured with ultrasound. In the absence of renal cysts, a length difference greater than 1.5 cm implies predominantly unilateral renal disease, and, in the context of hypertension, this is usually renal artery stenosis. Second, the peak systolic blood flow velocity is measured in the aorta and along the renal arteries. A threefold increase in velocity in a renal artery above that recorded in the aorta suggests renal artery stenosis. This noninvasive test is used for screening and to follow up patients after intervention to correct renal artery stenosis. Its accuracy depends on the skill, experience, and time taken by the operator.

Diagnostic Tests for Renal Artery Stenosis

Renal artery stenosis is diagnosed by angiography. The quantity of dye injected is reduced by a computerized enhancement method, termed digital subtraction. To cause significant renal ischemia, a stenosis must usually occlude 65% of the arterial lumen. However, the demonstration of an anatomic stenosis does not prove that it is the cause of the hypertension. Therefore, arteriography is performed on patients selected by a prior functional screening test such as a captopril-PRA or an ACEI-renogram.

Treatment

The goal is to improve or cure hypertension and to delay the progression to ischemic nephropathy that can occur in artherosclerotic renal artery stenosis.

Percutaneous transluminal renal angioplasty (PTRA) is successful in 80% of nonostial lesions. Stenting provides a similar rate of success for osteal lesions. These procedures are invasive and can cause arterial rupture or dissection, atheroemboli to the kidney or lower limbs, acute renal failure from contrast-induced nephropathy, bleeding at the puncture site, or, very rarely, death.

Surgical revascularization is reserved for those who have failed PTRA and stenting and for those with concomitant disease of the abdominal aorta requiring surgery. Patients with a small, minimally functioning kidney and severe, poorly controlled hypertension may benefit from a laparascopic nephrectomy.

PHEOCHROMOCYTOMA

Hypertension is caused by a tumor that secretes catecholamines. More than 90% are benign.

Pathophysiology

Neural crest cells are found in the adrenal medulla, autonomic ganglia, organs of Zuckendal (lying anterior to the aortic bifurcation), and bladder. Pheochromocytomas may form at any of these sites, but 90% are found in the adrenal gland. Tumors are bilateral in 10% to 20%. Pheochromocytoma may be inherited as an autosomal dominant trait either alone or as part of the syndromes of multiple endocrine neoplasia type 2 (MEN-2: medullary thyroid carcinoma, pheochromocytoma, and parathyroid hyperplasia), Von Hipple-Lindau syndrome (retinal and cerebellar hemangioblastomas, renal cell carcinoma, and pheochromocytoma), Von Reckling-hausen's syndrome (neurofibromatosis and café-au-lait skin pigmentation), or tuberous sclerosis (mental deficiency, tumors, and pheochromocytomas).

Clinical Features

Hypertension is the most common clinical manifestation. It is sustained in about 60% of patients. A paroxysm, caused by the sudden release of catecholamines, is accompanied by severe hypertension, headache, sweating, and palpitations. Paroxysms may be precipitated by exercise, urination, defecation, sexual intercourse, anesthesia, contrast agents, or certain drugs, including vasodilators. Other clinical features include weight loss, fever, anxiety, tremors, psychotic illness, and glucose intolerance. Orthostatic hypotension is secondary to diminished plasma volume and blunted sympathetic reflexes.

Screening Tests

The clinical features that suggest the need to screen for pheochromocytoma are:

- Hypertension and at least two of: headache, palpitations, or sweating
- Paroxysmal hypertension
- Sustained diastolic blood pressure over 120 mm Hg
- Hypertension and unexplained orthostatic hypotension

Currently, the preferred screening test is a measurement of plasma catecholamines while the patient is hypertensive. Levels increased more than three- to fivefold above normal are almost diagnostic of pheochromocytoma, whereas less severe elevations are also seen in patients with anxiety, pain, hypoglycemia, or hypoxemia.

Diagnostic Tests

Clonidine inhibits the sympathetic outflow from the brain. It reduces the plasma catecholamine levels in normal subjects and those with elevated levels caused by physiologic simulation from anxiety but not in those with an autonomously secreting pheochromocytoma. The clonidine suppression test is performed as follows:

1. Withhold β-blockers and diuretics for 2 weeks before testing.
2. Hold antihypertensives on the day of the test.
3. Patient is recumbent with an IV cannula 30 minutes before and during the test.
4. Administer 0.3 mg of oral clonidine.
5. Obtain plasma for catecholamines before and 3 hours after.
6. The test is positive if plasma total catecholamines remain above 500 pg/ml or fail to fall by at least 50%.
7. The sensitivity for detecting pheochromocytoma is >95%.

Localization Tests

A computed tomography (CT) scan, magnetic resonance imaging (MRI), or selective adrenal venous sampling for catecholamines are localization tests. The MRI is preferred because it is noninvasive and accurate in localizing tumors larger than 0.5 cm. It can discriminate between pheochromocytomas and other adrenal tumors or cysts. Slices of 0.5 cm should be taken through the regions of the adrenals, the anterior aspect of the aortic bifurcation, the superior aspect of the bladder, the chest, and the neck. These are all sites for pheochromocytomas that are multiple in 10% to 20% of patients.

Management

Surgical excision cures most patients. Preoperative stabilization with α-blockade and volume expansion is essential. Acute pheochromocytoma crisis responds to intravenous α-blockade with phentolamine. Prolonged, predictable α-blockade is achieved with the noncompetitive antagonist phenoxybenzamine. After hypertension is controlled, a β-antagonist can be administered to control tachycardia. The shorter-acting combined α- and β-blocker labetalol is useful for mildly hypertensive subjects.

PRIMARY HYPERALDOSTERONISM

Hypertension is caused by excess aldosterone secretion without renin activation.

Pathophysiology

Aldosterone-producing adenomas (APA) of the zona glomerulosa cells, also called Conn's syndrome, account for 60% of cases. Bilateral glomerulosa cell hyperplasia, also called idiopathic hyperaldosteronism (IHA), accounts for most of the remainder. Multiple adenomas occur in 10%. Rarer causes include glucocorticoid-remediable hyperaldosteronism (GRH). This dominant condition is diagnosed from the reversal of hyperaldosteronism and hypertension after suppression of ACTH secretion with dexamethasone. In all cases, the excessive production of aldosterone results in renal sodium retention, causing extracellular fluid volume expansion and hypertension. Aldosterone also enhances the excretion of K^+ and H^+, leading to hypokalemic metabolic alkalosis.

Primary aldosteronism should be differentiated from secondary aldosteronism caused by excess renin secretion. This occurs in renovascular hypertension or edematous states. It must also be differentiated from pseudohyperaldosteronism. This is associated with excess intake of licorice and some types of chewing tobacco that contain glycyrrhizic acid or is seen as a familial condition associated with excessive reabsorption of Na^+ via the sodium channel in the collecting ducts (Liddle's syndrome). Patients with pseudohyperaldosteronism have the clinical and biochemical changes characteristic of primary hyperaldosteronism but have suppressed levels of plasma aldosterone.

Clinical Features

The hallmarks of hyperaldosteronism are hypertension, hypokalemic metabolic alkalosis, suppressed PRA, but elevated plasma aldosterone. The hypokalemia may cause:

- Glucose intolerance secondary to insulin resistance
- Polyuria and polydipsia secondary to defective urinary concentration
- Muscular weakness
- Cardiac arrhythmias and palpitations
- ECG changes of flattened T waves and U waves
- Orthostatic hypotension and autonomic dysfunction

Screening Tests

The features that should prompt screening for primary hyper-aldosteronism are:

- Unprovoked or diuretic-induced hypokalemia with alkalosis
- Resistance to therapy with two or more drugs and suppressed PRA

Screening should follow correction of potassium deficits because hypokalemia suppresses aldosterone secretion even from adenomas. Primary hyperaldosteronism is suggested by:

- 24-hour urine potassium >40 mEq despite hypokalemia
- Low basal or furosemide-stimulated PRA
- Elevated plasma aldosterone (PA) : PRA ratio above 50 to 100
- Excessive 24-hour aldosterone excretion

Diagnostic Tests

These tests confirm the diagnosis and distinguish between APAs and IHAs.

Saline Suppression Test

This tests the dependency of aldosterone secretion on Ang II. It is performed by infusing 1.25 L of 0.9% NaCl intravenously over 2 hours to suppress PRA and Ang II. Blood is drawn before and after the infusion for plasma cortisol and aldosterone. The APAs continue to secrete aldosterone independent of Ang II. Therefore, these patients have an elevated postsaline plasma aldosterone level and an aldosterone:cortisol ratio above 2.2, whereas those with normal adrenals and IHAs show a 50% reduction in these measurements.

Postural Stimulation Test

This tests the relative response of adrenal aldosterone secretion to Ang II or to adrenocorticotropic hormone (ACTH). Orthostasis stimulates PRA and Ang II. The test is initiated when ACTH and cortisol normally decline. After 1 hour of recumbency at 8 a.m., a blood sample is obtained for aldosterone, 18-hydroxy-corticosterone (18-OHB), PRA, and cortisol and repeated after 4 hours of upright ambulation. A decrease in cortisol confirms that ACTH has fallen over the test period. The diagnosis of APA is suggested by elevated plasma aldosterone and 18-OHB levels that fail to increase with standing. Normals and those with IHA show an orthostatic increase in plasma aldosterone, 18-OHB, and PRA despite a fall in cortisol.

Computed Tomography Scan
This is accurate to detect tumors that are larger than 1 cm.

Adrenal Venous Sampling
This is required when functional tests suggest an APA but no mass is seen on CT scan. It is technically difficult. The adrenal venous effluent is assayed for plasma aldosterone and cortisol before and during ACTH infusion. A high ratio of aldosterone:cortisol is found on the side of a tumor, whereas the contralateral side shows a low value. Patients with IHA have elevated levels in both adrenal veins.

Treatment

Any APAs should be removed surgically. Blood pressure is normalized in 50% to 75%, and the biochemical abnormalities are corrected in all patients. The IHA is managed with spironolactone or, in those who develop adverse effects, with high doses of amiloride.

TABLE 22.4   Additional Causes of Secondary Hypertension

Cause	Clinical features
Preeclampsia	Third-trimester pregnancy, proteinuria, and edema
Cushing's syndrome	Central obesity, hirsutism, glycosuria
Coarctation of the aorta	Delayed pulses in legs
Hyperparathyroidism	Increased calcium and PTH levels
Congenital adrenal hyperplasia	
11-Hydroxylase deficiency	Virilization
17-Hydroxylase deficiency	Abnormal sexual development
Sleep apnea	Obesity, snoring, somnolence
Hypothyroidism	Bradycardia, hair loss, amenorrhea
Hyperthyroidism	Tachycardia, systolic hypertension, tremor
Acromegaly	Excessive growth, glycosuria

TABLE 22.5   Drug-Induced Hypertension

Adrenergic agonists:
  Methylphenidate
  Neosynephrine
  Phenylephrine
  Phenylpropanolamine
  Pseudoephedrine
Hypertension after abrupt withdrawal:
  Clonidine
  Barbiturates
Catecholamine-releasing drugs:
  Amphetamine
  Cocaine
Other agents:
  Cyclosporine
  Disulfiram (plus alcohol)
  Ergotamine
  Estrogen and birth control pills (high doses)
  MAO inhibitors (plus tyramine)

OTHER CAUSES OF SECONDARY HYPERTENSION

Additional causes of hypertension are presented in Table 22.4, and drug-induced causes in Table 22.5.

Suggested Readings

Brady HR, Wilcox CS. *Therapy in nephrology and hypertension.* Philadelphia: WB Saunders, 1998.

Grossman E, Goldstein DS, Hoffman A, et al. Glucagon and clonidine testing in the diagnosis of pheochromocytoma. *Hypertension* 1991; 17:733–741.

Fredrickson E, Wilcox CS, Bucci CM, et al. A prospective evaluation of a simplified captopril test for the detection of renovascular hypertension. *Arch Intern Med* 1990;150:569–572.

Wilcox CS. Use of angiotensin-converting-enzyme inhibitors for diagnosing renovascular hypertension. *Nephrol Forum Kidney Int* 1993; 44:1379–1390.

Wilcox CS. *Atlas of diseases of the kidney, Vol 3,* Schrier RW, ed. Philadelphia: Current Medicine, 1998.

Wilcox CS. Renovascular hypertension. In: Massry SG, Glassock RJ, eds. *Textbook of nephrology, 4th ed.* Philadelphia: Lippincott Williams & Wilkins, 1999 (in press).

Chapter 23

Treatment of Hypertension

Wen-Ting Ouyang
Christopher S. Wilcox

The aim of controlling hypertension is to reduce the associated risk of stroke, myocardial infarction (MI), renal failure from nephrosclerosis, and congestive heart failure (CHF). The blood pressure (BP) should be reduced to below 140/90 mm Hg in uncomplicated hypertension. Stricter control of BP is advised in diabetic nephropathy, proteinuric chronic renal failure, and CHF. To ensure that goals are met, patients should be encouraged to measure and record their own BP at home at least once daily. Occasionally, ambulatory BP monitoring is required. Patients with decompensated neurologic deficits (evolving stroke, subarachnoid hemorrhage), severe fixed vascular obstruction, or evolving myocardial infarction need special care and a more gradual reduction of BP (see Chapter 24).

Primary prevention of hypertension, for example by using the DASH diet, may be beneficial for the general population, as described in detail in the report by the Joint National Committee on Detection, Evaluation and Treatment of High Blood Pressure (JNC) (see References). Life-style modification may avoid potential side effects of pharmacologic treatments and can often reduce the numbers or doses of agents used for treatment. Assessment and correction of other cardiovascular risk factors and risk stratification are important in deciding if, when, and how to start pharmacologic therapy for hypertension.

PRINCIPLES OF DRUG THERAPY

Treatment decisions for hypertension are based on the stage of BP (Table 23.1), risk stratification by the presence of target organ damage (TOD), clinical cardiovascular disease (CCD) (Tables 23.2 and 23.3), and comorbid conditions.

Step-Down Therapy

About 15% of patients whose hypertension is well controlled on one medication for 5 years remain normotensive for 5 years after therapy is discontinued. "Step-down" therapy is more successful if life-style modifications are achieved. Follow-up is important for those who have their medications discontinued.

Nonpharmacologic Therapy

Restriction of Dietary Salt Intake
A reduction of sodium intake to about 100 mmol/day (equivalent to 100 mEq/day) in hypertensive subjects lowers BP by an average of 6/2 mm Hg over several weeks. Salt restriction enhances the antihypertensive actions of all agents except calcium antagonists. It reduces diuretic-induced potassium wastage, may regress LVH, and diminishes osteoporosis and renal stone formation. Salt intake can be assessed from 24-hour Na^+ excretion, providing the patient is in steady state and has not started or stopped diuretic therapy in the last 2 weeks. Reasonable goals for daily Na^+ intake is <120 mmol for mild hypertension, <100 mmol for moderate hypertension, and <80 mmol for resistant hypertension.

TABLE 23.1   Classification of Blood Pressure for Adults Aged 18 Years and Older

Class	SBP (mm Hg)		DBP (mm Hg)
Optimal	<120	and	<80
Normal	<130	and	<85
High normal	130–139	or	85–89
Hypertension			
Stage 1	140–159	or	90–99
Stage 2	160–179	or	100–109
Stage 3	>180	or	>110

TABLE 23.2   Cardiovascular Risk Stratification

Major risk factors	TOD and/or CCD[a]
Smoking	Heart diseases:
Diabetes mellitus	Left ventricular hypertrophy
Dyslipidemia	Angina or prior MI
Gender (men and	Prior coronary revascularization
postmenopausal women)	Heart failure
Family history of early cardio-	Stroke or transient ischemic attack
vascular disease: women before	Nephropathy
65 or men before 55 years	Peripheral vascular disease
Age > 60 years	Retinopathy

[a] TOD, target organ damage; CCD, clinical cardiovascular disease.

Weight Loss

Loss of as little as 10 lb (4.5 kg) reduces BP in most overweight hypertensives. This also reduces dyslipidemia and diabetes mellitus (DM).

Other

Brisk walking for 30 to 45 minutes on at least 4 days of the week, or an equivalent degree of regular aerobic exercise, lowers BP. Blood pressure can be reduced, and cardiovascular health promoted, by a diet with a low content of saturated fat and an intake

TABLE 23.3   Risk Stratification and Treatment

Blood pressure stage (mm Hg)	Risk group A (no risk factors; no TOD/CCD)[a]	Risk group B (at least 1 risk factor; no DM; no TOD/CCD)	Risk group C (TOD/CCD and/or DM)
High normal (130–139/85–89)	Life-style modification	Life-style modification	Drug therapy[c]
Stage 1 (140–159/90–99)	Life-style modification (up to 12 mo)	Life-style modification (up to 6 mo)[b]	Drug therapy
Stage 2 or 3 (>160/>100)	Drug therapy	Drug therapy	Drug therapy

[a] TOD/CCD indicates target organ disease/clinical cardiovascular disease (see Table 23-2).

[b] For patients with multiple risk factors, the clinician should consider initial drug therapy plus life-style modifications.

[c] For those with heart failure, proteinuric renal insufficiency, or diabetes mellitus.

of 90 mmol/day of potassium in the form of fresh fruits and vegetables with a liberal intake of calcium and magnesium. Strict cessation of smoking is imperative. Alcohol intake should be limited to 2 to 4 oz daily.

Individualized Treatment

In uncomplicated essential hypertension, diuretics and/or β-blockers are drugs of first choice. β-Blockers, angiotensin-converting enzyme inhibitors (ACEIs), and angiotensin receptor blockers (ARBs) are more effective in young, white, and high-renin individuals; in contrast, elderly, African-Americans, and low-renin individuals and those with azotemia respond better to diuretics and calcium antagonists. If a diuretic is not selected as the first drug, it is usually indicated as the second-step agent because diuretics potentiate the antihypertensive actions of other agents. A combination of low doses of agents from different classes provides additional antihypertensive efficacy, yet minimizes dose-dependent adverse effects. Angiotension II type I (AT_1) receptor blockers (ARBs) are used for patients in whom ACEIs are indicated but who develop a dry cough or angioedema.

If the response to the initial drug of choice is inadequate, then:

- Add a second agent if the patient tolerates the first and has some response
- Substitute another if the patient has adverse effects or no response

Cost and Compliance

These must be considered. Most treatment failures are because of noncompliance. Once-a-day dosing is preferred.

Refractory Hypertension

This is defined as a BP > 140/90 mm Hg despite adherence to an adequate and appropriate triple drug regimen, which includes a diuretic. These patients frequently have a secondary cause for their hypertension, such as renal artery stenosis. They should be referred to a specialist.

INDIVIDUAL DRUG CATEGORIES

Diuretics

These drugs reduce BP gradually over 1 to 3 months, accompanied by a fall in peripheral resistance. To be effective, they must be given with a salt-restricted diet. A thiazide is proven to reduce the risk of stroke, myocardial infarction (MI), or congestive heart failure (CHF) in hypertension. However, the reduction in mortality from coronary artery disease (CAD) is less than that expected from the fall in BP. Isolated systolic hypertension in the elderly carries a high risk for stroke and MI. It is particularly responsive to thiazide therapy. Salt depletion therapy with diuretics and a salt-restricted diet enhances the efficacy of all other antihypertensive agents except calcium antagonists. Thus, unless there are compelling contraindications, a diuretic should be part of all multidrug regimens for treatment of hypertension. They are frequently the only drug required to treat uncomplicated mild hypertension. For details of individual agents, doses, clinical use, and adverse effects, see Chapter 25.

β-Adrenergic Blockers

These agents reduce BP by reducing cardiac output and later by reducing peripheral resistance. They reduce plasma renin activity. They can be first-line treatment, especially for younger white patients and those with high renin levels. They are indicated especially for patients with angina, idiopathic hypertrophic cardiomyopathy (IHSS), hyperdynamic circulation, essential tremor, and migraine. Nonselective β-blockers may increase plasma levels of triglycerides (TG) and reduce those of high-density lipoprotein (HDL)-cholesterol. However, clinical trials have proven that they decrease mortality and recurrence in survivors of acute myocardial infarction. Pindolol is as effective as propranolol. Nonselective β-blockers are contraindicated in asthma and chronic obstructive pulmonary disease. Other adverse effects includes lethargy, malaise, nightmares, depression, impotence, and decreased capacity for prolonged exercise. Short-acting β-blockers generally are metabolized by the liver. They are preferred in renal failure. Cardioselective agents, or those with intrinsic sympathomimetic activity (ISA), are less likely to induce bronchospasm or metabolic disturbances. See Table 23.4 for details of individual agents.

TABLE 23.4 Selected β-Blockers for Hypertension

Agents	Cardioselectivity	ISA	Half-life (hr)	Dose adjustments in renal failure	Initial dose (mg daily)	Dosing frequency (per day)	Dose range (mg/day)
Acebutolol (Sectral)	+	+	3–4[a]	Yes	200	Once	200–800
Atenolol (Tenormin)	++	0	6–9	Yes	25	Once or twice	25–100
Betaxolol (Kerlone)	++	0	15	Yes	5	Once	5–20
Bisprolol (Zebeta)	++	0	9–12	Yes	2.5	Once	2.5–10
Carteolol (Cartrol)	0	+	5–6[a]	Yes	2.5	Once	2.5–10
Celiprolol	0	0	5	No	200	Once	200–600
Metoprolol (Lopressor) (Toprol XL)	++	0	3–4	No	25	Twice	25–300
					20	Once	25–300
Nadolol (Corgard)	0	0	20–24	Yes	40	Once	40–320
Penbutolol (Levatol)	0	+	27[a]	Yes	10	Once	10–20
Pindolol (Visken)	0	++	3–4	Yes	10	Twice	10–60
Propranolol (Inderal) (Inderal LA)	0	0	3–4	No	40	Twice	40–480
				No	40	Once	40–480
Timolol (Blocadren)	0	0	4–5	No	20	Twice	20–60

[a] Active metabolites prolong effective half-life. For details of prescribing for patients with renal insufficiency, see Chapter 32.

α- and β-Adrenergic Blockers

Labetalol is a nonselective β-adrenergic blocker that possesses selective α_1-blocking and ISA activity. It is a very effective antihypertensive medication that is available in IV form for hypertensive emergencies. Carvedilol has no ISA activity but has significant antioxidant actions. It has been shown to reduce mortality and morbidity in patients with hypertension and stable moderate to severe heart failure. These agents are especially useful to counteract the effects of catecholamine excess (e.g., perioperative management of pheochromocytoma, clonidine withdrawal). Hepatotoxicity is a serious but uncommon side effect. Fatigue, dizziness, headache, GI symptoms, scalp tingling, postural hypotension, and ejaculatory failure are other side effects. They do not accumulate in patients with renal failure. Unlike simple β-blockers, they are often effective monotherapy in African-Americans and patients with low renin levels. See Table 23.5 for details of individual agents.

α-Adrenergic Blockers

These drugs reduce BP by blocking postsynaptic α-adrenergic receptors on vascular smooth muscle cells. Prazosin has a short duration of action and can cause first-dose hypotension or syncope. These agents affect plasma lipids favorably and regress prostatic hypertrophy. Side effects include orthostatic dizziness (usually transient), lethargy, fatigue, and palpitation. Priapism has been reported. They may exacerbate angina. Dose adjustment in renal failure is not usually required. See Table 23.6 for details on individual agents.

TABLE 23.5   Selected α/β-Adrenergic Blockers for Hypertension

Agents	Half-life (hr)	Initial dose (mg daily)	Dose frequency (per day)	Dose range (mg/day)
Carvedilol (Coreg)	2–8	12.5	Twice	12.5–50
Labetalol (Normodyne, Trandate)	4–6	200	Twice or three times	200–2,400

For details of prescribing for patients with renal insufficiency, see Chapter 32.

TABLE 23.6 Selected α-Blockers for Hypertension

Agents	Half-life (hr)	Initial dose (mg daily)	Dosing frequency (per day)	Dose range (mg/day)
Doxazosin (Cardura)	20	1	Once	1–16
Prazosin (Minipress)	3	1	Twice or three times	2–30
Terazosin (Hytrin)	12	1	Once	1–20

For details of prescribing for patients with renal insufficiency, see Chapter 32.

Central Sympatholytic Agents

These act in the brain. They reduce BP by reducing sympathetic tone. They are particularly useful for patients who have hypertension with anxiety. Sedation and dry mouth can be troublesome adverse effects. Depression may be severe. α-Methyldopa can cause hypersenstivity reactions, hepatitis, and a Coombs-positive hemolytic anemia. Clonidine withdrawal can give severe rebound hypertension that is accentuated by β-blockers. Clonidine is available as a skin patch (tts) that provides a steady drug delivery over a 1-week period. See Table 23.7 for details on individual agents.

TABLE 23.7 Central Sympatholytic Agents for Hypertension

Agents	Half-life (hr)	Initial dose (mg daily)	Dosing frequency (per day)	Dose range (mg/day)
α-Methyldopa (Aldomet)	2	500	Twice	500–3,000
Clonidine (Catapress)	12	0.2	Twice or three times	0.2–1.2
(Catapress TTS)		0.1	Once per week	0.1–0.3
Guanabenz (Wytensin)	4–6	8	Twice	8–48
Guanfacin (Tenex)	12–24	1	Once at night	1–3

For details of prescribing for patients with renal insufficiency, see Chapter 32.

Peripheral Sympatholytic Agents

These reduce BP by depleting sympathetic nerves of catecholamines. Reserpine can cause severe depression and peptic ulcer disease and may precipitate a hypertensive crisis in patients receiving monoamine oxidase inhibitors (MAOIs). Other side effects include diarrhea and retrograde ejaculation. These agents are not frequently prescribed in current medical practice.

Angiotensin-Converting Enzyme Inhibitors

They block the formation of the active angiotensin II (Ang II) from the inactive precursor, Ang I. In addition, they block the degradation of kinins. Therefore, they diminish the generation of vasoconstrictor Ang II and enhance the tissue levels of vasodilator kinins. They are less effective in the elderly or African-American patients who have lower values for plasma renin activity (PRA), unless prescribed with salt-depleting therapy of diuretic and low salt intake. These drugs do not impair exercise or sexual ability. They reduce proteinuria and slow the progression of diabetic nephropathy and proteinuric renal diseases, where they delay the time to reach end-stage renal disease. They are also used to control polycythemia after kidney transplantation. They may prolong renal graft survival. They improve symptoms and survival in patients with congestive heart failure due to systolic dysfunction. Side effects include a nonproductive cough in 5% to 20% of patients. Hyperkalemia can occur in patients with renal failure. Occasionally, patients develop an allergy. Dose adjustment is required in renal failure with most of these agents because they have significant renal excretion. Fosinopril is metabolized and does not require dose reduction. They are contraindicated in pregnancy and in patients with bilateral renal artery stenosis, in whom they may cause azotemia. See Table 23.8 for details of individual agents.

Angiotensin II Receptor Blockers

These agents block the AT_1 receptor that mediates most of the effects of Ang II on the cardiovascular and renal systems. Thus, they are effective in many of the conditions that have proven responsive to ACEIs. Most of these drugs are effective when given once daily. Diuretics and salt restriction enhance the BP reduc-

TABLE 23.8   Selected Angiotensin-Converting Enzyme Inhibitors for Hypertension

Agents	Half-life (hr)	Initial dose (mg daily)	Dosing frequency (per day)	Dose range (mg/day)
Benazepril (Lotensin)	10–11	5	Once or twice	5–40
Captopril (Capoten)	2	25–50	Twice or three times	25–150
Enalapril (Vasotec)	11	2.5–5	Once or twice	5–40
Fosinopril (Monopril)	12	10	Once	10–40
Lisinopril (Zestril, Prinivil)	12	5	Once	5–40
Moexipril (Univasc)	2–9	7.5	Twice	7.5–15
Quinapril (Accupril)	25	10	Once	5–80
Ramipril (Altace)	13–17	2.5	Once	1.25–20
Trandolapril (Mavik)	16–24	1	Once	1–4

For details of prescribing for patients with renal insufficiency, see Chapter 32.

tion. They do not cause cough. They are metabolized and generally do not require dose adjustment in renal failure. Although some are metabolized by the hepatic P_{450} system, clinically relevant drug interactions are uncommon. They are contraindicated in pregnancy and in patients with bilateral renovascular disease. Details of individual agents are shown in Table 23.9.

Dihydropyridine Calcium Antagonists

These agents reduce blood pressure by reducing calcium entry into vascular smooth muscle and thereby reduce the peripheral vascular resistance. They facilitate natriuresis. Amlodipine and felodipine are safe in systolic cardiac dysfunction. These agents are usually well tolerated but have dose-dependent side effects of headache, tachycardia, and edema. Dose adjustment for patients with renal failure generally is not required. Details of individual agents are shown in Table 23.10.

TABLE 23.9   Selected Angiotensin Receptor Blockers for Hypertension

Agents	Half-life (hr)	Initial dose (mg daily)	Dosing frequency	Dose range (mg/day)
Candersartan (Atacand)	7[a] (4–11)	8–16	Once	8–32
Eprosartan (Teveten)	7 (5–9)	400	Twice	400–800
Irbesartan (Avapro)	13 (11–15)	150	Once	150–300
Losartan (Cozaar)	2[a] (6–9)	25	Once or twice	25–100
Telmisartan (Micardis)	24	20–40	Once	40–80
Valsartan (Diovan)	9	80	Once	80–320

[a] Effective half life prolonged by the presence of active metabolites. For details of prescribing for patients with renal insufficiency, see Chapter 32.

TABLE 23.10   Selected Dihydropyridine Calcium Antagonists for Hypertension

Agents	Half-life (hr)	Initial dose (mg daily)	Dosing frequency (per day)	Dose range (mg/day)
Amlodipine (Norvasc)	30–50	2.5	Once	2.5–10
Felodipine (Plendil)	11–16	5	Once	2.5–20
Isradipine (DynaCirc)	1.5–2	2.5–5	Twice	5–20
(DynaCirc CR)	8	5	Once	5–20
Nicardipine (Cardene SR)	8.6	20–40	Twice	60–90
Nifedipine (ProcardiaXL, Adalat CC)	24	30	Once	30–90
Nisoldipine (Sular)	7–12	20	Once	20–60

For details of prescribing for patients with renal insufficiency, see Chapter 32.

Nondihydropyridine Calcium Antagonists

These agents reduce cardiac rate but generally do not have significant negative ionotropic action. However, they must be used with caution in patients receiving β-blockers. They reduce proteinuria in diabetic nephropathy. They may reduce reinfarction after a myocardial infarction and therefore can be used when β-blockers are not tolerated. Constipation is common with verapamil. Diltiazem can cause headache. Details on individual agents appear in Table 23.11.

Direct-Acting Vasodilators

These agents directly vasodilate resistance vessels. They are contraindicated in patients with coronary artery disease because of reflex activation of the sympathetic nervous system. They can cause flushing, headache, and palpitations and can induce fluid retention. Hydralazine can cause a lupus-like syndrome, particularly in slow acetylators who accumulate the drug, and in dose above 200–300 mg/ day. Minoxidil causes hirsutism, ST-segment depression, and T-wave flattening or inversion and may cause pericardial effusion or tamponade. It is restricted to patients with refractory hypertension. Minoxidil does not accumulate in renal failure. Hydralazine metabolites do accumulate in renal failure, and it is therefore best avoided. Details on individual agents are shown in Table 23.12.

TABLE 23.11   Selected Nondihydropyridine Calcium Antagonists for Hypertension

Agents	Half-life (hr)	Initial dose (mg daily)	Dosing frequency (per day)	Dose range (mg/day)
Diltiazem (Cardizem SR,	3.5–4	120	Twice	120–360
Cardizem CD, Dilacor XL, Tiazac)	20	120	Once	120–360
Verapamil (IsoptinSR, Calan SR,	4.5–12	120	Once	120–480
Verelan, CoveraHS)	14–16	180	Once	180–480

For details of prescribing for patients with renal insufficiency, see Chapter 32.

TABLE 23.12 Selected Direct-Acting Vasodilators for Hypertension

Agents	Half-life (hr)	Initial dose (mg daily)	Dosing frequency (per day)	Dose range (mg/day)
Hydralazine (Apresoline)	1	75	Three times	75–300
Minoxidil (Loniten)	3–4	5	Twice	5–100

For details of prescribing for patients with renal insufficiency, see Chapter 32.

Combination Drug Therapy

The efficacy of antihypertensive therapy is related to the degree of blood pressure reduction achieved. Selection of two or more agents from different classes used in moderate doses maximizes efficacy and limits dose-dependent toxicity. Combination therapy simplifies prescribing. Examples are given in Table 23.13.

TREATMENT OF HYPERTENSION IN SPECIAL POPULATIONS

Associated diseases or conditions often influence the choice of drug (Table 23.14).

TABLE 23.13 Selected Combined Antihypertensive Agents

Brand names	Drug components	Doses sizes (mg)
Apresazide	HCTZ[a]/hydralazine	25/25, 50/50, 50/100
Dyazide	HCTZ/triamterene	25/37.5
Hyzaar	HCTZ/losartan	12.5/50
Inderide-LA	HCTZ/Inderal-LA	50/80, 50/120, 50/160
Lexxel	Felodipine/enalapril	5/5
Lotrel	Amlodipine/benazepril	2.5/10, 5/10, 5/20
Maxzide-25	HCTZ/triamterene	25/37.5
Maxzide	HCTZ/triamterene	50/75
Moduretic	HCTZ/amiloride	50/5
Tenoretic	Chlorthalidone/atenolol	25/50, 25/100
Vaseretic	HCTZ/enalapril	25/10
Zestoretic/Prinizide	HCTZ/lisinopril	12.5/20, 25/20

[a] HCTZ, hydrochlorothiazide.

TABLE 23.14 Initial Therapy for Hypertension Based on Coexisting Conditions

Coexisting condition	Diuretic	ACEI or ARB	α-Blocker	β-Blocker	Nondihydro-pyridine calcium blocker	Dihydropyridine calcium blocker
Older age	+++	+/−	+	+/−	+	+
Black race	++	+/−	+	+/−	++	++
Angina pectoris	+	+	+	+++	++	+/−
Post–myocardial infarction	+	+++	+	+++	++	−
Congestive heart failure with systolic dysfunction	+++	+++	+	++	−	−
Cerebrovascular disease	+	+	+/−	+	+	+
Renal disease with proteinuria including diabetic nephropathy	++	+++[a]	+	+	++	+
Renal disease without proteinuria	+++	+[a]	+	+	+	+
Dyslipidemia	+	++	+++	+/−[b]	+	+
Prostatism	+	+	+++	+	+	+
Migraine	+	+	+	+++	+++	+
Supraventricular tachyarrhythmias	+	+	+	+++	+++	+/−
Senile tremor	+	+	+	+++	+	+

+++, Strongly indicated and supported by evidence from clinical trials or extensive clinical experience; ++, preferred; +, acceptable; +/−, acceptable with reservation; −, generally contraindicated.

[a] Hyperkalemia occurs more frequently in renal failure, and needs closer monitoring.

[b] Cardioselective β-blockers and those with intrinsic sympathomimetic activities generally do not worsen dyslipidemia (see Table 23-4).

Chronic Renal Failure

This is usually salt sensitive and responds well to salt restriction, diuretics, and calcium antagonists. Loop diuretics are required if serum creatinine levels exceed 2–4 mg/dl. ACEIs and/or ARBs are mandated in patients with diabetic nephropathy or those with microalbuminuria or renal failure with daily proteinuria above 1 gm. This group also should have a reduced BP goal of 125/75 mm Hg. Serum K^+ must be monitored.

Renovascular Hypertension

Percutaneous transluminal renal angioplasty (PTRA) with stenting, if required, is the treatment of choice. ACEIs and ARBs can reduce GFR and cause azotemia and are best avoided. Calcium antagonists are the drugs of choice.

Pheochromocytoma

Phenoxybenzamine is a noncompetative α-adrenergic antagonist. It is a drug of first choice. A β-blocker can be added later to control tachycardia. Before operation, the plasma volume must be expanded by saline infusion.

Hyperaldosteronism

Surgery is the definitive treatment for adrenal adenoma. Spironolactone is the drug of choice for bilateral adrenal hyperplasia or idiopathic hyperaldosteronism. Patients who develop adverse effects can often be managed with high doses of amiloride, but it is less effective in reversing hypertension.

Race

Diuretics, calcium antagonists, and α-blockers are most effective in African-Americans.

Gender

Men and women normally respond similarly to therapy. Special circumstance in the treatment of women include:

Hypertension with Oral Contraceptives
Usually BP is unchanged or rises only modestly with the current low-dose oral contraceptives.

Hypertension in Pregnancy

Methyldopa is the drug of choice because it is proven effective and does not damage the fetus or newborn. Patients whose hypertension is controlled on diuretics can have these agents continued during pregnancy. ACEIs and ARBs are contraindicated. β-Blockers are best avoided because they retard fetal development and can cause neonatal hypoglycemia. Hydralazine is quite effective and safe. Labetalol and calcium antagonists are reserved for refractory patients because their safety is not well studied;

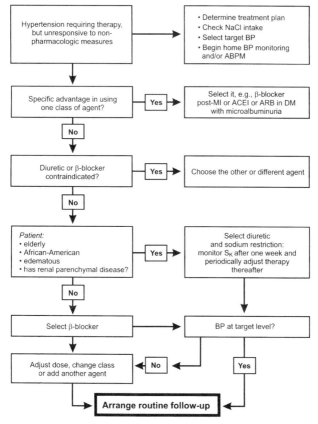

FIGURE 23.1 An algorithm for initiating antihypertensive treatment. ABPM, ambulatory blood pressure monitoring. After Unwin et al. (1998).

Hormone Replacement Therapy

This does not normally increase BP. Hypertension is not a contraindication to its use.

Age

Diuretics are drugs of choice in elderly patients with isolated systolic hypertension.

Patients Undergoing Surgery

For patients undergoing surgery, the BP should be reduced to normal if possible, and certainly <180/110 mm Hg. Cardioselective β-blockers are useful. Calcium antagonists increase surgical blood loss.

OVERVIEW

An algorithm for initiating antihypertensive therapy is presented in Fig. 23.1.

Suggested Readings

Frohlich E. Essential hypertension. *Med Clin North Am* 1997;81.
Izzo JL, Black HR. *Hypertension primer, 2nd ed.* Philadelphia: Lippincott, Williams & Wilkins for the American Heart Association, 1999.
Joint National Committee on Prevention, Detection, Evaluation, and Treatment of High Blood Pressure. Sixth report. *Arch Intern Med* 1997;157;2413–2441.
Kaplan N. Pharmacologic therapy. In: Brady HR, Wilcox CS, eds. *Therapy in nephrology and hypertension.* Philadelphia: WB Saunders, 1998:397–403.
Kaplan N, Gifford RW Jr. Choice of initial therapy for hypertension. *JAMA* 1996;20:1577–1580.
Krakoff L. Treatment decision for hypertension. In: Brady HR, Wilcox CS, eds. *Therapy in nephrology and hypertension.* Philadelphia: WB Saunders, 1998:387–391.
Unwin RJ, Capasso G, Wilcox CS. Therapeutic use of diuretics. In: Brady HR, Wilcox CS, eds. *Therapy in nephrology and hypertension.* Philadelphia: WB Saunders, 1998:654–664.
Weinberger M. Nonpharmacologic therapy. In: Brady HR, Wilcox CS, eds. *Therapy in nephrology and hypertension.* Philadelphia: WB Saunders, 1998:391–396.

Chapter 24

Hypertensive Crises

David T. Lowenthal
Christopher S. Wilcox

A *hypertensive crisis* implies a point at which the management of an acutely elevated BP plays a decisive role in the outcome. A *hypertensive urgency* implies a sudden rise in blood pressure without an acute deterioration in function of a critical target organ. Causes are given in Table 24.1. The clinical presentation includes headache, epistaxis, and psychomotor agitation. A *hypertensive emergency* implies a sudden rise in blood pressure with an acute deterioration in function of a critical target organ. Causes are given in Table 24.2. The clinical presentation may include anginal chest pain, dyspnea, and neurologic deficit. The most frequent consequences of end-organ damage are cerebral infarction, acute pulmonary edema, hypertensive encephalopathy, and cerebral hemorrhage.

PATHOPHYSIOLOGY

The range of normal cerebral autoregulation (mean arterial blood pressure, MABP, 60–160 mm Hg) increases to >200 mm Hg in patients with fixed systolic and diastolic hypertension. Acute rises in BP are especially dangerous because they may exceed the limits of autoregulation. The pathophysiology of hypertensive encephalopathy includes both an intense arteriolar spasm (overregulation) and a failure to autoregulate adequately (breakthrough). A sudden vasoconstriction, for example from cocaine abuse, can induce intense ischemia and neurologic manifestations. However, a sudden rise in blood pressure that exceeds the limit of cerebral autoregulation can also result in hyperemia, transudation of fluid through the blood–brain barrier, and cerebral edema. Pathologic changes

TABLE 24.1   Hypertensive Urgencies

Accelerated or malignant hypertension
Hypertension with left ventricular failure (LVF)
Hypertension with angina
Perioperative hypertension
Preeclampsia
Acute glomerulonephritis
Scleroderma renal crisis
Severe uncomplicated hypertension

include cerebral edema, petechial hemorrhages, vascular necrosis, and cerebral infarction. The neurologic manifestations include papilledema, transient ischemic attacks, seizures, and coma.

The renal circulation also may fail to regulate normally to an abrupt rise in BP because of structural vascular damage and inappropriate release of renin from ischemic nephrons. The hypertension induces a pressure natriuresis that can lead to blood volume depletion, further renin release and worsening renal vasoconstriction. The result is a vicious cycle of escalating angiotensin-dependent hypertension, azotemia, proteinuria, and progressive renal damage, as seen in malignant hypertension.

PRINCIPLES OF BLOOD PRESSURE REDUCTION

The blood pressure of most patients with a hypertensive crisis must be reduced without delay, but caution is needed because the blood flow to critical organs may be dependent on the perfusion pressure. Even in an emergency, the MABP should not be reduced by more than 25% within 2 hours. Thereafter, it can be reduced fur-

TABLE 24.2   Hypertensive Emergencies

Hypertensive encephalopathy
Hypertension with intracranial hemorrhage
Hypertension with stroke
Hypertension with pulmonary edema
Hypertension with acute myocardial infarction (MI) or coronary ischemia
Hyperadrenergic crisis from pheochromocytoma or drugs
Dissecting aortic aneurysm
Eclampsia
Perioperative hypertension with evolving organ dysfunction
Severe epistaxis

ther to about 160/100 mm Hg over the next 4 hours. The physician must articulate the BP goals clearly in the charts and order the neurologic and CVS observations and biochemical monitoring that are required before initiating therapy. As each goal is achieved, the patient must be reevaluated, fresh goals defined, and new orders written. Patients in hypertensive crisis are clinically precarious. If they show deterioration in neurologic or CVS function during BP reductions, it is necessary to return rapidly to BP levels that were tolerated previously. A rapid reduction in BP in patients with renal damage frequently worsens azotemia over the initial days or weeks. However, patients usually accommodate to the normalized BP with an improvement in renal function after a few days or weeks. Therefore, worsening of azotemia during initial therapy should not necessarily require a change in management strategy.

A hypertensive urgency can be managed in the clinic with oral agents. A hypertensive emergency mandates admission to an intensive care unit with continuous monitoring of BP and critical function and the use of short-acting intravenous drugs.

HYPERTENSIVE URGENCIES

Malignant Hypertension

The *definition* is severe hypertension (BP > 180/110 mm Hg) accompanied by advanced retinopathy with papilledema, progressive impairment of renal function with proteinuria and often worsening azotemia, and frequently widespread endothelial dysfunction evidenced by microangiopathic hemolytic anemia with schistocytes seen on blood smear examination, thrombotic thrombocytopenic purpura, pancreatitis, or multiorgan dysfunction. There may be intravascular coagulation and platelet consumption. It has a distinctive pathology that includes intense onion-skin proliferation of myoendothelial cells of resistance vessels, fibrinoid necrosis of arterioles and capillaries, and ischemia or infarction of end organs. If it is complicated by hypertensive encephalopathy or vital organ dysfunction, it becomes a hypertensive emergency.

The *incidence* is approximately 1% of hypertensives. It is more frequent in men, in Asians and African-Americans, and in those of poor socioeconomic background. Most underlying *secondary causes* reside in renal parenchymal or renovascular disease. The *clinical presentation* includes a rapid rise in BP, usually superimposed on preexisting hypertension. Most patients have left ventricular hypertrophy, and some have acute left ventricular failure. The initial neurologic features are usually nonspecific. They include headache, dizziness, and/or transient ischemic attacks. These are manifestations of *hypertensive encephalopathy*. If untreated, there is progressive azotemia and proteinuria. A urinalysis frequently shows red blood cells and may reveal an underlying primary renal disease. Electrolyte disturbances include hypokalemic metabolic alkalosis from volume depletion, renin secretion, and secondary hyperaldosteronism.

The *management* includes a gradual reduction of blood pressure to prevent cerebral or cardiac ischemia. Patients with prior neurologic deficits are at greater risk of rapid BP reduction. If malignant hypertension is complicated by evolving organ failure, BP must be reduced more rapidly with parenteral medications. Patients are often volume depleted; therefore, diuretics should be avoided in the acute phase. ACEIs are logical and effective therapy. The *prognosis* is surprisingly good if patients are diagnosed and treated promptly because the vascular lesions heal as the BP is normalized.

Other Categories

Hypertension with LVF, coronary ischemia, and perioperative hypertension are associated with pain, anxiety, and activation of sympathetic reflexes. The hypertension responds to sympatholytic agents such as labetalol. Hypertension with preeclampsia does not necessarily require treatment. The emphasis is placed on preparing for early delivery. However, hypertension in preeclampsia or acute glomerulonephritis carries a high risk of encephalopathy, even at relatively low BP levels, because the acute elevation in BP precludes effective resetting of cerebral autoregulation. The pathology of acute scleroderma crisis mimics malignant hypertension. It can progress rapidly to renal failure.

HYPERTENSIVE EMERGENCIES

The features of *hypertensive encephalopathy* were described under malignant hypertension. Hypertension with *intracranial hemorrhage* requires an abrupt reduction in BP to limit life-threatening bleeding. In contrast, hypertension with *cerebral infarction* requires much more moderate and gradual reductions in BP. A BP as high as 160/105 mm Hg may be tolerated during the first days of a thrombotic stroke, with gradual and controlled reductions thereafter.

Hypertension with acute LVF responds rapidly to a reduction in peripheral resistance with a direct-acting vasodilator. Intravenous furosemide, like intravenous nitrates, reduces venous compliance and alleviates pulmonary congestion.

Acute aortic dissection requires specific measures to reduce the vessel wall shear stress. Shear stress depends on blood flow rather than on BP. Therefore, the initial therapy must be a profound and sustained inhibition of cardiac contractility and rate with high-dose, long-acting β-blockers. Thereafter, BP can be reduced safely with a direct-acting vasodilator such as sodium nitroprusside.

PHARMACOLOGIC MANAGEMENT OF HYPERTENSIVE CRISES

Table 24.3 lists hypertensive crises and the drugs that are of special value. Table 24.4 details these agents. Short-acting calcium

TABLE 24.3 Drugs for the Treatment of Specific Hypertensive Crises

Clinical or associated condition	Drugs of choice	Contraindicated[a]
Hypertensive encephalopathy, intracerebral or subarachnoid hemorrhage	Sodium nitroprusside	Centrally acting drugs[b]
Renal failure	Sodium nitroprusside Labetalol Fenoldopam	
Eclampsia	Magnesium sulfate[c] Hydralazine Labetalol	ACEIs ARBs Diuretics
Acute congestive cardiac failure, acute left ventricular failure	Sodium nitroprusside Nitroglycerin Labetalol	Drugs that activate sympathetic reflexes[d]
Intra- and postoperative hypertension (cardiac and noncardiac)	Esmolol Sodium nitroprusside Fenoldopam Lebatalol	Centrally acting drugs[b]

(*continued*)

TABLE 24.3 *Continued*

Clinical or associated condition	Drugs of choice	Contraindicated[a]
Pheochromocytoma or release of catecholamines with MAOIs	Phentolamine β-Blockers (after α-blockade) Labetalol	Drugs that activate sympathetic reflexes[d]
Acute dissecting aneurysm of the aorta	β-Blockade, then sodium nitroprusside	Drugs that activate sympathetic reflexes[d]

[a] Contraindicated implies drugs to be avoided or used with special caution.

[b] These include clonidine, α-methyldopa, guanabenz, guanfacine, and reserpine.

[c] Magnesium sulfate is a drug of first choice for eclampsia but has little effect on BP.

[d] These include direct vasodilators such as diazoxide, hydralazine, and minoxidil, and short-acting calcium antagonists.

ACEIs, angiotensin-converting enzyme inhibitors; ARBs, angiotensin receptor blockers.

TABLE 24.4   **Parenteral Drugs for Hypertensive Emergencies**

Drug	Mechanism of action	Comments
Sodium nitroprusside	Vasodilates arterioles > veins	Rapid acting; thiocyanate toxicity (plasma levels > 10 mg/dl) causes CNS disturbance
Nitroglycerin	Vasodilates veins > coronary arteries > arterioles	Preferred in coronary ischemia; tolerance with prolonged use
Metoprolol, esmolol	β_1-Selective receptor antagonists	Metoprolol by bolus injection; esmolol by infusion; can cause bronchospasm and bradyarrhythmias
Phentolamine	Nonselective α-receptor blocker	For pheochromocytoma or adrenergic crisis; tachycardia problematic
Labetalol	β-/α-Receptor blocker	For hyperadrenergic syndromes
Enalaprilat	ACE inhibition	Effective in high-renin states; causes azotemia in bilateral RAS or ECV depletion[a]
Fenoldopam	Dopamine DA_1-receptor agonist	Renal and systemic vasodilator; may cause adrenergic activation
Furosemide	Rapidly acting loop diuretic with veno-dilation after IV use	Effective in acute LVF and pulmonary edema

[a] RAS, renal artery stenosis; ECV, extracellular fluid volume.

TABLE 24.5 Doses, Onset, and Duration of Action of Selected Drugs

Drug	Route and dose	Onset (min)	Duration
Sodium nitroprusside	IV infusion, 0.5–10 μg/kg/min	<1	3–5 min
Nitroglycerin	IV infusion, 5–100 μg/min	2–5	5–10 min
Labetalol	IV bolus, 20 mg over 2 min, then 40–80 mg per 10 min (300 mg max) PO dose; 100–200 mg	5	6–10 hr
Enalaprilat	IV bolus, 1.25–5 mg per 6 hr	15	6–12 hr
Fenoldopam	IV infusion, 0.1–1.6 μg/kg/min	4–5	10 min
Clonidine	PO dose, 0.1–0.3 mg	15	3–6 hr

antagonists cause sympathetic activation and an abrupt and unpredictable fall in BP. Therefore, they are not recommended. Table 24.5 lists the recommended drug dosages. Oral antihypertensive treatment should be instituted once neurologic or cardiovascular signs and symptoms clear.

Angiotensin-converting enzyme inhibitors (ACEIs) or angiotensin receptor blockers (ARBs) are of considerable value in the postcrisis management of patients with scleroderma renal crisis, malignant hypertension, cardiac failure, MI, or those with proteinuric renal failure. Patients who have had an acute MI require lifelong therapy with a β-blocker, an ACEI or an ARB, and low-dose aspirin unless these treatments are contraindicated. Further details of long-term therapy are given in Chapter 23.

Suggested Readings

Burris J, Freis ED. Hypertensive emergencies. In: Messerli F, ed. *Cardiovascular drug therapy, 2nd ed.* Philadelphia: WB Saunders, 1996: 148–160.

Joint National Committee on Prevention, Detection, Evaluation and Treatment of High Blood Pressure. Sixth report. *Arch Intern Med* 1997;157:2413–2446.

Mann SJ, Atlas SA. Hypertensive emergencies. In: Brady HR, Wilcox CS, eds. *Therapy in nephrology and hypertension.* Philadelphia: WB Saunders, 1998:404–411.

Nolan CR. Hypertensive crises. In: Wilcox CS, ed. *Atlas of diseases of the kidney, Vol III.* Philadelphia: Current Medicine, 1998:8.13–8.30.

Chapter 25

Clinical Use of Diuretics

David S. Amrose
Christopher S. Wilcox

Diuretics are proven effective in reducing blood pressure (BP), abolishing all the increased risk of stroke, and reducing the increased risk of myocardial infarction (MI) by approximately one-half. They are inexpensive and are well tolerated. It is not yet clear whether new antihypertensive drugs can provide the same long-term benefit in the primary prevention of cardiovascular disease as can diuretics. Therefore, diuretics remain the drugs of choice for treating hypertension.

SITES AND MECHANISMS OF ACTION

Osmotic Diuretics

They are freely filtered but are not reabsorbed. Fluid absorption from the proximal tubule and thin limbs of the loop of Henle increases the concentration of the osmotic diuretic sufficiently to diminish fluid absorption. These agents cause a rapid and substantial increase in the excretion of fluid, NaCl, and other ions.

Loop Diuretics

These drugs act on the thick ascending limb (TAL) of the loop of Henle, where they inhibit the luminal $Na^+–2Cl^-–K^+$ cotransporter (Fig. 25.1). Energy is provided by the $3Na^+/2K^+$-ATPase, which maintains a low intracellular $[Na^+]$. Reabsorbed K^+ is recycled via a K^+ channel in the luminal membrane. Therefore, the net effect of loop diuretics is to inhibit the absorption of Na^+ and Cl^-. A compensatory increase in Na^+ reabsorption occurs in the

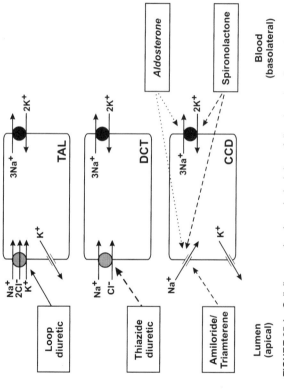

FIGURE 25.1 Cell diagram showing principal sites of diuretic action. For explanation, see text. Reproduced with permission from Unwin et al. (1998).

distal tubule and collecting ducts. Loop diuretics hyperpolarize the cell and decrease the electromotive force for Ca^{2+} and Mg^{2+} absorption. Because the medullary concentration gradient depends on NaCl reabsorption in the TAL, loop diuretics abolish urine concentration and dilution. The increase in distal flow increases K^+ and H^+ secretion and thereby predisposes to hypokalemia and alkalosis. The fractional excretion of Na^+ can increase to 15% to 20% during maximal loop diuretic therapy.

Thiazide Diuretics

These act primarily in the early distal convoluted tubule (DCT), where they inhibit the luminal Na^+–Cl^- cotransporter (Fig. 25.1). Because NaCl reabsorption in the DCT further dilutes the tubular fluid, thiazides impair urinary dilution and predispose to hyponatremia but, contrary to loop diuretics, do not disrupt the medullary concentration gradient and therefore do not inhibit urinary concentration. Also in contrast to loop diuretics, thiazides increase distal Ca^{2+} reabsorption. The blockade of luminal Na^+–Cl^- entry by thiazides reduces the $[Na^+]$ in the early distal convoluted tubule cell, thereby increasing the gradient for Na^+ entry in exchange for Ca^{2+} exit (Na^+/Ca^{2+} exchange) on the basolateral membrane. The consequence is enhanced Ca^{2+} reabsorption and reduced Ca^{2+} excretion.

Potassium-Sparing Diuretics and Aldosterone Antagonists

Potassium-sparing diuretics such as amiloride and triamterene decrease the hypokalemia and metabolic alkalosis that accompany the use of loop and thiazide diuretics. They act by inhibiting the luminal Na^+ channel on the principal cells of the collecting ducts (CCD) (Fig. 25.1). This channel, and the $3Na^+/2K^+$-ATPase, are activated by aldosterone. The inhibition of Na^+ entry by these drugs and by aldosterone antagonists such as spironolactone reduces the lumen-negative potential, thereby reducing the electrical gradient for secretion of positively charged K^+ and H^+ ions.

PHARMACOKINETICS, DRUG INTERACTIONS, AND INDIVIDUAL AGENTS

Loop Diuretics

These agents are readily absorbed and strongly bound to albumin, which prevents their glomerular filtration. They are secreted in the

S_2 and S_3 segments of the proximal tubule to reach their luminal sites of action. They compete for secretion with other organic acids, which are increased in renal failure. The doses of diuretic must therefore be increased in renal failure because of the decrease in GFR and competition for proximal secretion. Loop diuretics are bound to filtered albumin in the tubular fluid of patients with the nephrotic syndrome. This reduces the active, free fraction of diuretic in the tubular fluid to interact with the luminal Na^+–K^+–$2Cl^-$ cotransporter. Hypoalbuminemia also increases the volume of distribution of loop diuretics, thereby reducing the plasma delivery to the kidney. Furthermore, hypoalbuminemia reduces the secretion of loop diuretics by the S_2 and S_3 segments of the proximal tubule but enhances the uptake and metabolism to inactive glucuronides by the S_1 segment. Therefore, hypoalbuminemic patients require increased doses of loop diuretics. Nonsteroidal antiinflammatory agents (NSAIAs) block cyclooxygenase and hence reduce prostaglandin E_2 production. This blunts the natriuretic effect of the diuretic.

Individual drugs and doses follow:

- Furosemide (Lasix, initially 20–40 mg once or twice daily).
- Bumetanide (Bumex, initially 1–2 mg once or twice daily).
- Ethacrynic acid (Edecrin, initially 25–50 mg once or twice daily).
- Torsemide (Demadex, initially 5 mg once or twice daily).

Thiazide Diuretics

They are secreted by the S_2 and S_3 segments of the proximal tubule. They become less effective with advancing renal failure (plasma creatinine 2–4 mg/dl).

Individual drugs and doses follow:

- Hydrochlorothiazide (Hydrodiuril, initially 12.5–25 mg daily, duration 6–10 hours)
- Chlorthalidone (Hygroton, initially 12.5–25 mg daily, duration 24–36 hours)
- Metalozone (Zaroxolyn, initially 2.5–5 mg daily); has some additional action on the proximal nephron and may be more effective in patients with renal impairment

Distal K^+-Sparing Diuretics and Aldosterone Antagonists

These agents are secreted by the S_2 and S_3 portions of the proximal tubule. *Triamterene* is partly metabolized by the liver and accumulates in cirrhosis. *Amiloride* is excreted by the kidney in active form. Both drugs accumulate in renal failure. *Spironolactone* has active metabolites that require 24 to 48 hours for maximal action.

Individual drugs and doses follow:

- Triamterene (Dyrenium, 50–100 mg once or twice daily)
- Amiloride (Midamor, 5–10 mg daily)
- Spironolactone (Aldactone, 50–100 mg daily); doses up to 600 mg daily are sometimes required in patients with severe hyperaldosteronism.

Combination of these drugs with a thiazide is convenient [e.g., Maxzide and Dyazide (hydrochlorothiazide and triamterene), Moduretic (hydrochlorothiazide and amiloride), and Aldactazide (hydrochlorothiazide and spironolactone)].

CLINICAL INDICATIONS

Hypertension

Diuretics are drugs of first choice for treatment of hypertension (see Chapter 23).

Edematous States

Congestive Heart Failure

Mild chronic CHF can be managed by dietary salt restriction (goal: Na^+ intake of 80–120 mEq/day) and a thiazide. Because the risks of hypokalemia and hypomagnesemia are increased, particularly in those receiving digitalis glycosides, thiazides should be combined with a distal K^+-sparing diuretic. More severe CHF, particularly when complicated by decreased renal function, requires therapy with loop diuretics, which are often combined with distal K^+-sparing agents. An ACE inhibitor or AT_1 receptor antagonist is indicated for patients with heart failure. They increase cardiac output and decrease mortality in mild, moderate, and severe cardiac failure and in patients who have had a myocardial infarction. These drugs are often prescribed with diuretics. However, this combination can cause prolonged hypotension, hyperkalemia, and prerenal azotemia. Thus, therapy should be initiated with small doses of a short-acting agent (e.g., captopril, 6.25 mg twice daily) under close surveillance. Later, the patient can be switched to longer-duration drugs such as lisinopril, benazepril, ramipril, trandolapril, quinapril, enalapril, or fosinopril (ACEIs) or the angiotensin receptor blockers (ARBs) valsartan, irbesartan, or candesartan. An ARB is required if the patient develops a cough with ACEI therapy. Both ACEIs and ARBs usually improve renal function in patients with hypertension. Renal failure occurs in the setting of an abrupt or severe fall in BP, excessive volume depletion, or renal artery stenosis affecting both kidneys.

Nephrotic Syndrome

Nephrotic edema is best managed by dietary salt and fluid restriction. With more severe edema, especially in the presence of renal failure, loop diuretics are required. Overvigorous diuresis can reduce renal function further. Albumin infusions are not effective in increasing serum albumin significantly or in promoting diuresis. They are expensive. Premixing of furosemide with 25 g of albumin in the syringe before IV injection diminishes the volume of distribution of the diuretic and increases its effectiveness. The same effect can be achieved more conveniently by doubling the diuretic dose. Therefore, albumin is not recommended for hypoalbuminemic patients.

Cirrhosis and Ascites

A salt-restricted diet is sufficient for mild cirrhosis and ascites. However, more severe ascites requires diuretic therapy. Because these patients almost always have elevated aldosterone levels, and loop diuretic–induced hypokalemia and alkalosis can precipitate hepatic encephalopathy, spironalactone (25–100 mg daily) is preferred. Loop diuretics are added only for intractable edema that limits mobility or breathing. Large-volume paracentesis with IV albumin infusion is preferred for refractory ascites because it is more effective and causes fewer cardiovascular or electrolyte abnormalities than diuretics.

Electrolyte Abnormalities

- Hypercalcemia: Loop diuretics with IV hydration increase renal Ca^{2+} excretion
- Hyponatremia/SIADH: Loop diuretics with hypertonic saline treat acute, symptomatic hyponatremia
- Hyperkalemia and distal RTA: Loop diuretics and salt are given to patients with hyperkalemic distal RTA (type IV); patients who are not hypertensive can be managed with fludrocortisone

Nephrolithiasis

Thiazides prevent recurrent nephrolithiasis, especially in patients with idiopathic hypercalciuria.

Diabetes Insipidus

In the presence of Na^+ restriction, thiazides decrease urine volume in both central and nephrogenic diabetes insipidus.

Acute Renal Failure

High doses of loop diuretics can be used with osmotic diuretics (mannitol) to convert oliguric to nonoliguric acute renal failure. Although this may not diminish the progression of renal failure or decrease morbidity and mortality, it does decrease fluid overload and reduces the need for dialysis. Loop diuretics do not decrease the incidence of contrast nephropathy. Rather, the treatment of choice remains adequate pre- and postprocedure hydration with 0. 075 M saline at 2 ml/min.

ADVERSE EFFECTS OF DIURETICS

Azotemia

A rise in blood urea nitrogen (BUN) usually implies that the diuresis has been too abrupt or extensive and requires some ECV reexpansion (by decreasing diuretic dosage and liberalizing salt and fluid intake). Occasionally, azotemia with proteinuria indicates loop diuretic–induced interstitial nephritis.

Hyponatremia

Thiazides promote Na^+ loss and diminish urinary dilution. Severe hyponatremia ($S_{Na} < 120$ mEq/L) can occur particularly in elderly women with well-preserved renal function who drink substantial amounts of fluid. Such patients can develop hyponatremia on rechallenge with thiazides.

Hypokalemia

Serum K^+ (S_K) falls by an average of 0.6 mEq/L in hypertensive patients receiving thiazides. KCl supplementation reduces this fall. Loop diuretics and thiazides increase tubular fluid flow through the terminal nephron, which stimulates K^+ secretion.

The increased secretion of angiotensin and aldosterone promotes distal K^+ secretion further. Severe hypokalemia ($S_K < 3.0$ mEq/L) is associated with dangerous ventricular ectopy. Milder hypokalemia (S_K 3.0–3.5 mEq/L) may cause dangerous arrhythmias in patients with myocardial ischemia or in those receiving cardiac glycosides. Hypokalemia may contribute to diuretic-induced carbohydrate intolerance and hyperlipidemia. Therefore, most physicians maintain S_K above 3.5 mEq/L. Diuretic-induced hypokalemia can be managed by administration of two to six tablets of KCl daily. The ACEIs or ARBs, which blunt diuretic-induced increases in angiotensin II (Ang II) concentration or action, can potentiate the antihypertensive and salt-depleting actions of diuretics and diminish hypokalemia. Therefore, their careful use with diuretics can enhance efficacy and decrease toxicity.

Hyperkalemia

Distal K^+-sparing diuretics can cause hyperkalemia in renal failure.

Hypomagnesemia

Loop diuretics and thiazides increase Mg^{2+} excretion. Occasional patients develop overt hypomagnesemia and manifest depression, muscular weakness, and cardiac arrhythmias or failure. Distal K^+-sparing agents, and probably spironolactone, diminish Mg^{2+} excretion. The resulting Mg^{2+} depletion causes ongoing renal K^+ excretion and thereby maintains hypokalemia.

Metabolic Alkalosis

The plasma [HCO_3^-] usually increases 2–5 mEq/L or more with thiazides or loop diuretics. Alkalosis predisposes to cardiac arrhythmias and diminishes ventilatory drive in patients with chronic obstructive pulmonary disease. It is best managed by administration of KCl or a distal K^+-sparing diuretic.

Hyperglycemia and Hyperlipidemia

Loop diuretics and thiazides can impair carbohydrate tolerance. This has been ascribed to hypokalemia, which impairs insulin release and glucose uptake into skeletal muscle. However, the effects are usually mild or absent at clinically relevant doses. Patients with diabetes mellitus should receive diuretics as necessary, with special care to prevent hypokalemia. Hyperlipidemia normally is not a problem during long-term therapy.

Hyperuricemia

Loop diuretics and thiazides increase plasma urate levels by 1 to 3 mg/dl. They should be avoided in patients with gout. They can be combined with xanthine oxidase inhibitors, e.g., allopurinol.

Other Effects

Thiazides are a frequent cause of impotence in hypertensive patients. This can be managed by sildenafil (Viagra, 50 mg initially). Occasional patients receiving loop or thiazide diuretics develop an allergy manifested as skin rash, fever, and eosinophilia. Others develop interstitial nephritis with loop diuretics. Allergic effects are best managed by changing to the non-sulfur-containing diuretic ethacrynic acid.

CAUSES OF DIURETIC RESISTANCE

Diuretic resistance implies an inadequate fluid depletion produced by a full dose of diuretic.

Incorrect Diagnosis

Diuretics do not clear lympathic or venous edema.

Inadequate Diuretic Reaching the Tubule Lumen

- Poor compliance: Check with measurement of diuretic in urine
- Inadequate dose: Increased doses are required during regular therapy to counteract the compensatory increases in distal NaCl reabsorption
- Renal failure: Doses of loop diuretics must be increased in proportion to the reduction in creatinine clearance; thiazides are ineffective at a plasma creatinine above 2–4 mg/dl.

Inadequate Tubular Response to the Diuretic

- Nonsteroidal antiinflammatory drugs (NSAIDs): Such drugs (e.g., aspirin, indomethacin) impair the response to all diuretics, particularly in volume-depleted edemous patients

- Inappropriate dietary salt intake: Even powerful loop diuretics require dietary salt restriction. Therefore, salt intake should be assessed from measurements of 24-hour renal Na^+ excretion and restricted severely (80 mEq daily) in patients with resistant edema
- Advanced edema: Patients with uncompensated CHF, cirrhosis, or nephrosis are resistant to diuretics and require increased doses
- Physiologic adaption to diuretics: Prolonged therapy with one diuretic leads to humoral and renal adaptations that limit the response; however, patients remain very responsive to diuretics of a different class

MANAGEMENT

When an obvious cause for diuretic resistance is not discovered, it can be managed by addition of a second drug. Administration of a thiazide to therapy with a loop diuretic is often highly effective but can precipitate severe fluid and electrolyte depletion, notably hypokalemia. Administration of a distal K^+-sparing diuretic or spironolactone to therapy with a thiazide or loop diuretic produces less hypokalemia and alkalosis. When diuretic resistance is caused by overactivity of the renin–angiotensin–aldosterone system, addition of an ACEI or ARB is logical. However, there is an increased risk of hypotension and prerenal azotemia. Combined drug administration requires close surveillance.

Suggested Readings

Bleich M, Greger R. Mechanism of action of diuretics. *Kidney Int* 1997;51 (Suppl 59):S11–S15.

Ellison DH, Wilcox CS. Diuretic resistance. In: Brady HR, Wilcox CS, eds. *Therapy in nephrology and hypertension*. Philadelphia: WB Saunders, 1998:665–674.

Unwin RJ, Capasso G, Wilcox CS. Therapeutic use of diuretics. In: Brady HR, Wilcox CS, eds. *Therapy in nephrology and hypertension*. Philadelphia: WB Saunders, 1998:654–664.

Wilcox CS. Diuretics. In: Brenner BM, ed. *The kidney*. Philadelphia: WB Saunders, 1995:2299–2330.

Chapter 26

Acute Renal Failure

Nicolas J. Guzman

Acute renal failure (ARF) is an abrupt decrease in renal excretion of nitrogenous wastes, resulting in azotemia. It may be prerenal, parenchymal, or postrenal.

PRERENAL ACUTE RENAL FAILURE

Prerenal ARF is a rapidly reversible decrease in glomerular filtration rate (GFR) caused by renal hypoperfusion. It causes 50% of the cases of ARF.

Pathophysiology

Renal autoregulation maintains normal GFR and capillary hydrostatic pressure between a mean arterial pressure of 60 and 120 mm Hg. However, systemic hypotension also stimulates the renin–angiotensin–aldosterone axis, antidiuretic hormone release, and the sympathetic nervous system. The urine volume and sodium output decline, and the osmolality increases. Blood urea nitrogen (BUN) increases more than serum creatinine (S_{Cr}). If renal hypoperfusion is sustained or severe, acute tubular necrosis (ATN) may ensue, as summarized in Table 26.1.

Presentation and Management

The clinical presentation is reviewed in Table 26.2. Rapid volume replacement is essential to prevent ATN. A fluid challenge of 300 to 500 ml of isotonic saline can be given IV over 30 to 60 minutes or infused at 100 to 150 ml/hr in the elderly or when the cardio-

TABLE 26.1 Etiology of Prerenal Acute Renal Failure

Intravascular volume depletion

Hemorrhage	Skin loss of sweat
Gastrointestinal fluid losses	Sequestration of fluid in third spaces
Renal fluid losses	Inadequate fluid replacement
	Inappropriate diuretic therapy

Reduced cardiac output

Cardiogenic shock	Pericardial tamponade
Congestive heart failure	Massive pulmonary embolism

Systemic vasodilatation

Anaphylaxis	Sepsis
Antihypertensive drugs	Drug overdose

Renal vasoconstriction

Anesthesia
α-Adrenergic agonists or high-dose dopamine
Hepatorenal syndrome
Surgery

Hyperviscosity syndromes

Multiple myeloma or macroglobulinemia

TABLE 26.2 Clinical Presentation of Prerenal Acute Renal Failure

History and symptoms
  History of fluid losses (vomiting, diarrhea, polyuria, burns)
  Use of nonsteroidal antiinflammatory drugs or angiotensin-converting
    enzyme inhibitors
  Fluid deficit by intake–output balance (output greater than intake)
  Thirst
Signs
  Weight loss (catabolic patients may lose > 1 lb/day)
  Oliguria
  Orthostatic hypotension
  Tachycardia
  Flat neck veins in supine position
  Dry skin and mucosa with loss of skin turgor
Laboratory tests
  Hemoconcentration (increased albumin and hematocrit)
  Serum BUN/Cr > 20 (also occurs with increased protein catabolism)
  Urine specific gravity > 1.030
  Urine osmolality > 500 mOsm/kg H_2O
  Urinary sodium < 20 mEq/L
  Fractional excretion of sodium (FE_{Na}) < 1%
    where
$$FE_{Na} = \left[\frac{U_{Na} \times P_{cr}}{P_{Na} \times U_{cr}} \right] \times 100$$

vascular status is tenuous. This may be repeated twice at hourly intervals while the urine output and cardiovascular status are monitored. Thereafter, the aim of fluid replacement is to maintain the urine output at 1 to 2 ml/min. If there are doubts regarding the patient's cardiovascular status, a Swan-Ganz catheter should be inserted to monitor central venous pressure, pulmonary capillary wedge pressure, and cardiac output. In patients with prerenal azotemia from causes other than volume depletion (e, g., congestive heart failure, pericardial tamponade, drug overdose), the underlying disorder must be corrected.

ACUTE PARENCHYMAL RENAL FAILURE: ACUTE TUBULAR NECROSIS

Acute tubular necrosis (ATN) is an abrupt decrease in GFR caused by tubular cell damage from renal hypoperfusion, nephrotoxic injury, or severe tubulointerstitial nephritis. The incidence of ATN is 50% in patients undergoing emergency abdominal aortic surgery. Although ATN is usually accompanied by oliguria (urine output < 500 ml/24 hr), some patients continue to excrete 1 to 2 L of urine/day. The hallmark of ATN is the acute onset or worsening of azotemia, which is not immediately reversible after withdrawal of the causative agent or fluid replacement.

Etiology

Ischemic damage may occur without overt hypotension. The ATN may be caused by nephrotoxicity from either exogenous or endogenous toxins (Table 26.3). Most patients with ATN will have more than one etiology.

Aminoglycosides

Acute tubular necrosis occurs in 10% to 26% of patients receiving gentamicin, tobramycin, or amikacin, even with therapeutic plasma levels. Nephrotoxicity correlates with the total cumulative aminoglycoside dose. ATN, which is usually nonoliguric, becomes clinically apparent after 5 to 10 days of therapy. The following predispose to ATN during aminoglycoside therapy: advanced age, preexisting renal disease, volume depletion, and recent exposure to other nephrotoxins. Early findings include isosthenuria caused by nephrogenic diabetes insipidus, tubular

TABLE 26.3   Some Toxic Causes of ATN

Exogenous
    Antibiotics (e.g., aminoglycosides, cephalosporins, tetracyclines,
        amphotericin B, pentamidine)
    Radiographic contrast (contrast-associated nephropathy or CAN)
    Heavy metals (e.g., mercury, lead, arsenic, bismuth)
    Chemotherapeutic agents (e.g., cisplatin, methotrexate, mitomycin)
    Immunosuppressive agents (e.g., cyclosporine)
    Organic solvents (e.g., ethylene glycol)
Endogenous
    Myoglobin
    Hemoglobin
    Calcium phosphate precipitation

proteinuria, and Fanconi's syndrome with proximal renal tubular acidosis, glycosuria, and aminoaciduria. Magnesium and potassium wasting may lead to hypomagnesemia and hypokalemia. With more severe nephrotoxicity, azotemia ensues. Recovery may be slow (months) or incomplete. Tobramycin appears to be as nephrotoxic as gentamicin.

Amphotericin B

Nephrotoxicity is rare with cumulative doses below 600 mg. Distal nephron damage is manifested as polyuria with isosthenuria (nephrogenic diabetes insipidus), hypokalemia, hypomagnesemia, and distal renal tubular acidosis. Salt repletion and mannitol may be protective. Lyophilized formulations appear less nephrotoxic.

Radiographic Contrast Agents

The incidence of ATN with contrast agents is as high as 50% in high-risk patients. Renal failure usually occurs 1 to 2 days after exposure and is characterized by a persistent nephrogram, a low FE_{Na} and a high urine specific gravity. ATN can be prevented by adequate hydration and volume expansion with 0.45% saline administered before and during the contrast load to maintain a urine flow of 2 ml/min. The administration of diuretics can be detrimental. New nonionic agents are preferable in patients with preexisting renal insufficiency, particularly in the setting of diabetes mellitus. Risk factors for contrast-associated nephropathy ATN include renal insufficiency, volume depletion or any other prerenal state, diabetes mellitus, multiple myeloma, repeated doses of a radiographic contrast agent, and recent exposure to other nephrotoxic agents.

Cisplatin

Cisplatin nephrotoxicity usually causes severe magnesium wasting. ATN and chronic renal insufficiency can be reduced by hydration, mannitol, and a slow infusion of cisplatin in chloride-containing solutions. Carboplatin and iproplatin appear to be less nephrotoxic.

Organic Compounds

Renal failure from ethylene glycol results from tubular deposition of calcium oxalate crystals. It can be diagnosed by identifying these crystals in the urine. Treatment includes hemodialysis together with ethanol infusion to block ethylene glycol metabolism.

Endogenous Nephrotoxins

Pigments

Rhabdomyolysis sufficient to cause ATN can be caused by:

- Direct muscle damage (e. g., trauma, crush injury, burns)
- Ischemia and/or increased muscle metabolism (e. g., seizures, exercise, heat stroke, hyperthermia, shock, vascular occlusion)
- Metabolic disorders (e. g., ketoacidosis, hypokalemia, hypophosphatemia)
- Toxins (e. g., alcohol, heroin, CO poisoning, snake bite)
- Severe infections

The clinical features of rhabdomyolytic ATN include muscle pain, dark brown urine, a positive *ortho*-toluidine urine test for blood, hyperkalemia, hyperphosphatemia, hyperuricemia, early hypocalcemia, and late hypercalcemia. Serum creatine phosphokinase and myoglobin levels indicate rhabdomyolysis.

ATN can be prevented by vigorous volume replacement with isotonic saline (200–300 ml/hr), followed by intravenous mannitol (12.5–25 g in 30 minutes) or furosemide (40–300 mg every 4–6 hours) to maintain a urine output of 100 to 200 ml/hr and urine alkalinization to a pH above 7 with intravenous sodium bicarbonate (1 mEq/kg/dose). Alkalinization may induce tetany in hypocalcemic patients. When ATN develops, the patient is usually so severely hypercatabolic that early and frequent hemodialysis is often required. The prognosis for recovery of renal function is good.

Crystals

Acute tubular necrosis may result from intratubular deposition of uric acid crystals during chemotherapy for malignancies with high cell turnover (e, g., leukemia, lymphoproliferative and germ cell neoplasms). Hemodialysis is the treatment of choice. Preventive measures include vigorous hydration, alkaline diuresis, and allopurinol. These measures should be initiated several days before chemotherapy and maintained during induction. Hyperkalemia and hyperphosphatemia commonly complicate hyperuricemic ATN.

Multiple Myeloma

Acute tubular necrosis occurs from tubular damage by light chains, from intratubular casts, or from complications such as hypercalcemia, hyperviscosity, and volume depletion. They are susceptible to CAN.

Pregnancy

Acute tubular necrosis can occur early after septic abortion or during late pregnancy in association with eclampsia, abruptio placentae, peripartum hemorrhage, amniotic fluid embolism, or prolonged intrauterine fetal death. The pathogenesis includes a combination of renal hypoperfusion from vasospasm and formation of fibrin thrombi inside the glomerular capillaries. Disseminated intravascular coagulation is seen frequently. Cortical necrosis leading to end-stage renal failure can occur.

Rare forms of pregnancy-associated ARF include acute fatty liver with ATN and postpartum ARF. In the former, the only effective treatment is termination of the pregnancy. Postpartum ARF is a form of thrombotic microangiopathy. There is no effective therapy.

Hepatorenal Syndrome

This is a progressive decline in renal function in patients with advanced liver disease (usually cirrhosis) in the absence of other identifiable causes. There is marked renal vasoconstriction with oliguria. Usually the U_{Na} is less than 10 mEq/L, and FE_{Na} is less than 1% (and remains low after a volume challenge). The syndrome often develops in the hospital after aggressive diuretic therapy, surgery, or gastrointestinal bleeding. Paracentesis with removal of ascitic fluid in conjunction with salt-free IV albumin replacement may lead to improved diuresis. However, mortality remains very high (>95%) and is usually from liver failure, infection, or hemorrhage.

Pathophysiology

Loss of polarity of injured proximal tubular epithelial cells leads to abnormal apical integrin expression, which results in adhesion of tubular debris and tubular obstruction. Tubular fluid can leak back across a disrupted tubular epithelial barrier. Reduction in total renal blood flow, and its redistribution away from the outer cortex, occurs in all types of ATN. Regardless of the pathogenetic mechanism, the final result is always impaired renal function with progressive azotemia and impaired water and electrolyte handling.

Clinical Presentation and Laboratory Findings

Most patients present with an acute rise in S_{Cr} and oliguria. Some, particularly those with nephrotoxic injury, are nonoliguric initially. Complete anuria rarely occurs in ATN. Its presence suggests urinary obstruction, bilateral cortical necrosis, vascular occlusion, or rapidly progressive glomerulonephritis. Some present with volume overload or uremia. Frequently, patients will have marked electrolyte disturbances consisting of severe azotemia, hyperkalemia, high anion gap metabolic acidosis, and hyponatremia. The daily rate of rise in serum creatinine with total renal failure is 0.5 to 1.0 mg/dl. A more rapid increase suggests a hypercatabolic state or massive muscle destruction. Other metabolic abnormalities include hyperphosphatemia, hypermagnesemia, hypocalcemia, and hyperuricemia.

Examination of the urine sediment reveals renal tubular epithelial cells, cellular debris, and cellular and coarse granular casts. Hematuria and red blood cell casts are rare. White blood cells or white blood cell casts suggest acute interstitial nephritis.

In the setting of oliguria and acute azotemia, and in the absence of recent diuretic therapy, an FE_{Na} greater than 1%, a urine osmolality less than 350 mOsm/kg H_2O, and a urine sodium concentration over 40 mEq/L are characteristic of ATN. However, an FE_{Na} less than 1% can occur in nonoliguric ATN associated with radiocontrast agents, sepsis, burns, liver failure, and edematous states, in interstitial nephritis, in acute obstruction, and in acute poststreptococcal glomerulonephritis.

DIAGNOSIS OF ACUTE RENAL FAILURE

The first step is to exclude causes of spurious elevations in the S_{Cr}. The next step is to determine whether the ARF is acute or chronic (Tables 26.3 and 26.4).

The next step is to identify patients with pre- or postrenal ARF (Tables 26.1 and 26.5). Oliguric patients should have a single bladder catheterization. All patients should have a complete urinalysis and renal ultrasound to search for obstruction. If suspicion of obstruction is high, the ultrasound should be repeated, and further diagnostic tests (e.g., retrograde pyelogram, computed tomography, furosemide renogram) undertaken.

Acute Renovascular Disease

The presentation of acute renovascular disease (see Chapter 22) is given in Table 26.6. Its possible etiologies include the following:

- Aortic aneurysm (dissection, thrombosis)
- Renal artery dissection or thrombosis (trauma, angioplasty)
- Embolism (thrombus, cholesterol)
- Thrombotic microangiopathy
- Renal vein thrombosis

Acute Interstitial Nephritis

See Chapter 12 for a complete description of this condition.

Acute Glomerulonephritis and Vasculitis

Features suggestive of glomerulonephritis or vasculitis (see Chapters 8, 9, and 10) include fever, skin rash, arthralgias, or evidence of systemic disease or pulmonary involvement. Helpful laboratory findings include an elevated erythrocyte sedimenta-

---

TABLE 26.4   Features Suggestive of Chronic Renal Disease

Family history of renal disease (e.g., polycystic kidney disease)
History of chronic disease causing renal insufficiency (e.g., diabetes mellitus)
Polyuria, nocturia, or symptoms of chronic urinary obstruction or infections
Normocytic normochromic anemia
Radiologic evidence of renal osteodystrophy
Bilateral small (<10 cm) or scarred kidneys on ultrasound

TABLE 26.5   Features Suggestive of Obstructive Uropathy

Elderly man with acute or progressive renal failure
History of previous urinary tract obstruction or infections

Symptoms of bladder outflow obstruction (e.g., dysuria, nocturia, frequency, hesitation)

History of diseases known to predispose to papillary necrosis (e.g., diabetes mellitus, sickle cell disease, or analgesic abuse)

Pelvic or retroperitoneal disease or surgery
Complete anuria or wide variations in urine output
Normal urinalysis with progressive renal failure

tion rate, low complement levels, positive tests for collagen vascular disease, and hematuria or red blood cell casts.

Acute Tubular Necrosis

The diagnosis of ATN is made by exclusion of all other conditions. Renal biopsy should normally be performed in patients with suspected ATN in whom ARF persists beyond 4 weeks in the absence of a known etiology.

Clinical Course
The clinical course of ATN can be divided into three phases:

1. Initiating phase. This period between the onset of decreased renal function and established renal failure is usually reversible by treating the underlying disorder.
2. Maintenance phase. Renal failure is not immediately reversible. The duration is hours to several weeks. Renal function usually improves spontaneously after 10 to 16 days in oliguric patients and 5 to 8 days in nonoliguric patients.
3. Recovery phase. The BUN and S_{Cr} return toward normal. Patients may enter a polyuric phase that can cause fluid and electrolyte imbalances. Recovery of renal function usually occurs within 4 weeks but may be incomplete.

Management
First, reversible factors must be sought and treated rapidly and exhaustively. Conversion of oliguric to nonoliguric ATN facili-

tates management but does not reduce mortality. This may be achieved with a loop diuretic such as furosemide (80–400 mg IV, repeated once after 1 hour). High doses of loop diuretics may impair hearing and should not be administered indiscriminately. Administration of furosemide as an IV infusion (10–15 mg/hr) may be more effective than single doses. Complications can be prevented by close monitoring of fluid and electrolyte balance and by serial assessment of clinical and biochemical parameters, as indicated below.

Fluid Intake   Restrict fluids (<1 L/day in oliguria) to match measurable plus insensible losses.

Electrolytes   Restrict intake to match measured losses. This is usually less than 2 g or 86 mEq/day for sodium and less than 1.5 g or 40 mEq/day for potassium.

Diet   Restrict protein to 0.6 g/kg/day (high biological value). Provide at least 35 kcal/kg nonprotein calories. Allow for weight loss of 0.5 lb/day through catabolism. Consider hyperalimentation early, especially in catabolic patients.

Biochemical Monitoring

- Serum sodium. Avoid hyponatremia by restricting free water.
- Serum potassium. Treat hyperkalemia with glucose plus insulin, sodium bicarbonate, Kayexalate, or dialysis. Use calcium gluconate for cardiac effects (see Chapter 16).
- Serum bicarbonate. Maintain serum pH above 7.20 and bicarbonate above 20 mEq/L.
- Serum phosphate. Control hyperphosphatemia with phosphate binders (see Chapter 18).
- Serum calcium. Hypocalcemia rarely requires therapy; treat only if symptomatic.

Drugs   Avoid magnesium-containing medications. Adjust drug dosages for level of renal function (see Chapter 32).

Dialysis   Early dialysis simplifies management and nutritional support. Hemodialysis, continuous renal replacement therapy, and peritoneal dialysis are all effective (see Chapters 28 and 29). Indications are given in Chapter 28. The predialysis BUN and S_{Cr} should be maintained below 100 and 8 mg/dl, respectively.

TABLE 26.6   Features Suggestive of Acute Renovascular Disease

Hypertension (new onset or accelerated)

Aortic or renal arterial disease (aneurysm, abdominal bruits, reduced femoral pulses)

Vascular disease elsewhere (peripheral, cerebral)

Source for arterial embolization (infective endocarditis, atrial fibrillation, recent MI)

Cholesterol embolization (recent aortic catheterization, livedo reticularis, elevated erythrocyte sedimentation rate, peripheral eosinophilia, reduced complement, thrombocytopenia)

Evidence of thrombotic microangiopathy (thrombocytopenia, microangiopathic anemia, fever, neurologic abnormalities)

Nephrotic syndrome with proximal dysfunction (suggests renal vein thrombosis)

Prognosis

Mortality from ATN is 20% to 50% for medical patients and 60% to 70% for surgical patients. Factors associated with an increased mortality include advanced age, severe underlying disease, and multiple organ failure. Leading causes of death are infections, progression of the underlying disease, gastrointestinal hemorrhage, and fluid and electrolyte disturbances. Mortality has not changed during the past 20 years.

Suggested Readings

Agmon Y, Brezis M. Acute renal failure: a multifactorial syndrome. Pathogenesis and prevention strategies. *Contrib Nephrol* 1993;102:23–36.

Davda RJ, Guzman NJ. Acute renal failure: prompt diagnosis is key to effective management. *Postgrad Med J* 1994;96:89–101.

Hays SR. Ischemic renal failure. *Am J Med Sci* 1992;304:93–108.

Mehra MJ, Sharif K, Bode FR. Radiocontrast-induced nephropathy: prevention is better than cure. *Postgrad Med J* 1992;92:215–223.

Nolan CR, Anderson RJ. Hospital-acquired acute renal failure. *J Am Soc Nephrol* 1998;9:710–718.

Rabb H. Evaluation of urinary markers in acute renal failure. *Curr Opin Nephrol Hyperten* 1998; 7:681–685.

Solomon R, Werner C, Mann D, D'Elia J, Silva P. Effects of saline, mannitol, and furosemide on acute decreases in renal function induced by radiocontrast agents. *N Engl J Med* 1994;331:1416–1420.

Star RA. Treatment of acute renal failure. *Kidney Int* 1998;54:1817–1831.

Vijayan A, Miller SB. Acute renal failure: prevention and nondialytic therapy. *Semin Nephrol* 1998;18:523–532.

Chapter 27

Chronic Renal Failure

Abdul R. Amir
James F. Winchester

Chronic renal failure (CRF) is diminished renal function secondary to irreversible loss of functioning nephrons. End-stage renal disease (ESRD) is advanced CRF requiring dialysis or kidney transplantation.

PATHOPHYSIOLOGY

Loss of nephron mass results in structural and functional hypertrophy of the remaining nephrons. This restores the glomerular filtration rate (GFR). The single nephron glomerular capillary filtration coefficient (K_f), glomerular plasma flow, and intraglomerular pressure increase as a result of preferential vasodilation of the afferent arterioles. Proximal reabsorption of NaCl, fluid, and phosphate and collecting duct secretion of K^+ and H^+ are enhanced. However, the effective hyperfiltration response contributes to ongoing glomerular injury, resulting in an autodestructive process of progressive glomerular sclerosis and further loss of renal function.

Growth factors such as transforming growth factor β, platelet-derived growth factor, osteopontin, angiotensin II, and endothelin contribute to interstitial fibrosis. The reduction in GFR correlates with the degree of interstitial and tubular fibrosis.

CLINICAL PREDICTORS OF ACCELERATED PROGRESSION TO END-STAGE RENAL DISEASE

The Modification of Diet in Renal Disease (MDRD) study defined six independent risk factors for progressive loss of GFR (see References). These include black race, diagnosis of polycystic kidney disease, high mean arterial pressure, high-grade proteinuria, reduced serum transferrin (indicating malnutrition), and reduced high-density lipoprotein (HDL)-cholesterol (see Table 27.1).

INCIDENCE AND PREVALENCE OF END-STAGE RENAL DISEASE

The United States renal data system for the year 1996 reported 290,000 patients treated for ESRD. There are 75,000 new patients annually. Etiologies of ESRD are listed in Table 27.2.

UREMIC SYNDROME

Uremia is a constellation of signs and symptoms associated with CRF that result from retention of urea and end products of protein metabolism that are normally excreted in the urine. Uremic symptoms are not strictly related to the serum creatinine concentration (S_{Cr}) or the creatinine clearance (C_{Cr}). However, symptoms are common when the C_{Cr} falls below 10 ml/min. Diabetic patients may become symptomatic at a higher value of C_{Cr}.

Urea is synthesized in the liver from CO_2 and ammonia. Administration of urea to normal subjects results in only mild symptoms. Other potential uremic toxins include guanidine, guanidinosuccinic acid, β_2-microglobulin, hippurates, homocysteine, parathyroid hormone (PTH), phenols, phosphates, polyamines, and purines.

TABLE 27.1 Factors Contributing to Progression of CRF

The degree of systemic and intraglomerular hypertension
The degree of proteinuria
Glomerular hypertrophy with increase of wall stress
Intrarenal deposition of calcium phosphate or urate
Hyperlipidemia (increased low-density lipoprotein cholesterol, LDL)
Impaired prostaglandin generation with the use of NSAIDs
High-protein diet
Persistent metabolic acidosis and increased ammonia production
The extent of tubulointerstitial disease.

TABLE 27.2   Etiology of End-Stage Renal Disease

Condition	Fraction of total patients (%)
Diabetes mellitus	39
Hypertension and large-vessel disease	28
Glomerulonephritis, primary or secondary	13
Hereditary cystic and congenital renal diseases	4
Interstitial nephritis and pyelonephritis	4
Neoplasm/tumor	2
Unknown	4
Miscellaneous	3
Missing	3

METABOLIC AND ELECTROLYTE ABNORMALITIES IN CHRONIC RENAL FAILURE

Carbohydrate Intolerance

Insulin is degraded by the liver and by the kidneys. Its clearance is reduced in patients with CRF. This may explain the occasional episodes of hypoglycemia that these patients experience. However, the effects of a decrease in insulin clearance are generally more than offset by peripheral insulin resistance secondary to a postreceptor defect. Hyperparathyroidism inhibits insulin secretion and worsens any glucose intolerance. There is generally a decrease in requirements for insulin and oral hypoglycemic agents in diabetic patients as they develop renal failure.

Hyperlipidemia

Decreased plasma levels of high-density lipoprotein (HDL)-cholesterol and increased plasma levels of triglycerides and lipoprotein a antigen [Lp(a)] are common in CRF. These adverse lipid changes are usually mitigated by a decreased level of LDL cholesterol due to a decrease in lipoprotein lipase activity. The dyslipidemia can be ascribed primarily to hyperparathyroidism and insulin resistance.

Fluid and Electrolytes

There is an impaired ability to excrete free water rapidly because of a defect in tubular concentrating ability and a reduction in the

GFR. Normally, there is also an inability to excrete NaCl rapidly because of a defect in renal tubular regulatory mechanisms and a reduced GFR. The result is a subtle or overt expansion of the plasma and extracellular fluid volumes, leading to a high prevalence of salt-sensitive hypertension and edema as CRF progresses toward ESRD. Hyponatremia can result from failure to restrict free water to less than 1.5 L, leading to volume overload edema. Hypertension results from a failure to restrict Na^+ intake to 100 mEq/day.

In contrast, occasional patients, especially those with CRF caused by tubulointerstitial disease or primary diseases of the medulla, are unable to conserve NaCl and develop orthostatic hypotension and prerenal azotemia. These unusual patients with salt-losing nephropathy require stepwise increases in NaCl and fluid intake until these effects are reversed.

Potassium elimination in CRF is initially maintained by enhanced K^+ secretion by surviving nephrons and by colonic K^+ secretion. These adaptations are mediated hyperaldosteronism. However, as patients become oliguric and the GFR decreases to below 10ml/min, K^+ elimination is curtailed. Cellular K^+ uptake is also impaired in CRF. This is related to insulin resistance, β_2-adrenergic resistance, decreased Na^+/K^+-ATPase activity and metabolic acidosis. Therefore, hyperkalemia is frequent in CRF.

Acid–Base Abnormalities

Metabolic acidosis in CRF occurs primarily because of a defect in ammoniagenesis that limits distal tubular H^+ trapping as NH_4^+ and hence decreases renal bicarbonate regeneration. Additionally, there may be proximal HCO_3^- wasting or reduced distal H^+ secretion. Chronic metabolic acidosis should be corrected because it is accompanied by skeletal demineralization. As the GFR falls below 10 ml/min, there is a progressive retention of organic acids that raises the anion gap with a reciprocal fall in serum $[HCO_3^-]$.

Calcium and Phosphate Abnormalities and Renal Osteodystrophy

Phosphate retention begins when GFR is less than 25 to 50 ml/min. Metabolic acidosis increases bone resorption and raises the serum calcium (S_{Ca}) and phosphate concentrations. Hyperphosphatemia increases PTH secretion, reduces ionized S_{Ca}, and inhibits the renal hydroxylation of $25(OH)D_3$ to its active metabolite, $1,25(OH)_2D_3$.

This provides a further stimulus to PTH secretion. A decrease in active vitamin D decreases intestinal absorption and leads to hypocalcemia, which increases PTH further.

Renal osteodystrophy is classified in Table 27.3. Osteomalacia and adynamic bone disease can be caused by excessive aluminum deposition, which inhibits bone remodeling and mineralization. Adynamic bone disease is common in elderly diabetic patients and those receiving peritoneal dialysis. Patients with aluminum bone disease may have associated features of proximal muscle weakness, bone pain, resistant anemia, or dementia.

CARDIOVASCULAR ABNORMALITIES OF END-STAGE RENAL DISEASE

Hypertension

Hypertension occurs in 85% to 95% of patients with ESRD. It is ascribed primarily to excessive salt and water retention. Inappropriate secretion of renin and angiotensin and increased sympathetic tone often contribute. Blood vessels generate excessive quantities of the vasoconstrictor endothelin and diminished quantities of the vasodilator nitric oxide. Treatment of hypertension decreases the risk of cardiovascular mortality and slows the progression of renal failure in those with moderate or heavy proteinuria.

Cardiomyopathy and Pericarditis

The prevalence of left ventricular hypertrophy (LVH), coronary artery disease, and congestive heart failure (CHF) is increased two- to fivefold in ESRD. About half of all hemodialysis patients have

TABLE 27.3   Different Forms of Renal Osteodystrophy

Type of bone disease	Prevalence (%)
High-turnover bone disease	
Osteitis fibrosa cystica	53
Mixed uremic osteodystrophy	13
Low-turnover bone disease	
Adynamic bone disease	27
Osteomalacia	7

significant ischemic heart disease. Dyslipidemia, hypertension, hyperhomocysteinemia, diabetes mellitus, and insulin resistance are common in ESRD and may be risk factors for the development of atherosclerosis.

Diastolic dysfunction may present as heart failure and hypertension. This is more common in ESRD than systolic dysfunction with left ventricular dilation. Rarer causes of cardiac dysfunction include hyperparathyroidism, amyloidosis, and iron overload. Anemia aggravates LVH in patients with ESRD.

Pericarditis can present with a sharp pericardial chest pain that changes in its intensity with breathing or posture and is accompanied by a rub. Pericardial fluid is usually hemorrhagic, and tamponade can occur. Some patients have uremic pericarditis that responds to extra dialysis treatment.

NEUROMUSCULAR ABNORMALITIES

Changes in the function of the central nervous system (CNS) are characterized by decreased attention span, agitation, confusion, insomnia, and impaired memory. Patients may develop depression, hallucination, and delusion. Other symptoms or signs include hiccup, cramps, asterixis, myoclonus, fasciculations, and seizures.

Peripheral neuropathy is uncommon. It is usually symmetric and affects preferentially the lower extremities, with sensory involvement preceding motor dysfunction. Restless leg syndrome and burning feet are early phases of uremic peripheral neuropathy. Postural hypotension can be a manifestation of autonomic dysfunction.

HEMATOLOGIC ABNORMALITIES

Anemia

The anemia of CRF is normochromic and normocytic. The hematocrit falls as the S_{Cr} increases above 2 to 3 mg/dl. At the time of ESRD, the hematocrit is 15% to 30%. The primary cause of anemia is inadequate erythropoietin production by the diseased kidneys. Other causes include inhibition of erythroid production by retained uremic toxins, iron deficiency because of blood loss, and a short red blood cell life span because of a defect in Na^+/K^+-ATPase membrane pumps leading to mild hemolysis. Patients with renal disease are usually malnourished and may develop deficiencies of folic acid, thiamine, or pyridoxine. Therefore, patients with anemia and CRF require an assessment of iron nutrition and vitamin status, and erythropoietin therapy.

Uremic Bleeding Diathesis

This causes frequent bruising, ecchymoses, and bleeding from mucous membranes. Subdural hematomas can occur. There is a defect in platelet function that impairs platelet activation and adhesion to the endothelium. This has been ascribed to abnormalities of the von Willebrand factor (vWF), which facilitates the interaction between platelets and endothelium through its binding to platelet glycoprotein (GpIIb-IIIa) receptors. Other studies have implicated an abnormal formation of nitric oxide that inhibits platelet function by increasing cyclic guanosine monophosphate (cGMP) concentration. Anemia exacerbates uremic bleeding. Erythrocytes enhance platelet function by inactivating prostacyclin (PGI_2), which inhibits platelet aggregation by increasing the interaction of platelets with the vessel wall.

GASTROINTESTINAL ABNORMALITIES

Most patients with ESRD have gastrointestinal complaints. These include anorexia and early morning nausea and vomiting. As renal failure progresses, patients may develop uremic fetor, stomatitis, esophagitis, gastritis, duodenitis, and peptic ulcer disease. Gastrin is degraded by the liver and the kidney. Therefore, it has a prolonged half-life in patients with CRF. There is an increased incidence of gastroparesis and gastrointestinal bleeding because of vascular ectasia and peptic ulcer disease.

DERMATOLOGIC ABNORMALITIES

Uremic pruritus is related to calcium phosphate deposition as a consequence of secondary hyperparathyroidism, peripheral neuropathy, a dry skin, and anemia. It is usually resistant to treatment but may respond to naloxone. A yellow discoloration is related to the retention of urochrome pigments and urea.

EVALUATION OF CHRONIC RENAL FAILURE

The history should document the presence of uremic symptoms and possible etiology from conditions such as diabetes mellitus, hypertension, congestive heart failure, prolonged intake of nonsteroidal antiinflammatory drugs (NSAIDs), or multiple myeloma. A family history suggests the diagnosis of polycystic kidney disease or hereditary nephritis. A reduced kidney size by ultrasound imaging suggests CRF, although patients with diabetic nephropathy, amyloid, or multiple myeloma often have large kidneys. The degree of renal insufficiency may be determined by measuring BUN, S_{Cr}, and creatinine clearance or by nuclear medicine methods (Chapter 3). Volume depletion and obstructive nephropathy should be identified and treated promptly.

PREVENTION OF PROGRESSION OF RENAL DISEASE

Blood Pressure Control

The Multiple Risk Factor Intervention Trial (MRFIT) concluded that even mild hypertension is a risk for developing renal insufficiency. The Modification of Diet in Renal Disease (MDRD) randomized patients with CRF to a normal or low BP goal. Those randomized to a mean blood pressure of 92 mm Hg or less (125/75 mm Hg) had a slowing of the rate of progression of renal failure. This effect was confined to those with more than 1 to 3 g/24 hr of proteinuria. This blood pressure goal should be applied to all patients with proteinuria of more than 1 g/day.

Proteinuria

The degree of proteinuria is a reliable predictor of the rate of decline of renal function. Recent studies have indicated that the process of albumin filtration, reabsorption by the tubules, and metabolism elicits a cytokine response that may contribute to interstitial inflammation and fibrosis, which promote progressive loss of nephron function. Therefore, a reduction in proteinuria is now a treatment goal for patients with CRF.

Angiotensin-converting enzyme (ACE) inhibitors and angiotensin receptor blockers (ARBs) are the most effective agents in reducing proteinuria. Some studies also show that they are more effective than other antihypertensive agents in slowing the rate of loss of GFR in patients with CRF with or without diabetic nephropathy. Patients must be monitored for azotemia and hyperkalemia. Nondihydropyridine calcium channel blockers (diltiazem and verapamil) reduce proteinuria, but dihydropyridines are ineffective.

Dietary Protein and Restriction

Restricting dietary protein can ameliorate many of the symptoms of uremia and some of its metabolic complications. It also may slow the rate of progression of CRF by preventing glomerular hypertension and reducing angiotensin II and thromboxane formation. Protein restriction must provide adequate dietary intake to prevent malnutrition. Restriction to 0.6 g/kg/day is recommended for patients with moderate to severe CRF (GFR 5–25 ml/min). A more modest restriction to 0.8 to 1.0 g/kg/day can be prescribed for those with a GFR of 25–50 ml/min. For those with proteinuria, the daily protein intake is increased by the degree of measured 24-hour protein excretion. Compliance with dietary protein prescription is estimated by calculating the nitrogen intake (I_N) from 24-hour urinary urea nitrogen excretion (UUN):

$$\text{Nitrogen balance} = I_N - \left[\text{UUN} + \text{nonurea nitrogen} \right.$$
$$\left. \text{excretion} \left(\text{NUN}\right)\right]$$
$$\text{NUN} \left(g\right) = 0.031 \times \text{body weight} \left(kg\right)$$
$$I_N = \text{UUN} + \text{NUN}$$
$$\text{Daily protein consumption} \left(g\right) = I_N \times 6.25$$

These calculations assume that the patient is in steady state. Presently, the role of protein restriction is unresolved. The MDRD study detected no overall benefit of protein restriction in slowing the rate of loss of GFR in patients with moderate or severe CRF over 3 years. Protein restriction is difficult to achieve and requires the close cooperation of a nutritionist. It is not clear whether there are benefits of protein restriction in slowing progression of CRF above those that can be achieved by ACEIs, ARBs, and a reduced BP goal.

MANAGEMENT OF COMPLICATIONS OF CHRONIC RENAL FAILURE

Fluid and Electrolyte Disorders

Dietary NaCl restriction is required to control hypertension and prevent edema. The goal should be a daily Na^+ intake of less than 100 mEq. More severe restrictions to 80 mEq are needed for severe hypertension or diuretic resistance. Frequently, loop diuretics are also required (Chapter 25). Hyponatremia is treated by fluid restriction (1–1.5 L/day). Hyperkalemia is a life-threatening complication. Exogenous sources of potassium (foods with high K^+ content such as citrus fruits, chocolate, and salt substitutes) and medications that can cause hyperkalemia (ACEIs, ARBs, NSAIDs, K^+-sparing diuretics, β-blockers, and heparin) should be discontinued. Patients with hyperkalemia and electrocardiographic changes should be treated promptly with intravenous calcium gluconate or calcium chloride (10 ml of 10% solutions) followed by an infusion of 25 ml of 50% dextrose solutions with insulin. A $β_2$-adrenergic agonist (nebulized albuterol) is a useful adjunct to lower S_K. Bicarbonate administration lowers S_K more gradually over 6 to 24 hours. Oral alkali supplementation with sodium bicarbonate or citrate (650 mg or 8 mEq/tablet) should be instituted if the serum bicarbonate concentrations fall below 15 to 17 mEq/L. Sodium citrate should be avoided in patients taking aluminum-containing antacids, as it enhances intestinal aluminum absorption.

Hyperphosphatemia and Secondary Hyperparathyroidism

The dietary phosphorus intake of patients with moderate or severe CRF must be reduced to less than 10 mg/kg/day. Inadequate control of hyperphosphatemia requires institution of calcium-based phosphate binders in the form of calcium carbonate (Oscal, Tums), calcium acetate (Phoslo), or calcium citrate. These must be consumed with food because, if they are ingested on an empty stomach, they cause hypercalcemia. RenaGel is an alternative phosphate binder that rarely causes hypercalcemia.

Vitamin D (calcitriol) is usually required to replace decreased renal production of $1,25(OH)D_3$. It must be withheld until the serum phosphate concentration has been controlled to below 6 mg/dl because it may cause diffuse soft tissue calcification. The usual starting dose is 0.25 μg daily, which is increased in 2-to 4-week intervals to normalize the serum calcium concentration. Zemplar is a novel vitamin D analog (19-nor-1α, 25-dihdroxyvitamin D_2) that is reported to be effective in suppressing hyperparathyroidism but causes less hypercalcemia. Parathyroidectomy is indicated in patients with symptomatic soft tissue calcification and for severe secondary hyperparathyroidism that is refractory to calcitriol therapy.

Anemia

Correction of anemia with recombinant human erythropoietin (Epogen) improves cardiac function, exercise tolerance, sexual function, and psychological health. It should be initiated at a hematocrit of 30% or if the patient is symptomatic from anemia. The usual starting dose is 80 to 150 units/kg administered subcutaneously two to three times per week. The goal is to maintain the hematocrit at 33% to 36%. Failure to respond to erythropoietin suggests iron or vitamin deficiency, aluminum intoxication, severe hyperparathyroidism, an acute inflammatory process, or occult blood loss.

Hyperlipidemia

The goal of therapy should be to maintain the LDL-cholesterol below 130 mg/dl or, for patients at high risk, under 100 mg/dl. Patients should be started on a step I American Heart Association diet that provides less than 30% of total calories from fat and less than 300 mg cholesterol daily. After 2 months, if goals are not achieved, drug therapy with hydroxy-3-methylglutaryl coenzyme A (HMG-CoA) reductase inhibitors is usually indicated. In patients refractory to monotherapy, nicotinic acid may be added. Nicotinic acid specifically reduces the elevated levels of Lp(a) in CRF.

Suggested Readings

Kopple JD, Levey AS, Greene T, et al, for the Modification of Diet in Renal Disease Study Group. Effect of dietary protein restriction on nutritional status in the Modification of Diet in Renal Disease Study. *Kidney Int* 1997;52:778–791.

Lazarus JM, Bourgoignie JJ, Buckalew VM, et al. Achievement and safety of a low blood pressure goal in chronic renal disease. The Modification of Diet in Renal Disease Study Group. *Hypertension* 1997;29:641.

Martin KJ, Gonzalez E, Gellens M, Hamm LL, Abboud H, Lindberg J. 19-Nor-1α-25-dihydroxyvitamin D_2 (Paricalcitol) safely and effectively reduces the levels of intact parathyroid hormone in patients on hemodialysis. *J Am Soc Nephrol* 1998;9:1427.

Michael A. Hyperkalemia in end-stage renal disease: mechanisms and management. *J Am Soc Nephrol* 1995;6:1134–1142.

Remuzzi G, Minetti L. Anemia and coagulopathy. In: Brady HR, Wilcox CS, eds. *Therapy in nephrology and hypertension*. Philadelphia: WB Saunders, 1998:480–487.

Revicki DA, Brown RE, Feeny DH, et al. Health-related quality of life associated with recombinant human erythropoietin therapy for predialysis chronic renal disease patients. *Am J Kidney Dis* 1998;25:548.

Ruggenenti P, Perna A, Mosconi L, Pisoni R, Remuzzi G, on behalf of the 'Gruppo Italiono di Studi Epidemiologici in Nefrologia' (GISEN). Urinary protein excretion rate is the best independent predictor of ESRD in non-diabetic proteinuric chronic nephropathies. *Kidney Int* 1998;53: 1209–1216.

Striker GE, Klahr S. Clinical trials in progression of chronic renal failure. In: Schrier RW, Abboud FM, Baxter JD, Fauci AS, eds. *Advances in internal medicine, vol 42*. St Louis: CV Mosby, 1997:555–595.

United States Renal Data System. *USRDS 1998 Annual Data Report*. Bethesda, MD: National Institutes of Health, National Institutes of Diabetes and Digestive and Kidney Diseases, 1998.

Venkatesan J, Henrich WL. Anemia, hypertension, and myocardial dysfunction in end-stage renal disease. *Semin Nephrol* 1997;17:257–269.

Chapter 28

Hemodialysis and Continuous Therapies

Edward A. Ross
Leonid V. Yankulin

Hemodialysis is defined as the movement of solute and water from the patient's blood across a semipermeable membrane (the dialyzer) into the dialysate. The dialyzer may also be used to remove large volumes of fluid. This is accomplished by ultrafiltration, in which hydrostatic pressure causes the bulk flow of plasma water (with comparatively few solutes) through the membrane. With advances in vascular access, anticoagulation, and the production of reliable and efficient dialyzers, hemodialysis has become the predominant method of treatment for acute and chronic renal failure in the United States.

INDICATIONS FOR HEMODIALYSIS

Most patients with acute renal insufficiency are successfully managed without dialysis (see Chapter 26). Factors to be considered before initiating hemodialysis in patients with chronic renal failure should include comorbid conditions and patient preference. Timing of therapy is dictated by serum chemistries and symptoms. Hemodialysis is usually started when the creatinine clearance decreases below 10 ml/min, which typically corresponds to a serum creatinine of 8 to 10 mg/dl. However, more important than the absolute laboratory values is the presence of uremic symptoms. At present most patients who are not terminal from another progressive illness, or who are so mentally incompetent as to present a danger to themselves or others, are offered dialysis therapy (Table 28.1). Practice guidelines have been developed by the National Kidney Foundation for ESRD patients to

TABLE 28.1   Indications and Contraindications for Hemodialysis

Indications
  Relative
    Symptomatic azotemia including encephalopathy
    Dialyzable toxins (drug poisoning)
  Absolute
    Uremic pericarditis
    Hyperkalemia, severe (see Chapter 16)
    Diuretic unresponsive fluid overload (pulmonary edema)
    Intractable acidosis
Contraindications
  Relative
    Hypotension unresponsive to pressors
    Terminal illness
    Organic brain syndrome

assist in the choice of renal replacement therapy modality, creation of vascular access, administration of erythropoietin, and timing of the initiation of dialysis.

VASCULAR ACCESS

Provision of dialysis requires reliable repeated access to the patient's circulation that can provide blood flow of approximately 200 to 450 ml/min. Ideally, the access should be created well before the need for chronic dialysis, typically when the creatinine clearance falls below approximately 15 to 20 ml/min, depending on the tempo of the renal deterioration.

Acute Vascular Access

Internal jugular or femoral catheters have become the preferred method to obtain temporary vascular access for emergent dialysis and are useful until a more permanent access is ready. Although previously common, subclavian vein catheterization is now avoided for temporary access in all patients with chronic renal failure because of the risk of central venous stenosis, which may later cause problems establishing permanent dialysis access in the involved arm. Modern catheters with dual lumina can provide excellent bidirectional blood flow rates and can often be used in the internal jugular location for 2 to 3 weeks. Highly flexible silicone-based cuffed catheters, which are tunneled subcutaneously, may be used for much longer periods of time and have improved flow and infection rates. Femoral vein catheters, in comparison, are typically used for only 48 to 72 hours. They are not suitable for ambulatory patients, and long term use carries a significant risk of infection. Possible catheter complications include bleeding, infection, thrombosis or stenosis of the vessel, pneumothorax, and air embolus. Dialysis catheters should not be used as routine intravenous lines because breaks in sterile technique greatly increase the risk of infection and catheter thrombosis. Catheters obstructed by clot can often be successfully cleared using thrombolytic agents (streptokinase, urokinase).

In the presence of systemic bacteremia, temporary dialysis catheters should be removed, the appropriate cultures taken, including the catheter tip, and systemic antibiotics administered. The empirical antibiotic of choice is often vancomycin, which covers the most common gram-positive organisms. Effective blood levels may be maintained for up to 1 week with a single dose; however, close monitoring of blood levels is recommended, especially when high-flux dialysis is used.

Chronic Vascular Access

Arteriovenous Fistula
The arteriovenous fistula is the preferred vascular access for chronic hemodialysis and may last for years. When progression to end-stage renal failure is imminent, an effort should be made to spare the nondominant arm from venipuncture and arterial puncture. Fistulas are created by the surgical anastomosis of an artery and vein, most commonly the radial artery to the cephalic vein. Typically a new primary fistula should be allowed to mature for 2 to 4 months, during which time the vein enlarges ("arterializes") and is then used for cannulation by two needles (to and from the dialyzer). Examination of the functioning arteriovenous fistula reveals a palpable pulsation and a bruit by auscultation.

Arteriovenous Grafts
When the patient's own vessels are inadequate to create an arteriovenous fistula, native, bovine, or preferably polytetrafluoroethylene grafts (i.e., Gore-Tex) can be used to form a conduit from artery to vein. Antibiotic prophylaxis to safeguard synthetic grafts should precede procedures for which bacteremia is anticipated. Arteriovenous grafts should be placed at least 2 to 4 weeks before the anticipated need for hemodialysis.

Assessment of Vascular Access

In order to optimize dialysis delivery, it is important to assure that the access blood flow can match the desired extracorporeal pump rate. Inadequate blood supply would cause recirculation of a portion of the extracorporeal circuit and decrease dialysis effectiveness. It has been recommended that recirculation studies be performed at regular intervals, and if recirculation is greater than 10% to 15%, radiologic imaging was advised. Now, however, newer technologies allow direct measurement of intraaccess blood flow, which appears to be a superior monitoring method. Fistulograms are particularly helpful in studying an access, and in the presence of stenosis, angioplasty and stenting may correct the abnormality. In addition, imaging helps the surgeon to define the anatomy if revision is necessary.

Complications of chronic vascular access include:

- Stenosis leading to inadequate blood flow
- Thrombosis requiring surgical intervention in 24 to 48 hours
- Infection, skin erosion, or both
- Failure to develop adequate venous outflow
- Ischemic limb caused by vascular steal
- Venous hypertension syndrome
- High-output cardiac failure
- Pseudoaneurysms

HEMODIALYSIS: THE PROCEDURE

The equipment used for hemodialysis prepares the dialysate, regulates dialysate and blood flow past a semipermeable membrane, and monitors functions involving the dialysate and extracorporeal blood circuit. Heparin administration provides systemic anticoagulation.

Blood and dialysate are perfused on opposite sides of the semipermeable membrane in a countercurrent direction for maximal efficiency of solute removal. Dialysate composition, the characteristics and size of the membrane in the dialyzer, and blood and solute flow rates all affect solute removal.

Dialysate Composition

The standard glucose concentration of dialysate is 200 mg/dl. Sodium, potassium, magnesium, and calcium concentrations are prescribed as the clinical situation dictates. Low-calcium baths may be used in the acute and chronic therapy of hypercalcemia. Bicarbonate is used as the base buffer in modern dialysates, and its concentration can be changed as needed.

Dialyzers

Dialyzers are manufactured in hollow-fiber and parallel-plate configurations. Hollow-fiber dialyzers are composed of up to approximately 10,000 small-diameter fibers through which blood circulates. They have virtually replaced the parallel-plate dialyzers, which consist of a parallel arrangement of membrane sheets that form compartments for blood and dialysate. Commonly used membranes include cuprophane, cellulose acetate, and several high-porosity synthetic copolymer membranes (polyacrylonitrile, polymethylmethacrylate, and polysulfone). The nonsynthetic membranes are relatively bioincompatible in that they can activate the alternate complement pathway and lead to leukoagglutination and cytokine release. In comparison, the synthetic copolymer membranes exhibit better biocompatibility, improved ultrafiltration characteristics, and increased solute clearance, especially in the middle molecule (molecular mass 300–2,000 dalton) range. There are reports that in acute renal failure, outcomes are improved by use of biocompatible synthetic dialyzers. These membranes are also used in high-flux dialysis and hemofiltration. A disadvantage of the synthetic membranes is their high cost. Reprocessing or reuse of these dialyzers is commonly performed for chronic outpatient dialysis.

Allergic reactions, which may be caused by the membrane plastic compounds or disinfectants, are manifested by pruritus and respiratory distress on initiation of dialysis. Reactions may be prevented by rinsing the dialyzer; however, once they occur, cessation of dialysis, treatment with antihistamines, and expectant management of respiratory difficulty are required.

High-Flux Dialysis

High-flux dialysis has gained rapid acceptance and is accomplished using very permeable membranes that are also biocompatible. High blood and dialysate flow rates are used to further increase the efficiency of dialysis. These strategies may improve the clearance of larger metabolites and sometimes can permit shortening of the treatment time. Urea kinetic modeling is used to determine the adequacy of dialysis (see below).

AIMS OF DIALYTIC THERAPY

Incomplete understanding of the pathogenesis of uremic symptoms makes it difficult to define an optimum dialysis prescription. Although a predialysis blood urea nitrogen concentration of <80 mg/dl was once an aim of therapy, correlation of toxic manifestations of uremia with blood urea nitrogen is often poor. The National Cooperative Dialysis Study has shown low morbidity in chronic stable dialysis patients when time-averaged concentration urea levels are below 50 mg/dl. Time-averaged urea concentration is calculated from pre- and postdialysis blood urea nitrogen, dialysis time, and interdialytic time. More comprehensive mathematical approaches were then developed, and dialysis prescriptions are now guided by these methods of urea kinetic modeling. Key concepts in one model include the protein catabolic rate (a measure of the dietary protein intake), residual renal function, and the dimensionless parameter Kt/V_{urea}. The latter term expresses the fractional urea clearance, where K is dialyzer urea clearance, t is dialysis treatment time, and V is body urea distribution volume. This ratio determines the magnitude of decline of blood urea nitrogen during a dialysis, and it serves as a measure of the dose of dialysis related to urea removal. In practice, this parameter should be at least 1.2 to minimize uremic symptoms and is calculated using a complex set of equations. Alternatively, the more simplistic urea reduction ratio (i.e., target of a 65% reduction in BUN levels) provides much insight into dialysis adequacy. New technology for continuous monitoring of urea losses into dialysate may overcome the pitfalls of basing adequacy determination on just blood levels.

COMPLICATIONS OF HEMODIALYSIS

Hypotension

Hypotension, which is the most frequent complication during hemodialysis, has been related to prior use of acetate buffer dialysate, low-sodium dialysate (130–135 mEq/L), atherosclerotic heart disease, autonomic neuropathy, and excessive fluid weight gain. Prevention of symptomatic hypotension can be achieved by accurate determinations of dry weight, precise ultrafiltration with newer technology dialysis machines, biocompatible dialysis membranes, and reduction of antihypertensive medications immediately before dialysis.

Muscle Cramps

Muscle cramps occur commonly during rapid, high-volume ultrafiltration, causing plasma volume contraction and rapid sodium fluxes. Preventive measures include fluid restriction to gain no more than 2 kg between treatments, use of a transiently high sodium concentration in the dialysate (sodium modeling), stretching exercises, possibly carnitine supplementation, and, if clinically disabling, quinine sulfate administration (i.e., 325 mg PO before dialysis).

Dialysis Disequilibrium Syndrome

The dialysis disequilibrium syndrome is believed to result primarily from less rapid clearance of urea and other osmoles from the brain than from the blood, which results in an osmotic gradient between these compartments. This osmotic gradient leads to a net movement of water into the brain that results in cerebral edema. The syndrome is uncommon and is usually seen with the first dialytic treatments in severely azotemic patients. Other predisposing factors include severe metabolic acidosis, older age, pediatric patients, and the presence of other central nervous system disease such as a preexisting seizure disorder. Symptoms, which can occur during or after the procedure, include headache, lethargy, nausea, muscular twitching, and malaise, with rare progression to mental status changes, seizures, and even cardiorespiratory arrest. After recognition of high-risk patients, the use of smaller-surface-area dialyzers and lower blood flow rates will lessen osmotic shifts. Intradialysis mannitol infusion (25–50 g) may reduce the frequency and severity of symptoms but carries a risk of pulmonary edema.

Hypoxemia

Hypoxemia during dialysis is important in patients with compromised cardiopulmonary function. Research implicates membrane incompatibility, acid–base changes induced by the dialysate base buffer, and hypoventilation. Predisposed patients should be given supplemental oxygen and dialyzed with synthetic copolymer membranes using bicarbonate dialysate.

Arrhythmias

Hypoxemia, hypotension, removal of antiarrhythmic agents during dialysis, and rapid changes in serum bicarbonate, calcium, magnesium, and potassium (especially in patients taking digoxin) all contribute to arrhythmias in predisposed patients. Continuous electrocardiogram monitoring during dialysis is necessary in high-risk patients.

Bleeding

Uremia causes platelet dysfunction, which is best assessed by measuring the bleeding time. Heparin is typically used to prevent clotting of the extracorporeal circuit, and the dose is adjusted according to the clotting time. The action of heparin may be reversed by protamine sulfate, but if protamine sulfate is administered in excess, it has an anticoagulant effect. Dialysis may be attempted without heparin if indicated, using special protocols involving biocompatible membranes and saline rinses. Cryoprecipitate, 1-deamino-8-arginine vasopressin (DDAVP) (0.3 mg/kg body weight), and conjugated estrogen may prove successful when uremic bleeding is unresponsive to adequate dialysis.

Transfusion-Related Diseases

The incidence of hepatitis B infection has decreased dramatically since the screening of donor blood and implementation of isolation techniques. Hepatitis B vaccine induces seroconversion in 40% to 70% of hemodialysis patients. The incidence of non-A, non-B (hepatitis C) infection is also declining as blood donors are screened for hepatitis C virus antibodies. Other possible infections include human immunodeficiency virus and cytomegalovirus. Generally, fewer blood transfusions are required with the introduction of erythropoietin therapy, and this decreases the risk of blood-borne disorders.

Metabolic Bone Disease

The causes of metabolic bone disease include secondary hyperparathyroidism, oversuppression of parathyroid hormone, aluminum deposition (from aluminum-containing antacids used as phosphate binders), and a unique form of amyloid deposition (β_2-microglobulin). Clinical features common to dialysis bone disease include bone pain, arthralgias, fractures, bone cysts, and the carpal tunnel syndrome.

Acquired Renal Cystic Disease

Multiple renal cysts develop in the kidneys in up to 80% of dialysis patients treated for more than 3 years. Screening of hemodialysis patients by ultrasonography or computed tomography after 3 years on dialysis is recommended to detect malignant changes.

Pericarditis

Two distinct patterns of pericarditis are encountered in patients with renal failure. Pericarditis can occur in uremic nondialyzed patients and in those already receiving dialysis therapy. Uremic pericarditis usually responds to intensive daily dialysis, and a correlation between resolution of pericarditis and improvement in the uremia has been shown. Conversely, pericarditis that occurs in patients already on hemodialysis may be related to occult inadequate dialysis or concurrent illnesses, such as systemic lupus erythematosus or viral pericarditis. Treatment is intensive dialysis without heparin anticoagulation. The patient should be monitored clinically and by echocardiography for features suggestive of pericardial tamponade. A pericardiocentesis tray should be kept at the bedside. Patients need to be intensively monitored to detect hemodynamic instability, changes in pericardial friction rub, and pulsus paradoxus. If pericardial tamponade develops, percutaneous pericardiocentesis, placement of a pericardial window, or pericardiectomy may be necessary.

Anemia and Recombinant Human Erythropoietin

The causes of anemia in dialysis patients include decreased red blood cell production and survival and blood loss in the extracorporeal circuit. Recombinant human erythropoietin is used routinely to correct the anemia. The recommended starting dose in hemodialysis patients is typically 50 units/kg body weight IV or SC three times weekly. The dose is adjusted to keep the hematocrit between 30% and 36%. In addition to correction of anemia, recombinant human erythropoietin improves patient well-being, exercise tolerance, and cognitive function. Potential side effects include hypertension, seizures, thrombosis, iron deficiency, hyperkalemia, and flu-like symptoms. Resistance to recombinant human erythropoietin occurs in the presence of iron deficiency, aluminum toxicity, severe secondary hyperparathyroidism, infection, or other inflammatory diseases.

Dialytic Therapies in the Intensive Care Unit

Critically ill hemodynamically unstable ICU patients are typically the most challenging to treat with conventional dialytic modalities. The intermittent volume and solute fluxes may cause significant morbidity, which includes the worsening of hypotension and arrhythmias. Although there are yet to be convincing data that mortality can be improved, many investigators have proposed benefits from various forms of continuous renal replacement therapy (CRRT). Because acute peritoneal dialysis often cannot yield adequate solute removal or is precluded by abdominal surgery, peritoneal leaks, or peritonitis, a variety of blood clearance modalities were devised. The simplest of these methods utilizes hemofiltration, which relies on ultrafiltration (rather than diffusion) to move solutes across a high-porosity, semipermeable membrane. In continuous arteriovenous hemofiltration (CAVH), blood pressure alone provides the driving force for ultrafiltration. Large volumes of ultrafiltrate (up to 1, 200 ml/hr), with a composition similar to that of plasma water, can be generated (see Table 28.2 for indications). These losses are replaced by a balanced electrolyte solution (modified by the clinical situation and indicated in Table 28.3) in amounts determined by desired fluid losses or gains. The quantity of solute removed is a function of the amount of ultrafiltrate generated. Solute removal may be enhanced by continuously passing dialysate solution across the hemofilter using a pump. These techniques are known as continuous arteriovenous hemodialysis

TABLE 28.2   Indications for CAVH

Acute renal failure (with hemodynamic instability)
Need for parenteral nutrition in acute renal failure
Cardiogenic shock with pulmonary edema and inadequate urine output
Diuretic unresponsive congestive heart failure

TABLE 28.3   CAVH Replacement Solutions

Solution (connected by four-prong manifold)	
1 L 0.9% NaCl + 5.3 mL 10% CaCl$_2$	
1 L 0.9% NaCl + 0.8 mL 50% MgSO$_4$	
1 L 0.9% NaCl	
1 L D$_5$ W + 150 mEq NaHCO$_3$	
This yields (mEq/L)	
Na	153
K	0
Cl	119
HCO$_3$	37.5
Ca	2.4
Mg	2.0 mg/dL
Dextrose	1,250 mg/dL

(CAVHD) and hemodiafiltration (CAVHDF) and are particularly useful in catabolic patients. Arteriovenous access is obtained with large-bore catheters, most commonly in the femoral vessels. Systemic heparinization is usually required and necessitates regular monitoring. A frequent problem in continuous arteriovenous hemofiltration is a sudden decrease in ultrafiltrate production caused by kinked blood lines, improper elevation of the ultrafiltrate collection bag, hypotension, blood leaks, or hemoconcentration. A 50- to 100-ml bolus of normal saline (with the arterial line momentarily clamped) can be used to check for a clotted hemofilter. Advantages and disadvantages of continuous arteriovenous hemofiltration are listed in Table 28.4.

To overcome the blood flow limitations of CAVHD and avoid the need for arterial access, there has been the rapidly growing use of venovenous techniques (CVVH, CVVHD, CVVHDF). These have the disadvantage of the risks of continuous blood pumps but may offer the luxury of microprocessor-controlled fluid delivery and removal rates, user-friendly interfaces, and automated troubleshooting. At high pump speeds the daily solute and fluid clearance rates can match or even exceed those of daily conventional hemodialysis, which is particularly appropriate for very catabolic patients (i.e., those with sepsis or burns), who require high-dose or high-volume parenteral nutrition. Unfortunately, the complications from anticoagulating the extracorporeal circuit may limit the use of CVVH or necessitate complex protocols for regional anticoagulation (such as with citrate). These machines may also be used for fluid removal alone (slow continuous ultrafiltration, SCUF) for

TABLE 28.4 Advantages and Disadvantages of CAVH

Advantages
  Ease of initiation
  Gradual correction of uremia and electrolyte and acid–base abnormalities
  Precise fluid control
  Rare hypotension, less hemodynamic instability
  Large volumes of parenteral nutrition may be administered
  Technically less demanding
Disadvantages
  Intensive care unit setting only
  Poor emergent treatment for hyperkalemia and acidosis
  Systemic heparinization
  Possible inability to control nitrogen balance (intermittent hemodialysis needed)
  Requires adequate vascular (arterial) access
  Access site infection
  Requires strict fluid monitoring

renal support, as in select patients with severe congestive heart failure and inadequate urine volume. There is a growing appreciation that there are other special circumstances for which this modality may be particularly helpful, such as in neonates with congenital enzyme deficiencies, and hypo-and hyperthermia.

Because of the risks from continuous anticoagulation, the logistic difficulties in training large numbers of ICU nurses, the expense of new equipment and custom sterile fluids, and the difficulty in identifying patient subpopulations with improved outcomes from CVVH, recently some clinicians have returned to intermittent hemodialysis. They report satisfactory hemodynamic and clearance results using prolonged treatments (8 to 12 hours) with conventional machines slightly modified to deliver slow low-efficiency dialysis (SLED).

DIALYTIC TECHNIQUES IN DRUG OVERDOSE

Hemodialysis and a related technique, hemoperfusion, are occasionally helpful in the management of overdose or toxins. Charcoal hemoperfusion utilizes coated or uncoated charcoal particles to adsorb toxins or drugs. Complications are due to its bioincompatibility and include thrombocytopenia.

In acute poisonings, hemodialysis has the advantage of correcting any concurrent acid–base and electrolyte disturbances.

Table 28.5 gives a brief listing of medications removed by hemodialysis or hemoperfusion. Antidepressants and benzodiazapines are poorly removed by dialytic techniques. Dialysis for poisoning should be considered only when supportive measures are ineffective or there is impending irreversible organ toxicity.

OTHER CONSIDERATIONS IN CARE OF DIALYSIS PATIENTS

The following are important practical aspects in the care of hemodialysis patients that must be emphasized:

- Fluid intake should be limited to 1 to 1.5 L/day to avoid fluid overload because these patients are usually oligoanuric. For dietary therapy refer to Chapter 31.
- Phosphate binders, such as calcium carbonate, calcium acetate, sevelamer, and aluminum hydroxide, should be administered with meals.
- Many drugs, such as antibiotics and antiarrhythmics, are removed by hemodialysis. Therefore, alteration of dosage, supplemental doses, and monitoring of blood levels are frequently required. This may be especially problematic in patients undergoing hemofiltration.
- These patients are often on intravenous medications, such as recombinant human erythropoietin and vitamin D, as outpatients. These should be continued when the patients are admitted to the hospital.
- Magnesium-containing antacids and laxatives, or phosphorus-based (Fleets) enemas, should be avoided to prevent hypermagnesemia and hyperphosphatemia, respectively.
- If blood transfusions are required, they should be administered during hemodialysis to avoid fluid overload and hyperkalemia.

TABLE 28.5 Common Drugs and Toxins Removed by Hemodialysis

Alcohol (methanol)	Mannitol
Aspirin	Radiocontrast dye
Ethylene glycol	Theophylline[a]
Lithium	

[a] Hemodialysis or hemoperfusion is effective.

- Because these patients are immunosuppressed and frequently hypothermic, there should be a low threshold for an intensive work-up if they present with features suggestive of infection.
- Specific dialysis treatment goals, such as optimum fluid removal and target pulmonary capillary wedge pressure, should be discussed with the nephrologist.
- If invasive procedures are planned, the nephrologist should be informed in advance to modify the dialysis schedule, alter heparin dosage, and correct bleeding time abnormalities.

Suggested Readings

Couch P, Stumpf JL. Management of uremic bleeding. *Clin Pharmacol* 1990;9:673–681.

Daugirdas JT, Ing TS, eds. *Handbook of dialysis.* Boston: Little, Brown, 1994.

Forni LG, Hilton PJ. Continuous hemofiltration in the treatment of acute renal failure. *N Engl J Med* 1997;336:1303–1309.

Golper TA. Continuous arteriovenous hemofiltration in acute renal failure. *Am J Kidney Dis* 1985;6:373–386.

Hakim RM, Wingard RL, Parker RA. Effect of the dialysis membrane in the treatment of patients with acute renal failure. *N Engl J Med* 1994; 331:1338–1342.

Nissenson AR, Fine RN, Gentile DE, eds. *Clinical dialysis.* Norwalk, CT: Appleton & Lange, 1995.

Levin NW, Lazarus JM, Nissenson AR. National cooperative rHu erythropoietin study in patients with chronic renal failure an interim report. The National Cooperative rHu Erythropoietin Study Group. *Am J Kidney Dis* 1993;22(2 Suppl 1):3–12.

National Kidney Foundation. *NKF-DOQI, Clinical practice guidelines for vascular access.* New York: National Kidney Foundation, 1997.

National Kidney Foundation. *NKF-DOQI, Clinical practice guidelines for hemodialysis adequacy.* New York: National Kidney Foundation, 1997.

Ronco C, Bellomo R, eds. *Critical care nephrology.* Dordrecht, The Netherlands: Kluwer Academic Publishers, 1998.

Chapter 29

Peritoneal Dialysis

James F. Winchester

Modern peritoneal dialysis was introduced in 1968 by Popovich and Moncrief as continuous ambulatory peritoneal dialysis (CAPD). Currently, 14% of the 300,000 patients on renal replacement therapy in the United States receive peritoneal dialysis. CAPD was made possible with the development by Henry Tenckhoff of a Silastic catheter.

OVERVIEW

CAPD is a manual technique involving exchanges of 2 L of fresh dialysis fluid about four times a day. This maintains steady-state serum chemistries (BUN $\approx$ 70 mg/dl, serum creatinine $\approx$ 12 mg/dl) with a total fluid exchange of 10 L/day, which includes about 2 L of ultrafiltrate. A modification is continuous cyclic peritoneal dialysis (CCPD), where exchanges of dialysis fluid are made by a machine during the night. This technique is also called nocturnal intermittent peritoneal dialysis (NIPD). It can be combined with a daytime dwell of fluid. CCPD is more convenient but more costly than CAPD. The dialysis fluid contains hypertonic dextrose solution of various concentrations (1.5%, 2.5%, and 4.25%) to achieve fluid ultrafiltration. Other solutes (Ca, Mg, Na, lactate, chloride) are added to correct acidosis or replace deficiencies. The CAPD regimen consists of four exchanges of 1.5–3.0 L of warmed peritoneal dialysate infused into the abdominal cavity through a peritoneal catheter to dwell for 4 to 5 hours. The overnight exchange is longer (approximately 8 hours). With CCPD the exchange fluid is derived from two to three large-volume (5- to 6-L) bags and delivered by a machine at preselected volumes and dwell times. Patients must connect and disconnect themselves from the dialysis tubing using aseptic technique whether they are on CAPD or CCPD. They are instructed to flush one limb of a Y-shaped tubing set with spent dialysate to wash out any bacterial contamination (the "flush before fill" technique) before infusing the new dialysis fluid into the abdominal cavity. This maneuver has lowered the average frequency of peritonitis to once every 2 years.

PRINCIPLES OF SOLUTE AND FLUID REMOVAL

Solute Removal

Peritoneal dialysis is based on mathematical modeling. It achieves sufficient diffusive, convective, and osmotically derived solute transport to prevent uremia using the lowest quantity of dialysis fluid.

The accumulation of a metabolite such as urea is determined by its rate of generation less its rate of removal by residual renal function and dialysis. Therefore, as residual renal function declines, the importance of dialysis in preventing uremia increases. This mandates an increase in the frequency and volumes of dialysis. Exchanges are made when solutes such as urea have almost achieved equilibrium between plasma and dialysate. Solutes of higher molecular weight than urea, termed "middle molecules," are removed less effectively. However, the slow, continuous, convective transport provided by PD is more effective in clearing these molecules than the abrupt but relatively short periods of transport provided by conventional hemodialysis. Only expensive high-flux hemodialysis filters can surpass the efficiency of CAPD for removing middle molecules.

The adequacy of peritoneal dialysis is assessed by measurement of Kt/V. This is a dimensionless number derived from the calculated dialysis removal of urea (K), the time (t), and the volume of distribution of urea (V, or whole body water). Account is also made of the contribution from any residual renal function. A goal for weekly Kt/V for peritoneal dialysis is 2.2. The solute transport function of the peritoneal membrane can be assessed from the peritoneal equilibration test (PET). This measures the accumulation of urea and creatinine, and the disappearance of dextrose, over a 4-hour period of dialysis. It is used to adjust the dialysis prescription. Table 29.1 compares the clearances of urea and creatinine by peritoneal or hemodialysis.

Fluid Removal

Fluid balance is regulated by the osmotic influence of dextrose. Dextrose in concentrations of 1.5%, 2.5%, and 4.25% (equivalent to 347, 400, and 486 mOsm/kg H_2O) is adjusted to produce an ultrafiltration of about 300 to 1,000 ml per exchange. This provides a smooth control of fluid balance. Consequently, blood pressure control is better than that achieved by hemodialysis.

INDICATIONS FOR PERITONEAL DIALYSIS

The selection of a patient for CAPD or CCPD, compared to HD, is based on life-style requirements and medical suitability (Table 29.2). Relative indications for peritoneal dialysis include patients with cardiovascular or hemodynamic instability, patients for whom vascular access cannot be created, or those whose accesses have failed, patients living far from a dialysis center, and patients at high risk from the anticoagulation needed for hemodialysis. Contraindications to CAPD are listed in Table 29.3.

TECHNICAL ASPECTS OF PERITONEAL DIALYSIS

Catheters

These are flexible 25- to 30-cm-long tubules with distal perforations. They are often spiral to keep the tip in the pelvis and to prevent the pain experienced when dialysis fluid streams onto the rectal wall. The catheter is anchored with Dacron cuffs. About 15 cm of catheter is tunneled through the abdominal wall to the outside of the abdomen. The exit site is placed laterally below the belt

TABLE 29.1   Comparative Clearances Using Different Dialysis Techniques (L/wk)

	Dialysate volume	C_{urea}
CAPD/CCPD	56	67
HD	450	135

TABLE 29.2   Advantages and Disadvantages of Peritoneal Dialysis

Advantages	Disadvantages
Ease of performance	Low efficiency
High safety margin	Requires a dialysis catheter
Portability	Potential pulmonary compromise
Fewer dialysis-related symptoms	Potential protein loss and malnutrition
Better control of parathyroid hormone levels	Potential for infection
More liberal diet	Hypertriglyceridemia
No routine anticoagulation	
Fewer medications	
Better control of hypertension	

line. Catheters should not be used for 4 weeks following placement. This permits fibroblast ingrowth into the cuffs that seals the tunnel and prevents dialysis fluid from leaking into the abdominal wall.

TABLE 29.3   Contraindications to Peritoneal Dialysis

Absolute	Major	Minor
Peritoneal fibrosis (> 50%)	Colostomy or nephrostomy	Polycystic kidney disease
Pleuroperitoneal leak (hydrothorax)	Severe hypercatabolic state (e.g., burns)	Diverticulosis Obesity
	Fresh aortic prosthesis	Peripheral vascular disease
	Recent thoracic or abdominal surgery	
	Extensive abdominal adhesions	Hyperlipidemia
	Inguinal or abdominal hernia	Lack of a telephone for communication
	Blindness Quadriplegia Mental retardation	
	Poor motivation and compliance	
	Crippling arthritis	

Composition of Standard Dialysate Solution

Dialysate (see Table 29.4) is provided in premixed flexible plastic bags of 250 to 750 ml for children and 1 to 3 L for adults. Most adults tolerate 2-L volumes. Special formulations with low calcium and magnesium concentrations are available. Formulations containing amino acids are used for patients with malnutrition. A glucose polymer solution, which has prolonged ultrafiltration characteristics, is available in Europe.

Management of the Diabetic Patient Receiving Peritoneal Dialysis

Doses of regular insulin can be added to the dialysis solution of patients with diabetes mellitus. The dose must be decided empirically but is increased in proportion to the strength of the dextrose solution used for exchanges. A usual starting dose is 5 to 7 units per exchange.

COMPLICATIONS OF PERITONEAL DIALYSIS

Mechanical complications include pain with dialysate inflow or outflow, dialysate leakage (usually early after catheter placement), poor outflow drainage (omental wrapping and trapping of the catheter), scrotal edema (which usually indicates a patent processus vaginalis and need for hernia repair), hernias, catheter cuff extrusion, and lower back pain. Intestinal perforation is encountered only rarely.

Cardiovascular complications include fluid overload and hyper- and hypotension.

Pulmonary complications include atelectasis, hydrothorax, and hypoxemia in patients with severe chronic obstructive pulmonary disease.

TABLE 29.4   Peritoneal Dialysate Composition

Dialysate component	Concentration
Dextrose monohydrate	1.5%, 2.5%, 4.25%
Sodium	132 mEq/L
Calcium	2.5 mEq/L
Magnesium	1.5 mEq/L
Chloride	102 mEq/L
Lactate	35 mEq/L

Infectious and inflammatory complications include bacterial, fungal, and sclerosing peritonitis, catheter tunnel infections, catheter exit site infections, and pancreatitis.

Metabolic complications include hypertriglyceridemia and hyperglycemia.

PERITONITIS

Peritonitis presently occurs about once every 2 years. More frequent peritonitis should prompt a reevaluation of the exchange procedure and a consideration for retraining. Peritonitis is usually caused by a single organism, which is introduced by touch contamination. The finding of multiple organisms should prompt consideration of bowel perforation. Signs and symptoms of peritonitis are shown in Table 29.5.

Etiology

Infections with gram-positive organisms such as *Staphylococcus epidermidis* and *aureus* and *Streptococcus* species are common. Gram-negative organisms causing peritonitis include *Enterobacteriaceae, Proteus* species, *Escherichia coli, Klebsiella* species, *Enterobacter cloacae, Acinetobacter* species, and *Xanthomonas (Pseudomonas)* species. Other organisms that are encountered rarely include *Candida albicans, Nocardia asteroides, Aspergillus* species, *Fusarium* species, *Mycobacterium tuberculosis,* and nontuberculous mycobacteria.

Treatment

Vancomycin has been the mainstay of treatment. However, because of the emergence of vancomycin-resistant *Enterococcus* and *Staphylococcus,* it is reserved for the following situations: methicillin-resistant *Staphylococcus aureus;* β-lactam-resistant organisms; serious peritonitis in patients allergic to other antibiotics; and *Clostridium*

TABLE 29.5 Signs and Symptoms of Peritonitis

Cloudy dialysis fluid

A white blood cell count in PD fluid > 100/ml with > 50% polymorphonuclear leukocytes

Gastrointestinal symptoms (e.g., abdominal pain, cramps, constipation, diarrhea); these occur in 75% of patients

Gram stain of peritoneal fluid that demonstrates organisms

difficile enterocolitis unresponsive to metronidazole. Commonly selected antibiotic regimens for the treatment of peritonitis in PD patients are outlined in Table 29.6. The current recommendations for treating peritonitis and other infectious complications are available at the International Society for Peritoneal Dialysis web site at *http://www.ispd.org.*

There are three steps in the management that are usually performed on an outpatient basis over 2 weeks:

- Abdominal lavage with three rapid in-and-out flushes of dialysate fluid
- Empirical antibiotic coverage (intraperitoneal third-generation cephalosporin plus an aminoglycoside) until dialysate cultures and sensitivities allow specific antibiotic selection (Table 29.7). Rifampin is added in cases of *Staphylococcus aureus* peritonitis
- Catheter removal for fungal infection or if symptoms or dialysate cell counts fail to improve rapidly

Indications for hospitalization for peritonitis include the following:

- Infection that has not responded to routine therapy after 2 to 3 days

TABLE 29.6   Common Therapeutic Regimens for Peritonitis

Organism	Regimen
Gram-positive bacteria	Third-generation cephalosporin IP or vancomycin alone IP
Gram-negative bacteria	Aminoglycoside alone or a third-generation cephalosporin
Mixed organisms (suggests bowel perforation)	Third-generation cephalosporin IP or vancomycin (or ampicillin) + aminoglycoside + metronidazole (or clindamycin)
No organism present on Gram stain	Third-generation cephalosporin IP or vancomycin + aminoglycoside
Fungal forms	Intravenous or IP amphotericin or fluconazole IP

IP = intraperitoneal.

TABLE 29.7 Antibiotic Prescribing for Peritonitis in a PD Patient

Antibiotic	Loading dose/2-L bag[a]	Daily maintenance dose[a]
Cefazolin	500 once daily	125–250
Tobramycin	0.6 mg/kg	0.6 mg/kg once daily
Gentamicin	0.6 mg/kg	0.6 mg/kg once daily
Cefuroxime	1,000	125–250
Cefotaxime	2,000	250
Ceftazidime	1,000	125
Aztreonam	1,000	250
Fluconazole	150 mg IP	150 mg every other day
5-Flucytosine	2,000 mg PO	1,000 mg/day PO
Ciprofloxacin	500 mg PO	750 mg/12 hr PO; 25 mg/L
Amphotericin	NR	1–4 mg/L, 30 mg/day IV
Miconazole	200	50–100
Imipenem	500–1,000	50–100
Metronidazole	500 mg IV	500 mg IV every 8 hr
Isoniazid	300 mg PO	300 mg PO/day
Rifampin	600 mg PO	600 mg PO/day

[a] All doses are in milligrams per liter administered intraperitoneally unless specified otherwise. NR, not recommended.

- Unusually painful and severe peritonitis or the isolation of organisms such as *Pseudomonas (Xanthomonas),* fungi, and *Staphylococcus aureus* that are difficult to treat
- Suspicion of bowel perforation
- Failure to respond to initial antibiotic therapy
- Fecal or mycobacterial peritonitis

Suggested Readings

Gokal R, Mallick NP. Peritoneal dialysis. *Lancet* 1999;353:823–828.

Grapsa E, Oreopoulos DG. Dialysis in the elderly. In: Jacobs C, Kjellstrand CM, Koch KM, Winchester JF, eds. *Replacement of renal function.* Boston: Kluwer; Dordrecht: Dialysis, 1996:896–910.

Oreopoulos DG. The optimization of continuous ambulatory peritoneal dialysis. *Kidney Int* 1999;55:1131–1149.

Ronco C. Peritoneal dialysis: the state of the art in Europe. *Am J Kidney Dis* 1999;33:1–3.

United States Renal Data System. *USRDS 1998 Annual Data Report.* Bethesda, MD: The National Institutes of Health, National Institute of Diabetes and Digestive and Kidney Diseases, 1998.

Winchester JF, Rakowski TA. End-stage renal disease and its management in the elderly. *Clin Geriatr Med* 1998;14:255–265.

Chapter 30

Renal Transplantation

John R. Silkensen

Renal transplantation is the preferred modality for end-stage renal replacement therapy in the world at this time. In the United States, over 12,000 kidney transplants were performed in 1996, and the waiting list has increased from 13,000 in 1988 to 35,000 in 1997. Economically, it is a more feasible method of replacement therapy, an important factor in the face of increasing health care costs. In many countries, transplantation is the only option because nephrologists and technicians trained in dialytic techniques are relatively scarce. In terms of quality of life, most surveys indicate a clear preference for transplantation over other replacement therapies. Transplanted kidneys can come from cadaveric or living donors. Living donors have historically been related and more immunologically compatible, though living unrelated transplants are becoming more prevalent, with an increase greater than 45% from 1993 to 1996. Recent data showing superior graft survival of living unrelated versus cadaveric transplants has been the impetus for this increase. Current 1-year graft survival rates are 93% for living donor transplants and 87% for cadaveric transplants. Long-term survival, as measured by half-life, varies from 8.6 years for cadaveric transplants to 12.1 years for living related transplants. The beneficial effect of HLA matching is apparent by the half-life of 23.6 years in HLA-identical sibling transplants.

THE IMMUNE RESPONSE

The immune defense mechanism functions to protect the body against a host of foreign antigens including infections and, in the case of a transplanted organ, tissue that is recognized as "nonself." In fact, the process of organ rejection is quite similar in principle to the normal response of the body to a foreign antigen (infection) and to the abnormal response to "self" antigens that can manifest as autoimmune disease. Components of the immune system include the histocompatibility antigens, which are either class I or class II molecules, depending on their structure and cellular distribution. Class I molecules are named HLA (human leukocyte antigen)-A, HLA-B, and HLA-C, whereas class II molecules are designated HLA-DP, HLA-DQ, and HLA-DR. In clinical transplantation, A, B, and DR are considered the most important. Class I molecules are constitutively expressed by the plasma membranes of most cells and react with CD8+ (cytotoxic) T cells. Class I molecules are constitutively expressed on a smaller number of cell types including B lymphocytes, macrophages, and monocytes. They react with CD4+ (helper) T cells. HLA are coded by the short arm of chromosome 6, thus providing the basis by which a "0 antigen mismatch" transplant would have survival benefits over another transplant. The complex interaction among the histocompatibility antigens, T cells, B cells, macrophages, monocytes, endothelial cells, and cytokines will then determine whether rejection occurs. The use of immunosuppressive drugs permits manipulation of this system.

RECIPIENT EVALUATION

Because donor organs are in short supply, it is important that recipients are properly evaluated. In addition to the usual preoperative assessment, cardiac evaluation is important in these patients. The incidence of cardiovascular disease is increased in patients with end-stage renal failure, and cardiovascular disease remains the number-one cause of morbidity and mortality in renal transplant recipients. Furthermore, cardiovascular disease is one of the major limitations for graft survival. Special consideration must be given to diabetics undergoing evaluation for transplantation because of the high incidence of angiographically significant coronary disease in asymptomatic individuals.

Patients with active malignancies are unsuitable for transplantation. A careful history and physical exam are required to rule out an occult malignancy, and specific radiologic studies may be indicated if there is any suspicion of disease. In general, patients who have had a malignancy should be disease-free for at least 2 years before consideration for transplantation. In addition, immunosuppressive drugs predispose toward the development of other malignancies, especially skin cancer and lymphoproliferative disorders. Education regarding these possibilities should be an important part of the pretransplant evaluation.

Some centers have transplanted patients with the acquired immunodeficiency syndrome (AIDS), though results have been disappointing in part because of the need to use immunosuppressive medications. In general AIDS in a recipient is considered a relative contraindication to transplantation by most centers.

DONOR EVALUATION

Cadaveric Donor

Once an individual has been deemed an acceptable candidate for renal transplantation, he or she is placed on the United Network for Organ Sharing (UNOS) cadaveric waiting list or may obtain a transplant from a properly evaluated living donor. The great majority of transplants still come from cadaveric donors. An individual can be placed on the UNOS list when the GFR is less than 20 ml/min. There is a point system for kidney allocation that was devised by UNOS and takes into account time on the waiting list, number of B or DR antigen mismatches, and age, with pediatric patients receiving preference. In general, kidneys are offered locally, though a 0 antigen mismatch mandates shipping an organ anywhere in the United States. Individuals who fulfill the criteria for brain death are deemed potential donors. A donor should be free of HIV or any other systemic disease. Historically, donors have been younger than 65 years of age. With the increased need for organs, requirements for the donor have been relaxed. Older donors have been used, as have donors with hypertension or diabetes. Recently, non-heart-beating donors have been employed successfully, and this source will become increasingly important.

Living Donor

Potential living-related donors should be carefully screened in much the same way as cadaveric donors. Patients with familial renal disease require an even more careful evaluation for obvious reasons, but also because some diseases are more likely to recur in a related donor. Relative contraindications have included age over 65 years, advanced medical illness, severe hypertension, diabetes mellitus, preexisting renal disease, and active infection. The age requirements have been relaxed in some instances, though this remains a controversial issue. Follow-up studies of kidney donors and of patients with traumatic injuries to one kidney have shown no apparent decline in function of the remaining kidney for as long as 25 years after nephrectomy. However, there is a slight increase in the incidence of hypertension in this group and a modest degree of proteinuria, the significance of which is unclear.

IMMUNOSUPPRESSIVE DRUGS

Because transplantation involves the introduction of an immunologically dissimilar tissue into a new host, maintenance immunosuppression is necessary to prevent rejection of the allograft. The only exception is in the case of an identical twin transplant. Even with "0 antigen mismatches," some degree of immunosuppression is provided, often for life. So-called graft tolerance does develop in some individuals over time, but predicting this occurrence is difficult and unreliable. The strategy of immunosuppression generally involves three distinct phases: (a) *induction* is the period of time immediately after surgery when high doses of immunosuppressive drugs are used to initiate acceptance of the allograft; (b) *maintenance* involves continued drug therapy at tapered doses, ultimately allowing long-term immunosuppression with a minimum of side effects; and (c) *antirejection therapy* consists of higher doses of drugs employed to treat an episode of rejection. The most commonly used immunosuppressive protocol is a triple drug regimen consisting of corticosteroids, an antiproliferative drug (azathioprine or mycophenolate), and cyclosporine (CsA) or FK506 (tacrolimus). Some centers also use monoclonal or polyclonal antibodies for induction therapy (especially in high-risk patients) and for treatment of rejection.

Corticosteroids

Corticosteroids are the oldest of the drugs used to treat rejection and are employed in all phases of immunosuppressive therapy (induction, maintenance, and antirejection therapy). They have nonspecific antiinflammatory properties and also block the elaboration of interleukin-1, interleukin-6, and tumor necrosis factor by activated macrophages, an important step in T-cell activation. Prednisone is usually started at a dose of 0.5 to 2. 0 mg/kg/day and then gradually tapered to 10 mg/day within 3 to 6 months after transplantation.

Complications of corticosteroid therapy include impaired glucose metabolism, hyperlipidemia, weight gain, osteoporosis and osteonecrosis, cataracts, myopathy, easy bruisability, acne, hypertension, mood lability, and sleep disturbances. Wound healing may be delayed and/or impaired. Corticosteroids are, perhaps, the least popular drugs with transplant patients, and the complications with their use are considerable. Newer drug protocols have examined the effect of reducing or discontinuing corticosteroids, but a consensus opinion has not yet emerged.

Azathioprine

Long used as an immunosuppressive agent for transplantation and autoimmune disorders, azathioprine is an imidazole derivative of 6-mercaptopurine. The functional effect is dependent on its conversion in the liver to 6-mercaptopurine, the active metabolite. Azathioprine acts by reducing the availability of purines, thus impairing the ability of rapidly dividing cells to synthesize DNA.

Side effects associated with azathioprine include pancytopenia (more commonly leukopenia), megaloblastic erthropoiesis, hepatocellular injury, cholestatic jaundice, pancreatitis, pneumonitis, and alopecia. The dose of azathioprine should be lowered in the presence of hepatic injury because the route of elimination is disturbed. Special mention should be made of the potentially adverse interaction between azathioprine and allopurinol, especially in light of the increased incidence of gout in transplant patients on cyclosporine. Allopurinol inhibits the enzyme xanthine oxidase, which is critical in the degradation of azathioprine. Concomitant administration of these two drugs should be avoided to prevent profound bone marrow toxicity.

Mycophenolate Mofetil

Mycophenolate mofetil has a similar mode of action to azathioprine, though it is less likely to cause bone marrow suppression. This drug has gained favor in recent years because of studies showing fewer acute rejection episodes than associated with azathioprine. However, graft survival at 1 and 3 years is unchanged, and it remains to be seen whether a more prolonged benefit will be realized.

Cyclosporine

Introduced in the early 1980s, cyclosporine (CsA) revolutionized the field of transplantation, and it remains the mainstay of immuno-suppression at most centers. Cyclosporine inhibits the transcription of interleukin-2 mRNA, leading to decreased production of interleukin-2 and other cytokines critical to T-cell activation and proliferation. The major route of elimination is via biliary excretion. Monitoring of CsA trough levels should be employed as a guide to dosing changes because of significant interpatient and intrapatient variability in both its absorption after oral administration and its enterohepatic recirculation.

The usual oral starting dose is 8 to 10 mg/kg/day, and the usual intravenous starting dose is 3 mg/kg/day. There is considerable variability between centers in the use of oral versus intravenous CsA, and some centers avoid its use completely until renal function has clearly improved, a decision based on the nephrotoxic effects of CsA. Generally, when CsA is held, a polyclonal or monoclonal antibody is used for early immunosuppression. This technique is termed sequential immunosuppression, and the benefits of one technique over the other are a matter of some debate. Following the induction phase of immunosuppression, approximately 6 months after transplantation, the dose of CsA is gradually tapered to a maintenance dose of 3 to 6 mg/kg/day (given in two divided doses). Ultimately, trough levels should take precedence over drug quantity because of the variability described previously.

The major complication of CsA, and its "Achilles' heel," is nephrotoxicity. An acute decline in renal function is the most common finding, probably the result of renal vasoconstriction leading to impairment in glomerular hemodynamics. This complication is usually responsive to reductions in drug dose. Less commonly, CsA may cause a clinical picture resembling the hemolytic–uremic syndrome. This situation may respond to dose reduction or discontinuation of CsA. Additionally, chronic CsA nephrotoxicity manifested by small vessel obliteration with glomerular ischemia and sclerosis, tubular atrophy, and interstitial fibrosis may be seen. These histologic findings may be irreversible despite CsA dose reduction.

Other side effects associated with the use of CsA include hyperkalemia, hypomagnesemia, and hyperuricemia with gout. Hypertension is quite common and is characterized as salt-sensitive hypertension. Neurotoxicity manifesting as tremor or paresthesias is usually dose related. Hirsutism and gingival hyperplasia are bothersome cosmetic effects, though the hyperplasia can be very severe and may be exacerbated by the concomitant use of nifedipine for blood pressure control.

It is important to recognize the many drug interactions that affect CsA blood levels. Drugs that increase CsA levels through inhibition of hepatic P_{450} activity may result in nephrotoxicity, whereas drugs that induce P_{450} activity (lowering CsA levels) could place a transplant patient at risk for rejection. Furthermore, some drugs, such as cholestyramine, can affect levels by interfering with the intestinal absorption of CsA. Transplant patients must be well educated regarding the possibility of drug interactions. A partial listing of drugs that interact with CsA appears in Table 30.1.

FK506 (Tacrolimus) and Rapamycin (Sirolimus)

FK506 is a macrolide antibiotic resembling CsA in that it inhibits the activation of DNA-binding proteins necessary to activate the promoter sequence of the IL-2 gene. Nephrotoxicity is also the major side effect seen with FK506, and neurotoxicity, perhaps more severe than with CsA, is also a problem. One of the most serious side effects is drug-induced diabetes mellitus. Generally the diabetes is dose related, but in some cases it has been irreversible. Purported benefits over CsA include an absence of hirsutism and gingival hyperplasia. Though used originally in liver transplant recipients, FK506 has been used with increasing frequency in kidney transplantation.

TABLE 30.1   Drugs That Affect Level of Cyclosporine A

Increase	Decrease
Diltiazem	Carbamazepine
Erythromycin	Isoniazid (INH)
Fluconazole	Phenobarbital
Metoclopramide	Rifampin
Nicardipine	
Verapamil	
Ciprofloxacin	

Rapamycin is a macrolide antibiotic similar to FK506. In contrast to FK506, however, it does not block the transcription of IL-2. Instead, it blocks the signal generated by IL-2 through binding to the IL-2 receptor. Early reports showing a lower incidence of nephrotoxicity than with either CsA or FK506 make this a promising drug for further investigation.

Polyclonal and Monoclonal Antibodies

Polyclonal antibodies raised against animal lymphoblasts or thymocytes have been available for use in transplantation for over 25 years. Minnesota antilymphocyte globulin (MALG) is no longer available, but equine antithymocyte globulin (ATG) is still used in many centers for induction therapy and for treatment of steroid-resistant rejection. Because of their immunoglobulin nature, a serum sickness syndrome can occur in up to 15% of treated individuals.

The murine monoclonal antibody OKT3 is directed against the CD3 antigen complex found on all mature human T cells. It is a highly effective drug for use as an induction agent and as rescue therapy for steroid-resistant rejection. After initial lymphocyte activation, this drug modulates the antigen recognition structure, rendering the lymphocyte incapable of recognizing and responding to alloantigens. This early lymphocyte activation is the cause of a first-dose effect characterized by fever, chills, pulmonary edema secondary to a capillary leak phenomenon, and, occasionally, aseptic meningitis. The potential danger with the use of this drug mandates careful consideration for its use, and aggressive volume control is important in lessening the problems related to capillary leakage.

In addition to the early and severe side effects of the antibodies, especially OKT3, late complications of both polyclonal and monoclonal antibodies include an increased incidence of viral infections (herpes, CMV, Epstein-Barr) and posttransplant lymphoproliferative disease. More recent drugs, including the humanized monoclonal antibody daclizumab and the chimeric monoclonal antibody basiliximab, have shown promising results with fewer side effects.

SURGICAL PROCEDURE

The renal allograft is placed retroperitoneally in the iliac fossa. The right side is most commonly chosen because the accessibility of the iliac vein on the right makes the surgery easier. The renal artery is usually anastomosed to the internal iliac artery, and the renal vein with the external iliac vein. The ureter is implanted into the bladder by creating a submucosal tunnel to prevent reflux. In general, the surgery has become relatively routine, although the immunosuppressive drugs result in a delay in wound healing and an increase in propensity for infection.

EARLY POSTOPERATIVE COURSE

Intraoperatively, it is important to maintain adequate hydration so the newly transplanted kidney is perfused. A bladder catheter is usually left in place for 3 to 5 days, and the patient should have fluid intake and output measured scrupulously. In the case of delayed graft function, an occurrence in 10% to 50% of cadaveric transplants, medication dosages must be adjusted for the degree of renal dysfunction, and the dietary intake of potassium, phosphorus and magnesium should be decreased. Occasionally, a patient will require dialysis until renal function improves. These patients should be assessed on a daily basis for dialysis indications, and the dialysis prescription should avoid excessive ultrafiltration and a subsequent drop in blood pressure, a situation that could prolong allograft dysfunction. Obviously, wound management is an important part of the postoperative care. The incidence of wound infections, however, has dramatically decreased with the decrease in the amount of steroids that are used and the administration of intraoperative antibiotics.

ALLOGRAFT DYSFUNCTION

Etiology

As with all cases of renal failure, a comprehensive evaluation to eliminate prerenal, parenchymal, postrenal, and vascular etiologies needs to be performed. However, immunologic rejection, complications related to the surgical procedure, and nephrotoxicity by either CsA or FK506 are unique problems in the transplant recipient.

Prerenal Disease

Prerenal azotemia is fairly common and can occur as a result of excessive fluid losses from diuretic administration or an osmotic diuresis related to hyperglycemia or uremia. The diagnosis should be apparent from daily weights, assessing fluid intake and output, and evaluating the patient for orthostatic changes. Various laboratory parameters may provide some help, specifically a high plasma bicarbonate level seen with contraction alkalosis. An elevated BUN-to-creatinine ratio is less helpful in the transplant population because of their therapy with corticosteroids and the probability that the BUN will be elevated on this basis. Primary cardiac disease with diminished renal perfusion as well as impaired vascular tone should also be considered.

Parenchymal Disease

Acute Tubular Necrosis

The most common cause of parenchymal renal disease in the transplant recipient is acute tubular necrosis (ATN) caused by ischemia. ATN is also the most common cause of delayed graft function, which occurs in up to 50% of patients in some centers. A variety of factors are linked to the development of ATN, including a prolonged time interval between harvesting and engraftment, intraoperative hypotension, and adverse effects of the preservative solution used in the harvesting process. In addition to these factors, the transplanted kidney is subject to the same causes of ATN that lead to dysfunction in native kidneys, including nephrotoxic drugs and radiographic contrast agents. ATN should be managed with dialysis as indicated and with dose adjustments to all medications. Finally, one must not assume the diagnosis of ATN if function does not return. Many centers employ a protocol biopsy at approximately 1 week in a patient with delayed graft function secondary to presumed ATN. This is done to diagnose acute rejection, which is fairly common in patients with delayed graft function at 1 week.

Rejection

Immunologic rejection in the renal allograft is classified into four forms. These include hyperacute, accelerated, acute, and chronic rejection. The differentiation of these forms is based on timing, pathogenesis, and histologic features.

Hyperacute rejection, occurring minutes to hours after the transplant procedure, is caused by preexisting antibodies in the recipient directed against the donor tissue. These antibodies are directed against donor blood ABO or histocompatibility leukocyte antigens and interact with the transplant endothelium to cause complement activation and inflammatory cell infiltration. The resulting microvascular thrombosis and cortical necrosis almost invariably lead to graft loss and subsequent nephrectomy. Fortunately, more careful attention to ABO typing and the pretransplant cross-match have made this a rare problem.

Accelerated rejection is pathologically similar to hyperacute rejection and generally occurs in the first 2 to 4 days after engraftment. Either previously primed cellular (T cell) or humoral mechanisms (antibody) can mediate accelerated rejection. Clinically this form of rejection is characterized by either primary nonfunction or rapid deterioration following early initial function. The graft is usually lost.

Acute rejection usually occurs within the first 3 months following transplantation. It can be seen in the latter part of the first week of transplant, although typically it occurs somewhat later. When seen after 3 to 5 months, problems with medications (noncompliance or medication interactions) need to be considered. Acute rejection results from a primary response of the immune system with participation of both the cellular and humoral components. Infiltration of the interstitium with mononuclear cells and invasion of the tubular basement membrane and vessels with lymphocytes are seen on histologic examination. Acute rejection is seen in up to 40% of patients and is clinically characterized by a rise in the serum creatinine with or without diminished urine output. Sometimes low levels of either CsA or FK506 can point toward acute rejection as the cause of a serum creatinine elevation, and certain individuals are at increased immunologic risk of rejection (Table 30.2). The classic signs of fever and graft tenderness have become less pronounced in the CsA era, but with these signs a urinary tract infection must also be excluded.

Chronic rejection observed as early as a few weeks after transplantation is caused by immunologic and nonimmunologic insults.

TABLE 30.2   Characteristics of Recipients at Higher Risk for Rejection

High panel–reactive antibodies (>50%)
African-American race
Younger age
Second or subsequent transplant
Presence of delayed graft function

The relative contribution of each has remained a matter of debate, but it is clear that the number of acute rejection episodes strongly predicts the subsequent occurrence of chronic rejection. Conversely, since the widespread adoption of CsA in 1983, there has been a dramatic reduction in the incidence of acute rejection but not in chronic rejection. One of the purported nonimmunologic forms of damage, hyperfiltration injury, results from reduced nephron mass. Histologically, chronic rejection is characterized by glomerulosclerosis, thickening and reduplication of the glomerular basement membrane, tubular atrophy, interstitial fibrosis, and small vessel obliteration. Clinically there is progressive azotemia, proteinuria, and hypertension. Despite a role for immunologic damage in the pathogenesis of chronic rejection, intensification of immunosuppressive drug use provides no benefit. Hypertension should be aggressively managed, as with any renal disease, and some evidence suggests that use of ACE inhibitors may provide some advantage over other antihypertensive drugs.

Other Intrarenal Processes

Renal dysfunction associated with administration of antibiotics and other drugs can be seen in the renal allograft. ACE inhibitors can cause impairment in GFR, especially with transplant renal artery stenosis, which is analogous to bilateral renal artery stenosis in native kidneys. Also, nonsteroidal antiinflammatory agents are usually avoided in transplant patients because of the inhibition of vasodilatory prostaglandins that oppose the afferent arteriolar constriction induced by CsA or FK506.

In contrast to pyelonephritis in the native kidney, bacterial infection of the single functioning allograft is not an uncommon cause of graft dysfunction and should always be considered when a creatinine elevation is being investigated. Recurrence of the native kidney disease is another cause of graft dysfunction. Some renal diseases, such as diabetic nephropathy, will recur in 100% of patients with time (although most diabetics lose their allografts to other causes before recurrence becomes clinically important), whereas other diseases are less likely to recur. IgA nephropathy has been found to recur in 10% to 50% of transplants, with the higher numbers reported from centers that employ protocol biopsies. Rarely does recurrent IgA nephropathy result in graft failure. Other diseases that may recur include membranous glomerulopathy, focal segmental glomerulosclerosis, membranoproliferative glomerulonephritis, hemolytic uremic syndrome and, rarely, lupus nephritis.

Postrenal Disease

Interruption of urine flow by an obstruction of the collecting system (extrinsic or intrinsic) can result in renal dysfunction. A variety of fluid collections can result in extrinsic ureteral compression and subsequent hydronephrosis. Blood (hematoma) and urine (urinoma) can both cause obstruction. Lymph (lymphocele) can arise following interruption of lymphatic vessels around the surgical bed, and this complication is a relatively common finding (1–10% of patients). Most lymphoceles are small and inconsequential, but a large or strategically placed lymphocele can result in significant ureteral obstruction. Diagnosis of any of these processes is made by ultrasound, and analysis of the fluid can help determine the etiology. Lymph fluid has a high protein content and a creatinine equal to that of serum. Urine has a high creatinine, and reabsorption of the urine in the case of a urine leak without extrinsic obstruction can itself result in a rise in the serum creatinine. Intrinsic obstruction can result from blood clots, either postsurgical or postbiopsy. In fact, one of the first techniques employed for a sudden cessation in urine flow was irrigation of the bladder catheter. Other rarer causes include calculi or fungus balls. Bladder outlet problems caused by prostatic hypertrophy, neoplasms, and neurogenic bladder (especially in diabetics) can also result in postrenal disease.

Vascular Disease

Acute arterial or venous thrombosis occurs most often within the first 2 to 3 days after engraftment, although this complication may arise as long as 2 weeks after the procedure. Risk factors early include difficulty with the surgical procedure and recipient hypotension, while acute rejection is the most common cause for a later thrombosis. Most grafts with acute vascular thrombosis are not salvageable.

Renal artery stenosis is a relatively late complication of transplantation, occurring up to 2 years after the transplant but usually within the first 6 months. Observed in up to 12% of transplant recipients, the diagnosis is often suggested by hypertension and graft dysfunction, especially in the setting of ACE inhibition. An allograft bruit may be audible, though this is a fairly nonspecific clinical finding. Angioplasty offers the safest mode of treatment, though failure may necessitate surgical repair. The latter is associated with a significant incidence of graft loss (30%).

Diagnosis of Allograft Dysfunction

To evaluate a patient with allograft dysfunction, a thorough history must be obtained. Special attention needs to be directed toward any possible offending drugs (NSAIDS, diuretics), the timing of CsA or FK506 doses, and symptoms suggestive of rejection or infection. The physical examination should include orthostatic blood pressure readings as well as a careful manual evaluation of the allograft. Laboratory data should include electrolytes, blood urea nitrogen, serum creatinine, urine analysis and possibly culture, a complete blood count, and a trough CsA or FK506 level. If proteinuria is present, a 24-hour urine collection should be obtained for quantitation.

As mentioned earlier, patency of the urinary catheter should be ascertained when allograft dysfunction is noted. Unless contraindicated, and certainly if orthostatic, a fluid challenge can be prescribed. If the CsA or FK506 level is toxic, the dose should be decreased, and a repeat serum creatinine and drug level obtained in 2 to 3 days. A Doppler ultrasound is indicated if the above measures have not proven helpful. The ultrasound can detect hydronephrosis with or without a fluid collection. Hydronephrosis without a fluid collection is caused by obstruction within the collecting system. In the absence of bladder outlet obstruction, a retrograde pyelogram or antegrade pyelogram (after placement of a percutaneous nephrostomy tube to allow proximal drainage) should be attempted to localize the level of obstruction. If hydronephrosis with a fluid collection is discovered on ultrasound, the fluid can be sampled by needle aspiration and analyzed for creatinine. If the fluid and urine creatinine are equivalent, urine leak is likely. Conversely, if the fluid and serum creatinine are equivalent, a lymphocele is suggested. In addition to the above uses, Doppler ultrasound can be employed to assess blood flow to the graft. Vascular thrombosis is suggested by a lack of vascular pulsations. A renal nuclear scan or angiogram can confirm arterial thrombosis. Finally, if a correctable prerenal, postrenal, or vascular cause is excluded, an allograft biopsy is the next diagnostic procedure to pursue.

Management of Allograft Dysfunction

As in the nontransplant patient, prerenal azotemia is managed with volume repletion, discontinuation of diuretics, and optimization of cardiac function in the setting of congestive heart failure. Not infrequently, edema related to calcium channel-blocking agents can obscure the clinical picture and invite overly aggressive diuresis.

In the setting of ATN, dialytic therapy is provided until allograft function recovers. When primary nonfunction has occurred, presumably secondary to ATN, a biopsy may be appropriate at 7 to 10 days to exclude concurrent rejection, which may require therapy. As in all patients with ATN, avoidance of nephrotoxins and proper medication dosing is imperative. Pyelonephritis is treated with antibiotics.

Therapeutic options for patients with acute rejection include high-dose (pulse) corticosteroids and polyclonal or monoclonal antilymphocyte antibodies. High-dose steroids may be given either intravenously (methylprednisolone, 0.5 g every day for 3–4 days) or orally (prednisone, 100–200 mg every day for 3–5 days). Antithymocyte globulin or OKT3 is generally given as induction therapy in the very early transplant period (sometimes in an effort to avoid the nephrotoxins CsA or FK506 until allograft function improves) but also can be given for steroid-resistant or severe vascular rejection.

No specific therapy exists for chronic rejection, though baseline immunosuppressive drugs should be optimized and hypertension aggressively controlled. Protein restriction (0.6–0.8 g/kg/day) may be beneficial, especially in the presence of heavy proteinuria, and ACE inhibition may prove a unique drug in this population.

Drainage of fluid collections is attempted only if they are causing obstructive nephropathy or vascular occlusion. Not infrequently, lymphoceles will require creation of a peritoneal window for drainage if percutaneous attempts fail. A urinoma resulting from infarction of the ureter is managed by reimplantation or anastomosis of the viable portion of the ureter or renal pelvis to the bladder. Stent placement or reimplantation of the ureter into the bladder can correct obstruction caused by distal ureteral stenosis.

Vascular thrombosis of the artery or vein is generally a poor prognostic sign and usually leads to graft demise. Occasionally, surgical thrombectomy or antithrombolytic therapy may be successful. Stenosis of the transplant artery may require angioplasty or surgical revascularization, though the high incidence of graft loss with the latter must be considered.

LONG-TERM COMPLICATIONS OF TRANSPLANTATION

Infection

Infection has long been one of the most important medical complications of transplantation of all types. In the immediate postoperative period, the most common infections are bacterial and involve the urinary tract, the wound, the respiratory tract, and intravenous lines. Many infections can be avoided by common-sense measures such as prompt removal of the bladder catheter, prophylactic intraoperative antibiotics, meticulous wound management, and avoidance of prolonged use of intravenous lines. Opportunistic infections can arise at any time following transplantation but tend to occur following the first month, when the immunosuppressive effect is at its peak. The degree of immunosuppression is clearly linked to the development of opportunistic infections, and patients who have been treated for multiple rejection episodes or who have received a more aggressive regimen are definitely at higher risk.

Urinary tract infection is the most common infection in the transplant recipient and may present as pyelonephritis and septicemia. Graft dysfunction is not uncommon as the major presenting feature. Community-acquired infections such as the common cold, influenza, pneumococcal pneumonia, diarrheal syndromes, and sexually transmitted diseases can all affect the transplant recipient. It is critical that these routine infections be considered because there is a great temptation to focus on some of the more unusual possibilities, sometimes to the exclusion of the more common infections.

Reactivation of herpes simplex virus is frequently seen in transplant recipients, though less in patients treated with prophylactic acyclovir. Orolabial, esophageal, and genital involvement can occur, and treatment consists of acyclovir. Cytomegalovirus (CMV) is one of the most common and severe infections encountered in the first 6 months following transplantation. Acyclovir prophylaxis has been used historically, though the efficacy of this therapy in the prevention of disease is questionable. Many do feel that it can result in attenuation in disease severity and that its use is justified for that reason as well as its prophylactic effect on HSV. The most common clinical presentation for CMV is fever, malaise, and leukopenia. Other manifestations include chorioretinitis, pneumonitis, and gastrointestinal involvement (esophageal discomfort, cramping, diarrhea, and hepatitis). Patients at highest risk include CMV-seronegative recipients of CMV-seropositive donor kidneys. These individuals generally receive prophylactic acyclovir or CMV immune globulin. Because of the efficacy of oral ganciclovir in preventing retinitis in HIV-infected individuals, trials in transplant recipients have begun with promising results. In addition to primary CMV disease, reactivation disease in a seropositive recipient can be seen, though the severity of the illness is generally diminished. In patients with severe disease, usually those with sight-threatening retinitis or life-threatening systemic involvement (pulmonary, gastrointestinal, or hematologic), therapy with intravenous ganciclovir is initiated and immunosuppression reduced.

Other rarer diseases such as *Pneumocystis carinii, Listeria, Legionella, Nocardia, Toxoplasma,* and *Cryptococcus* can be seen in transplant patients, and it is important to consider these possibilities. With the routine prophylactic use of trimethoprim–sulfamethoxazole, however, the incidence of *P. carinii* has been markedly reduced. In patients allergic to sulfa, a combination of trimethoprim and dapsone or aerosolized pentamidine can be substituted. In obtaining a history from the patient, emphasis on travel and exposures may provide some clues to the ultimate diagnosis, especially in regard to fungal and mycobacterial infections.

All prospective transplant patients should receive vaccinations against hepatitis A and B, tetanus, diphtheria, and pneumococcal disease. Because these diseases have the potential of being much more serious in the immunosuppressed individual, the benefit of prevention is obvious. There is no vaccination at present for hepatitis C virus, and this disease has become a significant problem in the renal failure and renal transplant populations.

Cardiovascular Disease

Cardiovascular disease is now the most common cause of death following renal transplantation. Deaths over the years have not abated, and it is likely that the same epidemiologic risk factors for coronary artery disease in the normal population are operational in renal transplant recipients. Furthermore, factors unique to the transplant population may contribute to and, perhaps, increase the risk of coronary artery disease. Clearly, renal disease should now be considered a cardiac risk. Because transplant patients have been exposed to the uremic milieu for considerable amounts of time, they assume this particular risk factor. Progressive graft dysfunction, often accompanied by proteinuria, is one more insult to which many of these patients are exposed. Hyperlipidemia is a known cardiac risk factor that likely contributes to disease in the transplant population. It is a remarkably common problem posttransplant, and immunosuppressive drugs (corticosteroids and CsA) are clearly associated with hyperlipidemia, independent of the renal disease. Pharmacologic therapy may be necessary, and the HMG-CoA reductase inhibitors are probably the first choice in most centers. Previously, high-dose lovastatin was associated with an increased incidence of rhabdomyolysis in cardiac transplant patients. If liver function tests and creatine phosphokinase levels are followed periodically, and the patient is instructed about the possible symptoms of a myositis, the use of these drugs should be acceptable.

Because diabetes is the most common cause of ESRD in the United States, and the incidence of cardiac disease is much higher in this group, special attention needs to be given to the proper evaluation of these patients before transplantation. It has been clearly demonstrated that diabetics have a high incidence of asymptomatic coronary artery disease and that noninvasive stress tests in this group are not optimal. The appropriate cardiac evaluation, therefore, is somewhat controversial, though there is reasonable support for obtaining a coronary angiogram in all type I diabetics over age 45, even if asymptomatic. In patients younger than 45 years, multiple cardiac risk factors, a heavy smoking history, or an abnormal electrocardiogram should prompt the cardiologist to perform an angiogram, even in the absence of classic symptoms.

Malignancies

Immunosuppressive drugs induce alterations in the immune system that predispose transplant patients to develop certain tumors. Although there is no increased incidence of lung, breast, or colon cancer relative to the general population, transplant recipients are much more likely to develop skin cancer, especially squamous cell carcinoma. Though the insults predisposing an individual to skin cancer are cumulative and precede the transplant by years, it is important to educate the transplant patient about avoiding sun exposure and wearing sunscreen at all times. Other malignancies that occur at a rate higher than with the general population include non-Hodgkin's lymphoma (posttransplant lymphoproliferative disorder); Kaposi's sarcoma; and carcinomas of the cervix, uterus, vulva, perineum, and hepatobiliary system. General health screening similar to that with the general population is important, although Pap smears in particular are a necessity on a yearly basis.

The treatment of malignancies in the transplant patient may sometimes involve a reduction or cessation of the immunosuppressive regimen. This is particularly true for non-Hodgkin's lymphoma and Kaposi's sarcoma, where tumor regression and even cure can be seen.

Hypertension

Hypertension is very common in the transplant recipient, occurring in 50% to 60% of patients. As mentioned, hypertension can be caused or exacerbated by some of the immunosuppressive drugs, especially CsA and FK506. In addition, corticosteroids can contribute to this problem, especially when used in high doses for either induction or rejection therapy. Essential hypertension is still probably the major cause of hypertension in the transplant population, though transplant renal artery stenosis occurs not infrequently and should be suspected in a patient with worsening hypertension, a rise in the serum creatinine, and the presence of a graft systolic bruit. The last finding is fairly nonspecific, however, and should not by itself prompt a search for renal artery stenosis.

Calcium channel blockers have long been among the first line of drugs employed to combat hypertension in the transplant patient. This is partly because of the demonstration of a reversal in the reduction in renal plasma flow and GFR induced experimentally by CsA. Also, there is some suggestion that the calcium channel blockers may provide a direct immunosuppressive effect. In choosing a particular agent, it must be remembered that verapamil and diltiazem can cause an increase in CsA levels. Nifedipine and amlodipine do not alter CsA levels but are associated with a fairly high incidence of lower extremity edema and gingival hyperplasia.

Both α-and β-adrenergic blockers can be used safely in the transplant population. α-Adrenergic blockers have an added benefit in that they actually improve lipid parameters and may also cause a regression of prostatic hypertrophy. Finally, angiotensin-converting enzyme inhibitors have the added benefit of treating posttransplant erythrocytosis, a poorly understood problem in the transplant population. With these drugs, however, hyperkalemia may become a problem, especially with the concomitant use of CsA.

Bone Disease

Osteoporosis and osteonecrosis are a major concern and are caused to a large degree by the use of corticosteroids. Estrogen replacement for postmenopausal women and calcium supplementation are reasonable interventions at this time. The efficacy of drugs that reduce calcium mobilization (bisphosphonates) from bone remains to be seen. Despite problems incurred with transplantation, some of the beneficial effects on bone disease include healing of renal osteodystrophy and aluminum bone disease as well as eventual resolution of hyperparathyroidism.

Suggested Readings

Braun WE. Long-term complications of renal transplantation. *Kidney Int* 1990;37:1363–1378.

Hostetter TH. Chronic transplant rejection. *Kidney Int* 1994;46:266–279.

McKay DB, Milford EC, Sayegh MH. Clinical aspects of renal transplantation. In: Brenner BM, ed. *The kidney.* Philadelphia: WB Saunders, 1996, 2602–2652.

Ramos EL, Tisher CC. Recurrent diseases in the kidney transplant. *Am J Kidney Dis* 1994;24:142–154.

Chapter 31

Nutrition in Renal Failure

C. Peter Spies
Edward A. Ross

Patients with kidney disease have nutritional requirements that vary with the degree of renal insufficiency and proteinuria. The diet is restricted to reduce uremic symptoms from the accumulation of toxic metabolites, to facilitate electrolyte and water homeostasis, and to prevent renal osteodystrophy. Many patients with advanced chronic renal failure, however, ultimately develop protein-calorie malnutrition and require dietary supplementation.

GENERAL NUTRITIONAL CONCEPTS

Protein-Calorie Malnutrition

Patients with advanced renal insufficiency are at risk for malnutrition because uremic symptoms (anorexia, nausea, vomiting, and altered taste) are superimposed on the restricted diet, malabsorption, and urinary protein losses. This often results in hypoalbuminemia, abnormal profiles of blood amino acid levels, decreased protein and fat stores, and deranged white blood cell function. Institution of an appropriate diet or initiation of dialysis therapy may not correct these deficits, however. It is frequently necessary to enlist the aid of a renal dietitian to assist in an aggressive program of enteral or parenteral nutrition. This includes the careful monitoring of nutritional parameters such as serum albumin and transferrin levels, total lymphocyte counts, and anthropometric measurements of fat and muscle bulk (triceps skinfold thickness and midarm muscle circumference). Occasionally, impairment of gastric motility can lead to malnutrition in both diabetic and nondiabetic patients. Radionuclide studies can be used in such cases to assess gastric emptying and to test the therapeutic response of promotility agents such as metoclopramide and erythromycin.

Caloric Requirements

Patients with uncomplicated renal insufficiency have normal basal energy expenditure and caloric requirements. A diet containing at least 35 kcal/kg body weight is usually prescribed. Individuals who are catabolic or have proteinuria have greater requirements; without additional carbohydrate intake, they deplete their fat and protein stores.

Macronutrients

Protein

Stable patients with renal disease have normal minimum daily protein requirements. Protein restriction will delay the need for dialysis by preventing the uremic symptoms caused by nitrogenous wastes. The quantity of protein necessary to avoid malnutrition depends on the food's biological value (ratio of essential to nonessential amino acids). Fish, eggs, and milk are of higher biological value than poultry or beef, especially when compared with grains. Approximately 75% of the protein in renal diets should be of the high-biological-value type.

The amount of protein prescribed is based on the patient's renal function, proteinuria, type of dialysis, and body weight. As described below, the protein recommendation ranges from 0.6 to 1.5 g/kg/day. For edematous patients, the calculation should be based on the usual or estimated "dry" weight. For obese patients, calculate the "adjusted" body weight as the ideal body weight plus 25% of the excess weight. Generally, diets are reasonably tolerated if they contain at least 40 g of high-biological-value protein per day. Patients are usually in negative protein balance if their intake is restricted to 20 g/day unless they are provided with essential amino acid supplementation. α-Ketoanalogs (ketoacids) are experimental supplements that contain no nitrogen yet undergo liver transamination into the corresponding amino acid.

Intensive and repeated dietary counseling is helpful to improve compliance for protein restriction. A very useful monitor of dietary nitrogen intake (in grams) in a patient with stable renal function is to measure the 24-hour urine urea nitrogen ($U_{UN}V$):

$$I_N = U_{UN}V + NUN$$

where NUN is nonurea nitrogen excretion (in grams) and is estimated to be

$$NUN = 0.031 \times \text{body weight}$$

Daily nitrogen intake (I_N) is then converted to protein intake (in grams) as follows:

$$\text{Protein intake} = 6.25 \times I_N$$

As an example, consider a lean, nonedematous 70-kg man whose 24-hour urine reveals 5 g of urea N:

$$I_N = 5 \text{ g} + (0.031 \times 70 \text{ kg}) = 7.17$$

Estimated protein intake is $6.25 \times 7.17 = 48.8$ g/day, which is then compared with dietary protein prescription. In patients with significant proteinuria, the amount of protein lost in the urine also has to be taken into account, and the dietary protein prescription should be adjusted for this.

Lipids

Hyperlipidemia occurs in more than 50% of chronic renal failure patients and is of great concern because of the high mortality from atherosclerotic cardiovascular disease. Causes of the hypercholesterolemia and hypertriglyceridemia are multifactorial and include proteinuria in the nephrotic range, depressed lipoprotein lipase activity, decreased metabolism of remnant lipoproteins, and impaired cholesterol transport. Initiation of dialysis does not correct these disorders. Indeed, hypertriglyceridemia often worsens during peritoneal dialysis because of the absorption of large quantities of dextrose from the dialysate.

Dietary lipid guidelines and goals for renal patients are the same as those for nonuremic individuals. These include performing routine lipoprotein analyses, restricting fats to 30% of calories, substituting polyunsaturated fats for saturated fats, and reducing cholesterol intake to less than 300 mg/day. Reducing LDL-cholesterol levels is especially important in patients with cardiovascular risk factors because of the now well established increased mortality risk with poorly controlled lipid levels. However, it may be difficult to design a diet that provides adequate calories with concurrent fat and protein restrictions. Fruits (limited by their potassium content), sugars, and syrups are often useful.

Carbohydrates

Carbohydrates are a major source of calories in renal patients with multiple dietary restrictions and, thereby, are protein sparing. Sugars also permit the complete oxidation of fatty acids, which avoids ketone production. Grains, vegetables, and fruits are common sources of carbohydrate and have the added benefits of dietary fiber.

Micronutrients

Sodium and Chloride

Most patients with advancing renal insufficiency develop salt retention. This can be a management problem in patients with the nephrotic syndrome or oliguric renal failure. The dietary prescription is commonly expressed in either milliequivalents of NaCl or grams of sodium (100 mEq NaCl contains 2.3 g of sodium and 3.5 g of chloride).

Renal disease also may impair the patient's ability to conserve salt, which may lead to a superimposed prerenal azotemia. Many patients with acute renal failure have an initial oliguric phase when salt must be restricted and then a polyuric phase in which salt must be supplemented.

Potassium

The degree of dietary potassium restriction will depend on the amount of both renal and nonrenal losses. Foods high in potassium include citrus fruits, dairy products, and some vegetables and legumes. Because 40 g of protein contains 1 g (26 mEq) of potassium, a high-protein diet would preclude severe potassium restriction. In most patients, a diet limited to 1 mEq of potassium/kg body weight/day will prevent hyperkalemia. Additional potassium may need to be prescribed because of peritoneal dialysate or gastrointestinal losses.

Phosphorus

Hyperphosphatemia and secondary hyperparathyroidism develop with advancing renal insufficiency unless dietary phosphate is restricted concurrent with the use of phosphate binders. Patients on diets relatively high in protein will have an obligatory source of phosphorus and may require higher doses of binders. As noted in Chapter 28, calcium carbonate and calcium acetate are the preferred binders. However, these must be administered directly with the meals; a delay can lead to significant calcium absorption and cause hypercalcemia. Unless carefully specified in the physician orders, the proper timing of phosphate binders can be problematic in hospitalized patients because of variable meal schedules. The recently approved sevelamer hydrochloride (Renagel) is a nonabsorbed calcium-free and aluminum-free polymer resin that can be used in refractory hyperphosphatemia. It may become especially useful in hyperphosphatemic patients who have coexisting hypercalcemia, as it avoids the administration of aluminum hydroxide and its associated potential long-term toxic effects. Hypophosphatemia is rare in patients with renal failure unless accompanied by poor nutritional intake. An exception occurs in patients on continuous renal replacement therapies (such as CVVHD), which may cause hypophosphatemia by virtue of high dialysis phosphate clearance.

Vitamins and Minerals

Vitamin nutrition is complex in renal patients because some of these nutrients are deficient, whereas others can accumulate to the point of toxicity. The fat-soluble vitamins (A, E, and K) do not require supplementation, and excess vitamin A can be toxic in dialysis patients. The water-soluble vitamins, however, can become deficient because of losses into dialysate and decreased availability from the restricted diet, anorexia, or abnormal metabolism. For most water-soluble vitamins, supplementation should be 100% of the recommended daily intake (RDI). Vitamin C is not supplemented beyond the normal recommended daily requirement because its metabolite (oxalate) accumulates and contributes to secondary oxalosis in dialysis patients. An association between high levels of homocysteine and vascular morbidity (stroke, coronary artery disease, peripheral vascular disease) has recently emerged. Homocysteine levels rise with advancing renal failure and persist after initiation of dialysis. Studies have shown that although supplemental vitamin B_6, vitamin B_{12}, and folate can lower homocysteine levels in healthy patients, these agents unfortunately have a very attenuated effect in the end-stage renal disease population. It is unclear whether this resistance can be overcome with higher vitamin doses, and results from the use of two to five times the RDI of vitamin B_6 and folate have been disappointing. Because of the unique vitamin requirements of renal patients, routine multivitamin preparations are best avoided in preference for those formulated specifically for this population. Typical contents include folic acid, 1 mg; pyridoxine, 10 mg; thiamine, 1.4 to 1.6 mg; riboflavin, 1.6 to 2.0 mg; pantothenic acid, 5 to 10 mg; and ascorbic acid, 60 mg.

Carnitine

Carnitine is an important intermediate in fatty acid metabolism, and its deficiency has been associated with diverse and poorly characterized organ dysfunctional syndromes including cardiomyopathy, encephalopathy, infections, muscle weakness, and anemia refractory to erythropoietin. Benefits of carnitine repletion are often subjective and have not been shown to correlate well with plasma carnitine levels, as these may not reliably reflect tissue concentrations. If carnitine deficiency is suspected, it can be repleted at a dose of 20 mg/kg intravenously after dialysis or 330 mg PO tid.

Iron

Iron deficiency has become quite common in renal patients because of its increased utilization during erythropoietin therapy. Repetitive, albeit small, blood losses during hemodialysis also contribute to the iron deficit. Oral repletion is difficult in renal patients because of poor dietary intake of iron and decreased absorption when administered with phosphate-binding antacids. Even when oral iron is administered in high doses (65–150 mg of elemental iron) between meals, parenteral repletion is often necessary because of yearly requirements that may exceed 2g. The scheduled (i.e., weekly or monthly maintenance dosing) supplementation of parenteral iron is controversial and carries with it the theoretical risk of tissue and vascular damage mediated by toxic free radicals generated from transiently increased free iron levels. Similarly, raising the target levels for iron repletion (currently ferritin of 100 ng/ml or transferrin saturation of 20%) may enhance responsiveness to erythropoietin with the possible risk of additional iron toxicity.

Zinc

Zinc may become deficient in patients with advanced renal insufficiency because of decreased intake and absorption. This can be one of many causes of dysgeusia, alopecia, or impotence, and these may at least partially respond to zinc supplementation.

Magnesium

Because renal insufficiency decreases magnesium excretion, magnesium-containing laxatives and antacids should be avoided.

SPECIFIC RECOMMENDATIONS

Acute Renal Failure Patients Managed Without Dialysis

Macronutrients

The goal is to provide adequate nutrition without exceeding the patient's excretory capacity and inducing uremic symptoms. Caloric requirements typically increase with the stress of the acute illness to approximately 40 to 45 kcal/kg, reflecting a rise in the metabolic rate by over 20%. These extra calories are provided by a high-carbohydrate diet because protein must be limited to 0.6 to 0.8 g (high biological value)/kg/day. Patients who cannot tolerate oral feeding need parenteral nutrition with essential and nonessential amino acids, dextrose, and lipids.

Micronutrients

Oliguric patients at risk of volume overload need sodium to be restricted to 1 to 2 g/day and fluid intake decreased to 1.0 to 1.5 L/day. Depending on the degree of hyperkalemia, potassium may need to be limited to 50 mEq/day or less. Phosphate binders and a phosphorus intake of 0.6 to 1.0 g/day are necessary to prevent hyperphosphatemia. These restrictions must be liberalized in the setting of excessive nonrenal salt and water losses as well as after the onset of the diuretic phase of acute renal failure.

Chronic Renal Failure Patients: Predialysis

Macronutrients

Because of the risk of malnutrition from chronically restricted diets, careful monitoring with the assistance of a dietitian is necessary. Clinical studies have suggested that low-protein diets have a small benefit in slowing the decline of renal function in patients with moderate renal insufficiency. It is suggested that the daily protein intake be decreased to 0.6 to 0.8 g/kg with a diet containing approximately 35 kcal/kg. Compliance with the diet can be assessed by periodically measuring the urine urea nitrogen appearance rate, as described above. The nonprotein calories are provided by fats (such as poly- or monounsaturated vegetable oils) and simple carbohydrates. However, diabetic patients benefit from the use of complex carbohydrates. Once the glomerular filtration rate has fallen below approximately 15 ml/min, a 0.6- to 0.8-g protein/kg/day diet will clearly minimize uremic symptoms and permit a brief delay in the initiation of dialysis to establish appropriate vascular or peritoneal access.

Micronutrients

The degree of salt and water restriction needs to be individualized on the basis of the patient's residual renal function and associated electrolyte disorders (i.e., hyperkalemia, renal tubular acidosis). A daily 2- to 4-g sodium and 50- to 70-mEq potassium diet is often adequate in individuals retaining these salts. When the glomerular filtration rate declines below approximately 50 ml/min, patients benefit from a phosphate restriction of 0.8 to 1.2 g/day (later decreased to 0.6 to 0.8 g/day), phosphate binders, as well as monitoring of intact parathyroid hormone levels and initiating 1, 25-dihydroxyvitamin D therapy as necessary.

Patients with Nephrotic Syndrome

Macronutrients

Patients with the nephrotic syndrome present unique dietary problems because of the urinary protein losses, hypoalbuminemia, edema, and hyperlipidemia. Very-high-protein diets are generally ineffective in raising the serum albumin level and may exacerbate the proteinuria. There is recent evidence that dietary protein limited to 0.8 g/kg/day (supplemented with the amount lost in the urine) will provide adequate substrate for albumin synthesis and decrease proteinuria. Because of the associated lipid disorders, it is usually necessary to limit cholesterol intake to less than 300 mg/day with 30% of the dietary calories in fat (2:1 polyunsaturated-to-saturated fat ratio). The remainder of the 35 kcal/kg/day preferably consists of complex carbohydrates.

Micronutrients

The degree of sodium restriction will depend on the magnitude of edema and typically ranges from 2 to 4 g/day. Potassium and phosphorus are limited as necessary if glomerular filtration rate declines.

Patients on Hemodialysis

Macronutrients

Once hemodialysis is initiated, there will be small protein and amino acid losses into the dialysate, and the dialysis prescription should be adjusted periodically to optimize clearance of nitrogenous waste products. The dietary protein should be liberalized as indicated below with additional quantities prescribed to compensate for any residual renal losses. The Dialysis Outcomes Quality Initiative (DOQI) guidelines recommend assessing the dietary protein intake of dialysis patients by frequent (usually monthly) measurement of the protein catabolic rate (PCR), which is accomplished using urea kinetic modeling software programs. A dietary protein prescription that equals or exceeds the PCR is important to avoid negative nitrogen balance. The minimum PCR should be 0.8 g/kg/day, but a target of 1.0 to 1.2 g/kg/day has been associated with improved survival. In predialysis patients, a calculated spontaneous protein intake less than 0.8 g/kg/day may indicate such severe uremic symptoms that it can be used as a criterion to initiate hemodialysis independent of creatinine or urea clearance. Another important parameter to follow is the serum albumin concentration. Because a low serum albumin (especially less than 3.0 g/dl) at the commencement of dialytic therapy is associated with high patient morbidity and mortality, it is hoped that these individuals will benefit from very aggressive feeding. Various palatable dietary supplements are now commercially available for patients unable to consume standard meals because of anorexia, nausea, or vomiting. Intradialytic parenteral nutrition with solutions of 10% to 20% dextrose, 10% amino acids, and 20% lipids is reserved for those who cannot achieve adequate oral intake. The diet generally contains 35 kcal/kg/day, of which 35% to 50% of the calories are from carbohydrates and 30% from fat (2:1 polyunsaturated-to-saturated fat ratio). Cholesterol intake should be guided by periodic lipoprotein analyses. For anabolic patients gaining weight, calories must be increased with the use of fats and simple carbohydrates. Critically ill patients in an intensive care setting typically have increased caloric requirements and catabolic rates. Serial measurements of the PCR will best reflect their nutritional needs because protein requirements can vary widely and may exceed four times their basal values. Because parenteral nutritional supplementation often necessitates the administration of large fluid volumes, continuous renal replacement modalities (such as CVVHD) are sometimes superior to intermittent hemodialysis in order to assure adequate nutrition and volume removal.

Micronutrients

Sodium, potassium, and water restriction will depend on the residual renal function and urine output. Anuric patients typically require a daily restriction of 1.0 to 1.5 L fluid, 2 to 3 g sodium, and 70 mEq (1 mEq/kg) potassium. Phosphorus is limited to 0.8 to 1.0 g/day. Adherence to fluid restriction is important to avoid volume-dependent hypertension and adverse postdialytic symptoms associated with excess fluid removal (mainly cramping).

Vitamins

Dialysis patients should receive supplements of water-soluble vitamins because of the potential for increased removal of these vitamins, especially during high-flux dialysis. For most water-soluble vitamins, supplementation should be 100% of the recommended daily intake (RDI). The removal of fat-soluble vitamins by hemodialysis is negligible, and their supplementation is generally not recommended. Exceptions include treatment with vitamin D for renal osteodystrophy and possible supplementation of vitamin K in patients on long-term antibiotics.

Patients on Chronic Peritoneal Dialysis

Macronutrients

Malnutrition is a very common problem in peritoneal dialysis patients. Diminished appetite is mainly caused by the dialysate, which distends the abdomen, causes intermittent discomfort, and leads to dextrose absorption. The calories from dextrose are significant and can be estimated based on a 70% to 80% peritoneal absorption rate and 3.4 kcal/g. For example, 2 L of 4.25% dextrose will yield a total of 85 g, of which an estimated 80% (or 68 g) can be absorbed after a long dwell time. This would provide

68×3.4 or approximately 231 kcal. Protein nutrition is, however, much more of a problem because in some patients ("fast solute" transporters) more than 2g can be lost with each dialysate exchange. During episodes of peritonitis, the losses can exceed 15 g protein/day. For this reason, patients are placed on a 1.2- to 1.5-g protein/kg/day diet, which is increased during peritonitis. Balancing the types of nutrients to provide a total of 35 kcal/kg/day is further complicated when fat intake is limited because of hyperlipidemia. Dietary fat is usually reduced to 30% of the prescribed calories, with a 2:1 polyunsaturated-to-saturated fat ratio. Malnutrition is so common that it has led to the development of aggressive strategies for enteral food supplementation as well as the use of experimental dialysate solutions containing amino acids. As peritoneal dialysis adequacy targets are better defined, it has become apparent that poor nutritional intake is often linked to uremic symptoms associated with an inadequate dialysis prescription. Unfortunately, to achieve more rigorous solute clearance goals, the use of larger fill volumes can exacerbate early satiety, gastroesophageal reflux symptoms, and anorexia.

Micronutrients

Salt and water balance is less problematic than in hemodialysis because patients can compensate for their diet by adjusting the type and frequency of peritoneal dialysate exchanges. However, the chronic use of high dextrose concentrations to increase ultrafiltration may worsen the hyperlipidemia. Thus, sodium intake occasionally needs to be limited to 2 to 4 g/day in 1.0 to 1.5 L of fluid. Hyperkalemic patients should limit their potassium intake to 70 mEq/day. Hypokalemia occasionally occurs because of significant peritoneal potassium losses when patients fail to meet the protein intake targets. Cautious use of potassium supplementation with frequent monitoring of blood levels may be indicated in these situations. The high-protein prescription makes it difficult to decrease phosphorus to less than approximately 1.0 g/day.

Kidney Transplant Patients

Postoperative kidney transplant patients receiving glucocorticoids require close attention to assure they are receiving increased nutrients. Even if the allograft has initial nonfunction, these patients should receive 1.5 g protein/kg/day, and the increased protein and caloric intake commonly demands more intensive dialytic therapy.

Subsequent dietary guidelines depend on the degree of allograft function. Steroid-induced hyperglycemia may limit the permissible simple carbohydrate intake. Calcium intake should be monitored to achieve approximately 1 g/day. Particular attention should be focused on dietary modification for control of hyperlipidemia. In addition, potassium and magnesium intake may need to be adjusted because of the hyperkalemia and hypomagnesemia associated with cyclosporine therapy.

Suggested Readings

Anderson S. Low protein diets and diabetic nephropathy. *Semin Nephrol* 1990;10:287–293.

Consensus Group Statement. Role of *l*-carnitine in treating renal dialysis patients. *Dial Transplant* 1994;23:177–181.

Golper TA, Ahmad S. L-Carnitine administration to hemodialysis patients: has its time come? *Semin Dial* 1992;5:94.

Hoy WE, Sargent JA, Freeman RB, et al. The influence of glucocorticoid dose on protein catabolism after renal transplantation. *Am J Med Sci* 1986;291:241–247.

Kaysen GA. Effect of dietary protein intake on albumin homeostasis in nephrotic patients. *Kidney Int* 1986;29:572–577.

Klahr S, Levey AS, Beck GJ, et al. The effects of dietary protein restriction and blood-pressure control on the progression of chronic renal disease. *N Engl J Med* 1994;330:877–884.

Kopple JO, Blumenkrantz MJ. Nutritional requirements for patients undergoing continuous ambulatory peritoneal dialysis. *Kidney Int* 1983;24(Suppl 16):S295–S302.

Leverve X, Barnoud D. Stress metabolism and nutritional support in acute renal failure. *Kidney Int* 1998;53(Suppl 66):S62–S66.

Mitch WE. Dietary protein restriction in chronic renal failure: nutritional efficacy, compliance and progression of renal insufficiency. *J Am Soc Nephrol* 1991;2(Suppl 4):823–831.

Mitch WE, Klahr S. *Nutrition and the kidney, 2nd ed.* Boston: Little, Brown, 1993.

National Kidney Foundation. *Dialysis outcomes quality initiative (DOQI) guidelines.* 1997.

Rocco MV, Makoff R. Appropriate vitamin therapy for dialysis patients. *Semin Dialysis* 1997;10:272–277.

Chapter 32

Use of Drugs in Renal Failure

Abdul R. Amir
Nicolas J. Guzman

The activity of a drug is related to the concentration of free drug in the tissue compartment where the effect occurs (Fig. 32.1). The kidney is a major route of drug elimination through excretion and metabolism; therefore, patients with renal disease, and also the elderly, are more susceptible to adverse drug reactions and toxicity. Uremia alters drug pharmocokinetics, including absorption, volume of distribution, degree of protein binding, and biotransformation. It also reduces the hepatic elimination of certain drugs, which can result in accumulation of the parent drug and its active metabolites to toxic levels (e.g., acyclovir, captopril, codeine, meperidine, and procainamide). Some drugs may trigger or exacerbate an ongoing metabolic disorder that is secondary to renal disease. Others may accelerate the progression of renal failure by causing acute or chronic renal injury. The nephrotoxicity of commonly used drugs is discussed in Chapter 26.

DRUG BIOAVAILABILITY AND ABSORPTION

The bioavailability of a drug is the fraction present in the blood after a given time period following its administration. It depends on the route of administration and the presence of other medications that can bind drugs in the gut. Increased bioavailability of propranolol and dihydrocodeine occurs in patients with renal insufficiency because of decreased first-pass hepatic metabolism. Changes in the rate of drug absorption may lead to variations in

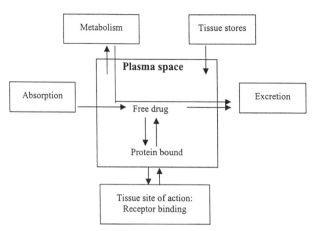

FIGURE 32.1 The relationships among absorption, distribution, protein binding, and excretion of a drug and its concentration at its site of action.

blood levels with subsequent therapeutic failure or toxicity. Several processes that impair gastrointestinal absorption of drugs in severe renal insufficiency are described below.

Uremia

Uremic patients may develop anorexia, nausea and vomiting, or gastroparesis. Because most drugs are absorbed in the proximal part of the small intestine, delayed gastric emptying can diminish total drug absorption and delay peak plasma levels.

Association of Renal Failure with Other Conditions That Impair Gastrointestinal Motility

Delayed drug absorption may occur in a diabetic patient with autonomic neuropathy and gastroparesis. Diarrhea and steatorrhea decrease contact time for intestinal absorption. Patients on peritoneal dialysis may develop peritonitis, which decreases intestinal peristalsis and drug absorption.

Adverse Drug Effects and Drug Interactions in Renal Failure

Gastric pH is frequently elevated as a result of the use of phosphate-binding antacids or histamine H_2 receptor blockers, which may result in delayed gastric emptying and impaired absorption of medications that require an acid milieu. Aluminum- or calcium-based phosphate binders may form nonabsorbable chelation products with certain drugs, such as digoxin or tetracycline, with impairment of their absorption. Aluminum-based antacids may also cause constipation, thereby increasing contact time for intestinal absorption and hence drug bioavailability. On the other hand, drugs that stimulate gastrointestinal transit, such as metoclopramide and cisapride, may accelerate gastric emptying and intestinal transit, resulting in earlier and higher peak plasma concentrations.

DRUG DISTRIBUTION

Factors that affect the extent of drug distribution in the body include molecular size, plasma protein binding, and drug tissue binding. The presence of edema and ascites increases the volume of distribution for hydrophilic and highly protein-bound agents. Decreased binding of acidic drugs to proteins in uremia increases the unbound drug levels and consequently their distribution and elimination. The alteration in protein binding may be caused by one of the following three mechanisms:

Decreased serum albumin concentration is seen in nephrotic syndrome, protein malnutrition, and patients receiving peritoneal dialysis.

Accumulation of substances in uremic plasma that displace acidic drugs from albumin binding sites. Endogenous organic acids that accumulate in uremia compete with acidic drugs for albumin binding sites. This increases the plasma free drug concentration and requires a reduction in drug dosage and/or frequency to prevent toxicity. On the other hand, basic drugs such as clonidine, imipramine, and lidocaine have increased binding to glycoproteins. This decreases the plasma free drug concentrations, diminishes the therapeutic effect, and requires an increase in the drug dosage or frequency.

Alteration in capacity of albumin to bind drugs results from uremia or acidosis. Reductions in the amount of albumin-bound drug decreases the total plasma drug concentration. Therefore, where a highly albumin-bound drug such as phenytoin has been displaced from its protein binding sites, total plasma drug concentrations underestimate free drug levels and therapeutic responses. There is a transient rise in free drug levels, but these later return to steady state as the total drug level decreases. The finding of a low total drug level may prompt the physician to increase drug dosage to reestablish "therapeutic" total plasma drug levels with the danger of drug toxicity. Measurement of plasma free drug concentrations avoids drug toxicity.

CLEARANCE

The total plasma clearance of a drug depends on renal elimination and hepatic metabolism and conjugation. Renal elimination of drugs is determined by the glomerular filtration rate (GFR), tubular secretion, and tubular reabsorption. The GFR can be estimated using the Cockcroft-Gault formula (see Chapter 3). Protein-bound drugs are poorly filtered, but they may be efficiently secreted by the proximal tubule. Unbound drugs are usually freely filtered through the glomerulus.

Drugs with hepatic elimination are preferable for patients with renal insufficiency. However, renal insufficiency may decrease hepatic acetylation, hydroxylation, demethylation, and conjugation of drugs and reduce drug metabolism by the cytochrome P_{450}IID6 isoenzymes.

PRESCRIBING FOR THE PATIENT WITH RENAL INSUFFICIENCY

Calculation of Initial Loading Dosage

Patients with renal failure and normal extracellular volume are given a normal loading dose, whereas those with edema or ascites require a larger loading dose.

Calculation of Maintenance Dosage

The fraction of the normal dose for a patient with renal insufficiency can be calculated from:

$$\text{Dose fraction} = \left(t_{\frac{1}{2}} \text{ normal}\right)\big/\left(t_{\frac{1}{2}} \text{ renal failure}\right)$$

where $t_{1/2}$ is the half-time for elimination. To calculate the dose of a drug, use:

Drug dose in renal failure patient = Normal drug dose

× Dose fraction

Alternatively, to maintain the usual drug dose, increase the dosage interval:

Drug interval in renal failure patient = (Normal dose

interval)/(Dose fraction)

HEMODIALYSIS OF DRUGS

The degree to which a drug is removed by hemodialysis (HD) is directly proportional to the plasma concentration of free drug and to the clearance characteristics of the dialysis membrane. The fraction of the drug removed by dialysis and the endogenous clearance of a drug in the interdialytic period determine the need for supplemental postdialytic or interdialytic dosing. For example, an arrhythmia may occur on dialysis in a patient receiving procainamide because the active metabolite, N-acetylprocainamide, is dialyzable. Opiates and ethanol are dialyzable; their removal can precipitate withdrawal symptoms.

PERITONEAL DIALYSIS OF DRUGS

Although drug removal by continuous ambulatory peritoneal dialysis is minimal, drug absorption following intraperitoneal (IP) administration may be substantial. Antibiotics are frequently used intraperitoneally to treat dialysis-related peritonitis.

DETAILS OF DRUG DOSING IN RENAL FAILURE

Figure 32.1 summarizes the factors that affect pharmacokinetics. Table 32.1 provides details of drugs that require dose adjustments in patients with renal insufficiency and those receiving dialysis.

TABLE 32.1 Details of Drugs Requiring Dose Adjustments in Patients with Renal Insufficiency and Those Receiving Dialysis

| Drug | Excreted unchanged (%) | Protein bound (%) | t₁/₂ Normal/ renal failure (hr) | Dose or frequency adjustment for GFR (ml/min) | | | Supplemental dose for | |
				GFR > 50	GFR 10–50	GFR < 10	Hemodialysis	PD
Antibiotics								
Aminoglycosides								
Amikacin	95	<5	2.3/17–150	60–90%	30–70%	20–30%	2/3 normal dose	15–20 mg/L/day
Gentamycin	95	<5	1.8/20–60	60–90% q8–12hr	30–70% q12h	20–30%	2/3 normal dose	3–4 mg/L/day
Streptomycin	70	35	2.5/100	q24hr	q24–72hr	q27–96hr	1/2 normal dose	20–40 mg/L/day
Tobramycin	95	<5		60–90% q8–12hr	30–70% q12hr	20–30% q24–48hr	2/3 normal dose	3–4 mg/L/day
Carbapenems								
Imipenem	20–70	13–21	1.0/4.0	100%	50%	25%	Dose after HD	dose for GFR<10
Cephalosporins								
Cefaclor	70	25	1.0/3.0	100%	50–100%	50%	250 mg post-HD	250 mg q8–12hr
Cefamandole	50–70	75	1.0/6–11	q6hr	q6–8hr	q12hr	0.5–1.0 g post-HD	0.5–1 g q12hr
Cefazolin	75–95	80	2/40–70	q8hr	q12hr	q24–48Hr	0.5–1 g post-HD	0.5 g q12hr
Cefixime	18–50	50	3.1/12	100%	75%	50%	300 mg post-HD	200 mg/day
Cefotaxime	60	37	1.0/15	q6hr	q8–12hr	q24hr	1 g post-HD	1 g/day
Cefotetan	75	85	3.5/13–25	100%	50%	25%	1 g post-HD	1 g/day
Cefoxitin	80	41–75	1.0/13–23	q8hr	q8–12hr	q24–48hr	1 g post-HD	1 g/day
Cefprozil	65	40	1.7/6	250 mg q12hr	250 mg q12–16hr	250 mg q24hr	250 mg post-HD	dose for GFR<10
Ceftazidime	60–85	17	1.2/13–25	q8–12hr	q12–24hr	q24hr	1 g post-HD	0.5 g/day
Ceftizoxime	57–100	28–50	1.4/35	q8–12hr	q12–24hr	q24hr	1 g post-HD	0.5–1 g/day
Ceftriaxone	30–65	90	7–9/12–24	100%	100%	100%	dose post-HD	750 mg q12hr
Cefuroxime	90	33	1.2/17	q8hr	q8–12hr	q12hr	dose post-HD	dose for GFR<10

(continued)

TABLE 32.1 *Continued*

Drug	Excreted unchanged (%)	Protein bound (%)	$t_{1/2}$ Normal/ renal failure (hr)	Dose or frequency adjustment for GFR (ml/min)			Supplemental dose for	
				GFR > 50	GFR 10-50	GFR < 10	Hemodialysis	PD
Cephalexin	98	20	0.7/16	q8hr	q12hr	q12hr	dose post-HD	Dose for GFR<10
Cephalothin	60-90	65	0.51/3-18	q6hr	q6-8hr	q12hr	dose post-HD	1 g q12hr
Fluroquinolones								
Ciprofloxacin	50-70	20-40	3-6/6-9	100%	50-75%	50%	250 mg q12hr	250 mg q12hr
Levofloxacin								
Ofloxacin	68-80	25	5-8/28-37	100%	50%	25-50%	100 mg q12hr	Dose for GFR<10
Trovafloxacin	6	75	9-12.2/?	100%	100%	100%	None	?
Macrolides								
Azithromycin	6-12	8.0-50	10-60/?	100%	100%	100%	None	None
Clarithromycin	15	70	2.3-6/?	100%	75%	50-70%	Dose post-HD	None
Erythromycin	15	60-90	1.4/5-6	100%	100%	50-70%	None	None
Miscellaneous								
Clindamycin	10	60-95	2-4/3-5	100%	100%	100%	None	None
Metronidazole	20	20	6-14/7-21	100%	100%	50%	Dose post-HD	Dose for GFR<10
Sulfamethoxazole	70	50	10/20-50	q12hr	q18hr	q24hr	1 g post-HD	1 g/day
Trimethoprim	40-70	30-70	9-13/20-49	q12hr	q18hr	q24hr	dose post-HD	dose for GFR<10
Vancomycin	90-100	10-50	6-8/200	500 mg q12hr	500 mg q24-48hr	500 mg q48-96hr	dose for GFR<10	dose for GFR<10
Penicillins								
Amoxicillin	50-70	15-25	2.3/5-20	q8hr	q8-12hr	q24hr	dose post-HD	250 mg q12hr
Ampicillin	30-70	20	1.5/7-20	q6hr	q6-12hr	q12-24hr	dose post-HD	250 mg q12hr
Aztreonam	75	45-60	2.9/6-8	100%	50-75%	25%	0.5 g post-HD	dose for GFR<10
Dicloxacillin	35-70	95	0.7/1-2	100%	100%	100%	None	None
Methicillin	25-80	35-60	0.5/1-4	q4-6hr	q6-8hr	q8-12hr	None	None
Mezlocillin	65	20-46	1.2/3-5.4	q4-6hr	q6-8hr	q8hr	None	None

Drug								
Penicillin G	60-85	<5	0.5/6-20	100% q4-6hr	75% q6-8hr	20-50% q8hr	dose post-HD	dose for GFR<10
Piperacillin	75-90	30	0.8-2/3-5.1	1-2 g q4hr	1-2 g q8hr	1-2 g q12hr	dose post-HD	dose for GFR<10
Ticarcillin	85	45-60	1.2/11-16	1-2 g q4hr	1-2 g q8hr	1-2 g q12hr	3 g post-HD	dose for GFR<10
Tetracyclines								
Doxycycline	35-45	80-90	20/18-25	100%	100%	100%	None	?
Minocycline	6-10	70	16/12-18	100%	100%	100%	None	None
Tetracycline	48-60	55-90	10/57-108	q8-12hr	q12-24hr	avoid	None	None
Antifungals								
Amphotericin B	5	90	24/unchanged	q24hr	q24hr	q24-36hr	None	dose for GFR<10
Fluconazole	70	12	22/?	100%	100%	100%	200 mg post-HD	dose for GFR<10
Fluocytosine	90	<10	6/75-200	q12hr	q16hr	q24hr	dose post-HD	0.5-1 g/day
Itraconazole	35	99	21/25	100%	100%	50%	100 mg q12-24hr	100 mg q12-24hr
Miconazole	1	90	24/unchanged	100%	100%	100%	None	None
Antiparasitic								
Chloroquine	40	50-65	4/5-50 days	100%	100%	50%	None	None
Pentamidine	20	69	29/118	q24hr	q24-36hr	q48hr	None	None
Quinine	5-20	70	16/unchanged	q8hr	q8-12hr	q24hr	dose post-HD	dose for GFR<10
Anti-TB								
Ethambutol	75-90	10-30	4.0-7/15	q24hr	q24-36hr	q48hr	dose post-HD	dose for GFR<10
Isoniazid	5-30	4.0-30	0.7-4/8-17	100%	100%	50%	dose post-HD	dose for GFR<10
Pyrazinamide	1-3	0.5	54/?	100%	avoid	avoid	avoid	avoid
Rifampin	15-30	60-90	1.5/1.8-11	100%	50-100%	50%	None	dose for GFR<10
Antiviral								
Acyclovir	40-70	15-30	2.1-3.8/20	5 mg/kg q8hr	5 mg/kg q12hr	5 mg/kg q24hr	dose post-HD	dose for GFR<10
Amantadine	90	60	12/500	q24-48hr	q48-72hr	q7 day	none	None
Didanosine	60	<5	1.3-1.6/4.5	q12hr	q24hr	q48hr	25% of daily dose	dose for GFR<10
Famciclovir	50-65	<25	1.6-2.9/10-22	q8hr	250 mg q12hr	250 mg q48hr	250 mg post-HD	?
Foscarnet	85	17	3/prolonged	28 mg/kg	15 mg/kg	6 mg/kg	dose post-HD	dose for GFR<10

(continued)

TABLE 32.1 *Continued*

| Drug | Excreted unchanged (%) | Protein bound (%) | $t_{1/2}$ Normal/ renal failure (hr) | Dose or frequency adjustment for GFR (ml/min) | | | Supplemental dose for | |
				GFR > 50	GFR 10–50	GFR < 10	Hemodialysis	PD
Ganciclovir	90–100	?	3.6/30	q12hr	q24–48hr	q48–96hr	dose post-HD	dose for GFR<10
Indinavir	Hepatic	60	1.8/?	?	?	?	?	?
Lamivudine	68–71	36	5–7/15–35	150 mg q12hr	100 mg qd	50 mg qd	dose post-HD	?
Ribavirin	10–40	0	30–60/?	100%	100%	50%	dose post-HD	dose for GFR<10
Rimantadine			13–65/ prolonged	100 mg q12hr	100 mg qd	100 mg qd	?	?
Ritonavir	Hepatic	98–99%	3–5/?	?	?	unknown	unknown	?
Squinavir	Hepatic	97%	1–2/?	?	?	?	?	?
Stavudine	40	<1	1–1.4/5.5–8	100%	50%	50% q24hr	dose post-HD	?
Valacyclovir			2.5/3.3	1 g q8hr	1 g q12–24hr	0.5 g 24hr	dose post-HD	dose for GFR<10
Zalcitabine	75	<4	0.75 mg q12hr	0.75 mg q8hr	0.75 mg q12hr	0.75 mg q24hr	dose post-HD	?
Zidovudine	8–25	10–30	1.1–1.4/1.4–3	200 mg q8hr	200 mg q8hr	100 mg q12hr	100 mg post-HD	dose for GFR<10
Cardiovascular drugs								
Adenosine	<5	0	<10 sec/ unchanged	100%	100%	100%	None	None
Amiodarone	<5	96	14–120 day/ unchanged	100%	100%	100%	None	None
Aminone	10–40	20–40	8.3/?	100%	100%	50–75%	?	?
Bertylium	75	6	13.6/16–32	100%	25–50%	25%	None	None
Digoxin	76–85	20–30	36–44/80–120	100% q24hr	25–75% q36hr	10–25% q48hr	None	None

(continued)

Drug								
Disopyramide	35–65	54–81	5.0–10/18	q8hr	q12–24hr	q24–40hr	None	None
Dobutamine	<10	?	2 min/?	100%	100%	100%	?	?
Esmolol	<10	55	7 min/unchanged	100%	100%	100%	None	None
Flecainide	25	52	12.0/19–26	100%	100%	50–75%	None	None
Lidocaine	10	60–66	2.2/3	100%	100%	100%	None	None
Mexiletine	10	70–75	8.0/13–16	100%	100%	50–75%	?	?
Milrinone	80–85	?	1/1.5–3	100%	100%	100%	?	?
Nitroglycerin	<1	?	2–4 min/unchanged	100%	100%	100%	?	?
Procainamide	50–60	15	4.9/5.3–5.9	q4hr	q6–12hr	q8–24hr	200 mg	None
Propafenone	<1	>95	12/?	100%	100%	100%	None	None
Quinidine	20	70–95	6.0/4–14	100%	100%	75%	100–200 mg	None
Sotalol	60	<1	?	100%	30%	15–30%	80 mg	None
Tocainide	40	10–20	14/22–27	100%	100%	50%	200 mg	None
ACE Inhibitors								
Benazepril	20	95	22/30	100%	75–100%	50%	25–30%	None
Captopril	30–40	25–30	1.9/21–32	100%	75%	50% q24hr	25–30%	None
Enalapril	43	50–60	24/34–60	q8–12hr 100%	q12–18hr 75–100%	50%	20–25%	None
Fosinopril	<1	95	11–12/12–20	100%	100%	75%	None	None
Lisinopril	80–90	0–10	12.6/40–50	100%	50–75%	25–50%	20%	None
Quinapril	30	97	1–2/6–15	100%	75–100%	50%	25%	None
Ramipril	10–21	55–70	5.8/15	100%	50–75%	25–50%	20%	None
Angiotensin receptor blockers								
Losartan	10	30	3.0/4	100%	100%	100%	None	None
Candesartan	33	99	9/?	?	?	?	?	?
Irbesartan	20	90	12–20/?	?	?	?	?	?
Valsartan	13.2	85–99	6.1/?	?	?	?	?	?
β-Blockers								
Acebutolol	55	20	7.0–9/7	100%	50%	30–50%	None	None

TABLE 32.1 *Continued*

Drug	Excreted unchanged (%)	Protein bound (%)	$t_{1/2}$ Normal/ renal failure (hr)	Dose or frequency adjustment for GFR (ml/min)			Supplemental dose for	
				GFR > 50	GFR 10–50	GFR < 10	Hemodialysis	PD
Atenolol	>90	3	6.7/15–35	100% q24hr	50% q48hr	30–50% q96hr	25–50 mg	None
Celiprolol	10	?	4.0–5/5	100%	100%	75%	?	None
Labetalol	<5	50	3–9/ unchanged	100%	100%	100%	None	None
Metaprolol	5	8	3.5/2.5–4.5	100%	100%	100%	50mg	None
Nadolol	90	28	19/45	100%	50%	25%	40 mg	None
Pindolol	40	50	2.5–4/3–4	100%	100%	100%	None	None
Propranolol	<5	93	2–6/1–6	100%	100%	100%	None	None
Timolol	15	60	2.7/4	100%	100%	100%	None	None
Calcium channel blockers								
Amlodipine	<10	>95	35–50/50	100%	100%	100%	None	None
Diltiazem	<10	98	2–8/3.5	100%	100%	100%	None	None
Fleodipine	<1	99	10–14/21–24	100%	100%	100%	None	None
Isradipine	<5	97	1.9–4.9/10	100%	100%	100%	None	None
Nicardipine	<1	98–99	5.0/5–7	100%	100%	100%	None	None
Nifidipine	<10	97	5.5/5–7	100%	100%	100%	None	None
Verapamil	<10	83–93	3–7/2.4–4	100%	100%	100%	None	None
Central agents								
Clonidine	45	20–40	6–23/38–42	100%	100%	100%	None	None
Methyldopa	25–40	<15	1.5–6/6–16	q8hr	q8–12hr	q12–24hr	250 mg	None
Diuretics								
Amiloride	50	30–40	6–8/10–144	100%	50%	avoid	?	?
Bumetanide	33	96	1.2–1.5/1.5	100%	100%	100%	None	None
Chlorthalidone	50	88–96	44–80/ unchanged	q24hr	q24hr	avoid	?	?

Ethacrynic acid	20	90	2–4/?	q8–12hr	q8–12hr	avoid	None	None
Furosemide	67	95	0.5–1.1/2–4	100%	100%	100%	None	None
Indapamide	<5	76–79	14–18/ unchanged	100%	100%	100%	None	None
Metolazone	70	95	4–20/?	100%	100%	100%	None	None
Thiazides	>95	40	6–8/12–20	100%	100%	avoid	?	?
Trimeterene	5.0–10	40–70	2.0–12/10	q12hr	q12hr	avoid	?	?
Vasodilators								
Hydralazine	5.0–10	87	2–4.5/7–16	q8hr	q8hr	q8–16hr	None	None
Minoxidil	15–20	0	2.8–4.2/ unchanged	100%	100%	100%	None	None
Prazasin	<5	97	2–3/2–3	100%	100%	100%	None	None
Terazosin	20–30	90–94	9–12/8–12	100%	100%	100%	?	?
Antiulcerative								
Cimetidine	50–70	20	1.5–2/5	100%	50%	25%	None	None
Famatidine	65–80	15–22	2.5–4/12–19	50%	25%	10%	None	None
Nizatidine	10–15	28–35	1.6/5.3–8.5	75%	50%	25%	?	?
Ranitidine	80	15	1.5–3/6–9	75%	50%	25%	50%	None
Antidepressant, Antiparkinsonian, Antipsychotic								
Amitriptyline	Hepatic	96	24–40/ unchanged	100%	100%	100%	None	?
Carbamzepine	2–3	75		100%	100%	100%	None	None
Carbidopa	30	?	2/?	100%	100%	100%	?	?
Clonazepam	Hepatic	47	18–50/?	?	?	?	?	?
Ethosuximide	17–40	10	35–55/ unchanged	100%	100%	100%	None	?
Fluoxetine	Hepatic	94.5	24–72/ unchanged	100%	100%	100%	?	?
Haloperidol	Hepatic	90–92	10–19/?	100%	100%	100%	None	None
Levodopa	None	5–8	0.8–1.6/?	100%	100%	100%	?	?
Lithium	Renal	None	14–28/40	100%	50–75%	25–50%	dose post-HD	None
Phenobarbital	Hep/Renal	40–60	60–150/ 117–160	q8–12hr	q8–12hr	q12–16hr	dose post-HD	50%

(*continued*)

TABLE 32.1 *Continued*

Drug	Excreted unchanged (%)	Protein bound (%)	$t_{1/2}$ Normal/ renal failure (hr)	Dose or frequency adjustment for GFR (ml/min)			Supplemental dose for	
				GFR > 50	GFR 10–50	GFR < 10	Hemodialysis	PD
Phenytoin	2	90	24/ unchanged	100%	100%	100%	none	None
Sertraline	Hepatic	97	24/?	?	?	?	?	?
Valproic acid	3–7	90	5–16/ unchanged	100%	100%	100%	None	None
Antidiabetic								
Chlorpropamide	47	91–99	24–48/50–200	50%	avoid	avoid	?	None
Glipizide	4.5–7	97	3–7/?	100%	100%	100%	?	?
Glyburide	50	99	1.4–2.9/?	?	avoid	avoid	None	None
Metformin	90–100	Negligible	1–5/ prolonged	50%	25%	avoid	?	?
Antihyperlipidemic								
Atorvastatin	<2	>98	14/?		?	?	?	?
Cholestyramine	None	None	not absorbed		100%	100%	None	None
Clofibrate	40–70	92–97	15/30–110	q6–12hr	q12–18hr	avoid	None	?
Fluvastatin	<1	?	0.5–1/?	100%	100%	100%	?	?
Gimfibrozil	None	97–99	7.6/	100%	100%	100%	None	?
Lovastatin	None	>95	1.1–1.7/ unchanged	100%	100%	100%	?	?
Niacin	None	?	0.5–1/?	100%	50%	25%	?	?
Pravastatin	<10	40–60	0.8–3.2/ unchanged	100%	100%	25%	?	?
Simvastatin	<0.5	>95	?	100%	100%	100%	?	?

?, Unknown; hepatic, predominantly eliminated by hepatic metabolism. Modified from Aronoff GR et al. (1999a, 1999b).

Suggested Readings

Aronoff GR, Berns JS, Brier ME, et al. *Drug prescribing in renal failure: dosing guidelines for adults, 4th ed.* Philadelphia: American College of Physicians, 1999a.

Aronoff GR, Erbeck KR, Brier M. Prescribing drugs for dialysisab patients. In: Henrich WL, ed. *Principles and practice of dialysis, 2nd ed.* Baltimore: Williams & Wilkins, 1999b.

Ateshkadi A. Principles of drug therapy in renal failure. In: Greenberg A, Cheung A, Coffmann T, Folk R, eds. *Primer on kidney diseases, 2nd ed.* San Diego: Academic Press, 1998.

Dudley MN. Clinical pharmcokinetics of nucleoside antireteroviral agents. *J Infect Dis* 1995;171:S99–S122.

Lam F, Banerji S, Hatfield C. Principles of drug administration in renal insufficiency. *Clin Pharmacokin* 1997;32:30–57.

Swan SK, Bennett WM. Drug dosing guidelines in patients with renal failure. *West J Med* 1992;156:633–638.

Subject Index

Note: Page numbers followed by f denote figures; those followed by t denote tables.